Handbook of
Pediatric
Surgery

Jessica L. Buicko, MD
Endocrine Surgery Fellow
Department of Surgery
Weill Cornell Medicine-New York Presbyterian Hospital
New York, NY

Michael A. Lopez, DO
Surgical Resident
Department of Surgery
University of Miami School of Medicine
JFK Hospital Surgical Residency Program
Atlantis, FL

Miguel A. Lopez-Viego, MD, FACS
Clinical Associate Professor of Surgery
University of Miami School of Medicine
JFK Hospital Surgical Residency Program
Atlantis, FL

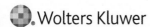. Wolters Kluwer

Philadelphia • Baltimore • New York • London
Buenos Aires • Hong Kong • Sydney • Tokyo

Acquisitions Editor: Keith Donnellan
Development Editor: Sean Buicko
Editorial Coordinator: Kerry McShane
Editorial Assistant: Levi Bentley
Marketing Manager: Julie Sikora
Production Project Manager: Bridgett Dougherty
Design Coordinator: Joan Wendt
Manufacturing Coordinator: Beth Welsh
Prepress Vendor: TNQ Technologies

9 8 7 6 5 4 3 2 1

Printed in China

Library of Congress Cataloging-in-Publication Data

Names: Buicko, Jessica L., author.
Title: Handbook of pediatric surgery / Jessica L. Buicko, MD, Endocrine Surgery Fellow, Department of Surgery, Weill Cornell Medicine-New York Presbyterian Hospital, New York, NY, Miguel A. Lopez, DO, Surgical Resident, Department of Surgery, University of Miami School of Medicine, JFK Hospital Surgical Residency Program, Atlantis, FL, Michael A. Lopez-Viego, MD, FACS, Clinical Associate Professor of Surgery, University of Miami School of Medicine, JFK Hospital Surgical Residency Program, Atlantis, FL.
Description: Philadelphia : Wolters Kluwer, [2019]
Identifiers: LCCN 2018040436 | ISBN 9781496388537 (paperback)
Subjects: LCSH: Children–Surgery–Handbooks, manuals, etc. | BISAC: MEDICAL / Surgery / General.
Classification: LCC RD137 .B85 2019 | DDC 617.9/8–dc23
LC record available at https://lccn.loc.gov/2018040436

shop.lww.com

To my family, for always supporting me,
To my friends, for always
keeping me grounded,
To my mentors, for always
inspiring me, and
To anyone who's ever told me
"you can't," for giving me the
opportunity to prove "I can."
Jessica L. Buicko, MD

Preface

The treatment of the surgical disorders that affect children is one of the most important and challenging fields in medicine. Children present with symptom complexes and conditions that can be difficult to diagnose and treacherous to manage. Any misdiagnosis or mismanagement of the surgical diseases of pediatric patients can result in decades of disability and a lifetime of unfulfilled potential.

Pediatric surgery is a rapidly evolving field focused on the modern treatment of ancient ailments of children. Only by understanding the applied anatomical and physiological basis of the mechanisms of disease of these maladies can the surgeon deliver the appropriate medical and surgical interventions to correct them. This book is a product of the thoughtful work of the residents and faculty of the Department of Surgery of the University of Miami at the JFK Medical Center in Palm Beach County, Florida, and the members of the Seacrest Surgical Society from around the country.

The book is dedicated to providing a contemporary and comprehensive source of information regarding the care of the pediatric surgery patient. It is focused on being an efficient and readily available resource for surgical residents, pediatric residents, emergency physicians, and medical students. It provides a thorough discussion of the presentation and management of all the major pediatric surgical diseases.

Nawara Alawa, MD, MPH
Pediatric Resident
Department of Pediatrics
Baylor College of Medicine
Texas Children's Hospital
Houston, TX

Bijan J. Ameri, DO
Orthopedic Resident
Department of Orthopedic Surgery
Broward Health Medical Center
Fort Lauderdale, FL

Fawaz M. Ashouri, MD
Ashouri Urology Clinic
Jacksonville, FL

Kenan Ashouri, MD
Urology Resident
Department of Urology
University of Florida
Gainesville, FL

Kara Baker, MD
Surgical Resident
Department of Surgery
University of Miami School of Medicine
JFK Hospital Surgical Residency Program
Atlantis, FL

Jessica L. Buicko, MD
Endocrine Surgery Fellow
Department of Surgery
Weill Cornell Medicine-New York Presbyterian Hospital
New York, NY

Carly M. Conway, BS Candidate
Department of Psychology
Georgetown University
Washington, DC

Erica Davanian, DO
Surgical Resident
Department of Surgery
University of Tennessee Health Science Center
Nashville, TN

Caroline R. Deyoe, BS Candidate
Department of Human Sciences
Florida State University
Tallahassee, FL

Marcus E. Eby, MD
Surgical Resident
Department of Surgery
University of Miami School of Medicine
JFK Hospital Surgical Residency Program
Atlantis, FL

Blaze D. Emerson, DO, MS
Orthopedic Resident
Department of Orthopedic Surgery
Broward Health Medical Center
Fort Lauderdale, FL

Paige E. Finkelstein, MD/MPH
Surgical Resident
Department of Surgery
Mount Sinai Medical Center
Miami, FL

Lukas Gaffney, MD/MPH Candidate
Miller School of Medicine
University of Miami
Miami, FL

Junyan Gu, MD, PhD
Surgical Resident
Department of Surgery
Florida Atlantic University
Boca Raton, FL

Arielle D. Henderson, MS, MD Candidate
Charles E. Schmidt College of Medicine
Florida Atlantic University
Boca Raton, FL

Ashley B. Hink, MD, MPH
Surgical Resident
Department of Surgery
Medical University of South Carolina
Charleston, SC

Kandace Kichler, MD
Advanced GI and Minimally Invasive Surgery Fellow
Department of Surgery
Cleveland Clinic Florida
Weston, FL

John H. Kimball, BS, MD/MPH Candidate
Miller School of Medicine
University of Miami
Miami, FL

Adam Michael Kravietz, MD, MPH
Otolaryngology Resident
Department of Otolaryngology - Head and
    Neck Surgery
New York University
New York, NY

Ann Alyssa Kurian, MD
Surgical Resident
Department of Surgery
University of Miami School of Medicine
JFK Hospital Surgical Residency Program
Atlantis, FL

Anne Marie Lopez, MD
Radiology Resident
Department of Radiology
University of Florida
Gainesville, FL

Michael A. Lopez, DO
Surgical Resident
Department of Surgery
University of Miami School of Medicine
JFK Hospital Surgical Residency Program
Atlantis, FL

Rennier A. Martinez, MD
Surgical Resident
Department of Surgery
University of Miami School of Medicine
JFK Hospital Surgical Residency Program
Atlantis, FL

Lacey P. MenkinSmith, MD
Assistant Professor
Department of Emergency Medicine
Medical University of South Carolina
Charleston, SC

Tyler Montgomery, BS, MD Candidate
Charles E. Schmidt College of Medicine
Florida Atlantic University
Boca Raton, FL

Alison M. Moody, MD, MPH
Surgical Resident
Department of Surgery
Louisiana State University
New Orleans, LA

Nadine Najjar, MD, MPH
Pediatric Resident
Department of Pediatrics
Emory University School of Medicine
Atlanta, GA

Hibbut-ur-Rauf Naseem, MD
Surgical Resident
Department of Surgery
Florida Atlantic University
Boca Raton, FL

Kenneth F. Newcomer Jr, MD
Surgical Resident
Department of Surgery
Washington University School of Medicine
Saint Louis, MO

Joshua P. Parreco, MD
Trauma and Critical Care Fellow
Department of Surgery
University of Miami
Miami, FL

Ann M. Polcari, MD, MPH, MS
Surgical Resident
Department of Surgery
The University of Chicago
Chicago, IL

Courtland Polley, MD
Surgical Resident
Department of Surgery
UT Southwestern Medical Center
Dallas, TX

Gina Prado, BS, MD Candidate
Charles E. Schmidt College of Medicine
Florida Atlantic University
Boca Raton, FL

Grace E. Pryor, MD, MPH
Pediatric Resident
Department of Pediatrics
UT Southwestern Medical Center
Dallas, TX

Sana Ahmad Qureshi, MBBS
Surgical Resident
Department of Surgery
Florida Atlantic University
Boca Raton, FL

Ryan D. Reusche, MD, MPH
Surgical Resident
Department of Surgery
Florida Atlantic University
Boca Raton, FL

Scott J. Revell, MD
Surgical Resident
Department of Surgery
University of Miami School of Medicine
JFK Hospital Surgical Residency Program
Atlantis, FL

Allison Rice, MD
Surgical Resident
Department of Surgery
University of Miami School of Medicine
JFK Hospital Surgical Residency Program
Atlantis, FL

Bradley Roche, BA, MD Candidate
Charles E. Schmidt College of Medicine
Florida Atlantic University
Boca Raton, FL

Reagan Lindsay Ross, MD, MPT, RPVI
Assistant Professor
Department of Surgery
JFK Medical Center
University of Miami
Atlantis, FL
Assistant Professor
Department of Surgery
Florida Atlantic University
Boca Raton, FL

Isolina R. Rossi, MD
Surgical Resident
Department of Surgery
Carolinas Medical Center
Charlotte, NC

David Rubay, MD
Surgical Resident
Department of Surgery
Florida Atlantic University
Boca Raton, FL

Stephanie Scurci, MD
Surgical Resident
Department of Surgery
University of Miami School of Medicine
JFK Hospital Surgical Residency Program
Atlantis, FL

Lauren P. Shapiro, MD
Emergency Medicine Resident
Department of Emergency Medicine
University of South Florida
Tampa, FL

Sarah Simko, MD/MPH Candidate
Miller School of Medicine
University of Miami
Miami, FL

Olga Zhadan, MD
Surgical Resident
Department of Surgery
Charles E. Schmidt College of Medicine
Florida Atlantic University
Boca Raton, FL

Contents

SECTION 3
Common Pediatric Surgical Problems

SECTION 1

Management of the Pediatric Surgical Patient

Chapter 1

Evaluation and Examination of the Pediatric Surgical Patient

Nicholas Cortolillo

- Assessment of the pediatric surgical patient requires in-depth knowledge of surgical diseases in children as well as an understanding of the spectrum of pediatric physiology and its derangements across several ages from newborns to infants, children, and adolescents.
- Surgeons and their trainees must also be aware of the unique challenges embedded into pediatric medicine.
- The care plan must take into account the patient, the problem, the anticipated prognosis, and the child's caretaker.[1]
- Substantial anxiety is usually present with the surgical evaluation of a child.
- Trust building with patients and their parent or guardian lays the foundation for an effective evaluation.
- Establishing rapport begins at the initial encounter and continues into the postoperative stages.
- Fears and knowledge gaps should be elicited and addressed by the pediatric surgeon through communication and education.
- Reviewing images, explaining models, and freehand drawings may be helpful toward this goal.
- Surgeons should be prepared to explain topics such as embryologic development, genetics, and oncology in layperson's terms.
- The size of the incision, the intervention, and the expected postoperative course should all be discussed.

HISTORICAL BACKGROUND

- An adequate history involves input from both the child and parents and forms the foundation of the relationship to follow.
- The chief complaint (CC) represents the reason why the patient presented for care.
- A history of present illness (HPI) should be methodical and include symptom onset, acuity, progression, severity, associated symptoms, and aggravating or alleviating factors.
- Pertinent positives and negatives should be documented in a thorough review of systems.[2]
- Birth history, developmental milestones, medical conditions, and previous surgeries, or interventions should be listed separately.
- Diligently note any unusual bleeding episodes or known bleeding disorders. Inquire about any previous exposure to anesthesia.[3]
- Review scheduled medications, "as needed" medications, and supplements that the child takes.
- Drug allergies, food allergies, and symptoms that occur with these reactions are important.
- For children with genetic diseases, congenital malformations, or malignancies, the social and family histories are requisite for a complete pediatric presentation.

THE EXAMINATION

- Every examination begins and ends with handwashing.
- Not only does this form the foundation for infection control, the routine also nonverbally reassures the parent that the surgeon promotes hygiene.
- It also helps to warm the surgeon's hands before touching the child.
- The physical examination may be performed according to a standard routine in older and more cooperative children.
- Improvisation and flexibility are required in the approach to young children and infants who may not cooperate.[4]
- Portions of the examination for young children and toddlers may occur within their parents' laps.
- It is advisable to perform the abdominal, rectal, and genital examinations on an examination table.
- Having the parent close by will help to reduce the child's anxiety (Figure 1.1). Infants should always be evaluated on the examination table.

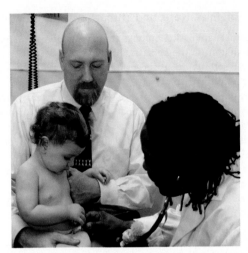

Figure 1.1 The child may feel more secure if the caregiver stays with the child during the physical examination. (Reprinted with permission from Hatfield NT, Kincheloe CA. *Hatfield Introductory Maternity and Pediatric Nursing.* 4th ed. Philadelphia, PA: Wolters Kluwer; 2018.)

Skin

- The pediatric surgeon is frequently asked to evaluate lumps and bumps and skin lesions.
- Complete description of any lesion includes size, shape, mobility, circumscription, and consistency.
- The remaining skin must be assessed for similar lesions, surgical scars, or rashes, which can key into autoimmune disorders or vasculitides.
- Bruises, redundant or irregular scars, and well-defined burns should raise concern for child abuse.[5]

Lymphatics

- In children, lymphadenopathy is most commonly infectious; therefore, searching for a source of infection in the examination is prudent.[6]
- Bacterial, viral, fungal, and protozoal culprits should be considered.
- Enlarged lymph nodes may represent primary malignancy (acute lymphoblastic leukemia [ALL] and Hodgkin and non-Hodgkin lymphoma) or metastatic malignancy.
- The axillary, cervical, inguinal, and epitrochlear basins are the most frequent locations for lymphadenopathy.

Head, Ear, Eyes, Nose, and Throat

- Physical examination findings among these organ systems are high-yielding in the pediatric population.
- Scleral icterus may suggest hepatic dysfunction, biliary obstruction, or hemolysis.
- Micro- or macrocephaly may signify an intracranial process.
- Abnormal fusion of coronal sutures is not considered normocephalic.
- Otitis media may be excluded if the tympanic membranes are clear and landmarks are visible.
- An inflamed oropharynx in the setting of rhinorrhea may signify an upper respiratory infection.
- Loose teeth are important to acknowledge for children who are to receive anesthesia.[7]

Chest Wall

- The evaluation of pectus excavatum (concave) and pectus carinatum (convex) is accompanied with heart and lung examinations.
- Ascertaining the degree of deformity and assessing its psychosocial effects are required.[8]
- Breast tissue is common in infants of both sexes because of a slow decline in maternal hormones in circulation.
- Male adolescents may also experience gynecomastia because of high hormonal activity during puberty.[9]
- In preadolescent girls, breast growth occurs at different rates, so one must be able to distinguish a breast mass from a breast bud.

Cardiovascular

- Age-appropriate exercise activity and feeding provide functional clues to the child's cardiac status.
- Rate and rhythm should be compared against age-appropriate norms.
- Color and respiratory effort should be assessed.
- The neck should be examined for prominent vessels, abnormal pulsations, and bruits.
- The lungs should be auscultated for crackles or wheezing, features which suggest cardiac asthma of congestive heart failure.
- Likewise, the abdomen should be assessed for hepatomegaly or ascites.
- Capillary refill should be under 3 seconds.
- Pulses in all 4 extremities should be strong and equal; any discrepancy warrants vascular evaluation.

- Many children will have a murmur between infancy and adolescence, most of which are innocent.
- Red flags that increase the likelihood of a pathologic murmur include a holosystolic or diastolic murmur, grade 3 or higher murmur, harsh quality, an abnormal S2, maximal murmur intensity at the upper left sternal border, a systolic click, or increased intensity when the patient stands.[10]

Lungs

- As in the cardiovascular examination, no layers of clothing should be present between the stethoscope and skin.
- All breath sounds should be clear and equal.
- Wheezes, rhonchi, and crackles are abnormal.

Abdomen

- A plethora of major pathology may be found here; thus a systematic approach is needed.
- First inspect the abdomen for scars and for shape.
- Scaphoid abdomens may occur in the setting of underfeeding or giant diaphragmatic hernias.
- Abdominal distention can occur secondary to ascites, tumor, intestinal obstruction, or organomegaly.
- Next, auscultate for bowel sounds.
- These may be diminished in peritonitis or high pitched in intestinal obstruction.[11]
- After auscultation, an efficient strategy is to assess for any tenderness with the stethoscope.
- Assess all 4 quadrants starting with the area farthest away from the reported pain.
- Use gentle palpation as you assess for peritoneal signs of rebound and guarding.
- Facial expressions, behavior, and tone or pitch of crying may signify the severity of these findings more so than verbal reports.
- Overly aggressive examination maneuvers may create fear in the child and compromise the remainder of the examination.

Inguinal Region

- Concurrent with abdominal and genital examination, the umbilical and bilateral inguinal regions should be associated for hernia and hydrocele (Figure 1.2).
- Valsalva maneuvers can be created with coughing or straining and increase the sensitivity of finding a hernia on examination. Infants often perform Valsalva with crying.[12]

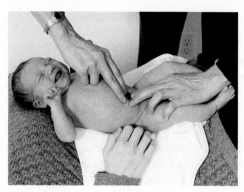

Figure 1.2 Examination for an umbilical hernia. (Reprinted with permission from Anrig CA, Plaugher G. *Pediatric Chiropractic.* Philadelphia, PA: Wolters Kluwer Health/Lippincott Williams & Wilkins; 2011.)

Genital Region

- For boys, examination of this region is necessary for hydrocele, undescended testes, and hernia.
- Lying down or standing are acceptable positions.
- Note the shape and size of the both testicles and the presence of any fluid in the scrotum. Be aware that retractile testes may mimic undescended testes.[13]
- Transillumination may assist with visualizing scrotal contents but should not form the basis of a diagnosis, especially in infants.
- Performing a female examination is relevant in the diagnosis of imperforate hymen, fused labia, and vaginal or perineal bleeding, among other diseases.
- Vaginal tears or vaginal discharge should raise concern for abuse or sexually transmitted infection.[14]
- Modesty is present in children as early as 2 years of age; therefore, special respect should be given to this point during the examination.
- A chaperone of the same sex as the child must be present.
- Note that for many patients this may be their first genital examination with lasting psychosocial consequences.

Rectum

- Speed and thoroughness are essential for this stressful portion of the examination.
- Explaining the process to the parent and the child may help to assuage intense fears.
- Spreading and inspection is enough to assess external pathology—such as skin tags, fissures, fistulas, and other lesions.

- Condyloma accuminata should raise concern for sexual abuse.
- Next, apply gentle pressure externally as you communicate to the patient; this may cause a transient relaxation in sphincter tone and facilitate passage into the anal canal.[15]
- Sphincter tone may be diminished after anoplasty, after traumatic injury to the sphincter, or after spinal cord injury.
- Palpate 360° within the anal canal and note the size and locations of any masses.
- Attempts should be made to differentiate discomfort from the examination from pain with examination, as can be seen with a low-lying inflamed appendix.[16]

Nervous and Psychiatric System

- A child who plays and interacts may be considered neurologically intact.[17]
- A thorough neurologic examination may be performed in short time with practice.
- Cranial nerves should be assessed in any child with disease of the head and neck. Cognition is frequently impaired in the acutely ill child.
- Motor and sensory reflexes require baseline assessment.

Spine and Back

- Vertebral tenderness may indicate trauma.
- Right costovertebral angle tenderness may be seen with pyelonephritis or inflammation of a retrocecal appendix.
- Scoliosis may be apparent.

Extremities

- Evaluate for muscle bulk and tone, as they are indicators of nutritional and functional status.
- Digital clubbing is observed in chronic illness, particularly in pulmonary disease.
- Edema usually suggests cardiac or renal dysfunction.

SPECIAL CONSIDERATIONS

Acutely Ill Child

- Care of the ill child is one of the most challenging and potentially rewarding facets of pediatric surgery.
- This includes children suffering from intra-abdominal emergencies, foreign ingestions, and trauma.

- In ABC fashion, the first priority is to secure and maintain the child's airway and ventilation.
- Second priority is to support perfusion to end organs.
- Children with burns, hemorrhage, peritonitis, bowel obstruction, vomiting, or diarrhea will suffer from intravascular volume depletion.
- An initial 20 mL/kg of warmed crystalloid bolus may be used to begin resuscitation, followed by serial reevaluation to guide additional resuscitation.
- Endpoints of resuscitation are restoration of skin color, skin turgor, good capillary refill, and 2 mL/kg per hour of urine output in infants and 1 mL/kg per hour of urine in older children.[18]
- These goals are crucial in pediatric surgery.
- Anesthetic agents will blunt a child's robust protective mechanisms against hypovolemia by causing vasodilation, resulting in life-threatening hypotension and end-organ ischemia.
- Acid-base disturbances and electrolyte derangements should be corrected promptly and reevaluated serially.

Chronically Ill Patient

- Managing chronically ill patients requires the best of the pediatric surgeon.
- Malnutrition, anemia, and growth delays may be seen in these frequently deconditioned children, many of whom are secondarily immunocompromised or coagulopathic.[19]
- In elective settings, chronically ill children should be optimized before any surgery.
- This includes optimizing nutritional status in malnourished children with extra protein and calories.
- Insulin-dependent patients require a change in their regimen with nil per os (NPO) status and surgical stress.
- Patients with short- and intermediate-acting insulin regimens should continue this until the morning of surgery.
- Patients on long-acting insulin should receive an intermediate-acting insulin the night before surgery.
- For patients on insulin pumps, it is essential to involve the patient's endocrinologist in perioperative management.[20]

Chronic Cardiac and Respiratory Disease Patients

- For children with complicated heart disease, involve the patient's cardiologist ahead of any planned surgery and make every effort to involve the cardiologist with unplanned emergent and urgent surgeries as well.
- Close electrolyte and volume management with diligent intake and output monitoring is necessary.

- Prosthetic heart valves or patches or native valvular abnormality should be given antibiotic prophylaxis to prevent bacterial endocarditis.
- Ampicillin and gentamicin are effective in patients for GI and GU surgery.
- Ampicillin prophylaxis is adequate for respiratory tract surgery.[21]
- For child with a penicillin allergy, cephalosporins, clindamycin, azithromycin, and clarithromycin are acceptable prophylaxes.[21]
- Frequently the pediatric surgeon will be called to see children with pulmonary disease. In these patients a preoperative chest X-ray is routine.
- In elective settings, children with asthma should be asymptomatic preoperatively, with good pharmacologic and environmental control in place.
- Medications should be continued up to the morning or day of surgery.
- Likewise, children with cystic fibrosis need to be in optimal condition before surgery working in concert with pulmonology.
- Neonates with hyaline membrane disease may progress into bronchopulmonary dysplasia, which increases CO_2 retention and atelectasis.[22]

Chronic Liver and Renal Failure Patients

- Hepatic failure in children may result from biliary atresia, cystic fibrosis, hepatitis, or liver injury.
- Try to avoid hepatically metabolized medications in this population.
- In patients with comorbid ascites or edema, restriction of sodium and diuretics is needed.
- Obtain baseline liver tests and coagulation profiles before surgery.
- Children with renal failure require diligent fluid and electrolyte balance monitoring in the perioperative setting.
- Careful attention to intake and output is needed.
- Hyperkalemia, acidosis, and hyperphosphatemia are seen with advanced failure.
- Some children cannot concentrate urine and depend on intake of sodium and free water, which can be problematic during NPO periods.
- As with liver failure, avoid agents that are metabolized renally.

PEARLS AND PITFALLS

- Pediatric surgical patients present unique challenges not seen in the care of adults.
- Its complexity requires surgeons who can wear multiple hats outside the operating room and guide the process of surgical care from evaluation to diagnosis, to communication, and to education.
- The history and physical examination of a sick child are truly an art.
- This key interaction forms the foundation for the relationship to follow between the surgeon and the child and parent or guardian.

REFERENCES

1. Ambulatory & office pediatrics. In: *Current Diagnosis & Treatment Pediatrics*. 23rd ed. AccessMedicine, McGraw-Hill Medical; 2006. Available at http://accessmedicine.mhmedical.com/content.aspx?bookid=1795&sectionid=125737347. Accessed February 4, 2018.
2. Section on Anesthesiology and Pain Medicine. The pediatrician's role in the evaluation and preparation of pediatric patients undergoing anesthesia. *Pediatrics*. 2014;134:634-641.
3. Serafini G, Ingelmo PM, Astuto M, et al. Preoperative evaluation in infants and children: recommendations of the Italian Society of Pediatric and Neonatal Anesthesia and Intensive Care (SARNePI). *Minerva Anestesiol*. 2014;80:461-469.
4. Evaluation and preparation of pediatric patients undergoing anesthesia. American Academy of Pediatrics. Section on Anesthesiology. *Pediatrics*. 1996;98:502-508.
5. Child abuse & neglect. In: *Current Diagnosis & Treatment Pediatrics*. 23rd ed. AccessMedicine, McGraw-Hill Medical; 2006. Available at http://accessmedicine.mhmedical.com/content.aspx?bookid=1795&sectionid=125737263. Accessed February 4, 2018.
6. Ghirardelli ML, Jemos V, Gobbi PG. Diagnostic approach to lymph node enlargement. *Haematologica*. 1999;84:242-247.
7. Ferrari LR. Preoperative evaluation of pediatric surgical patients with multisystem considerations. *Anesth Analg*. 2004;99:1058-1069.
8. Barness LA. *Manual of Pediatric Physical Diagnosis*. Mosby Inc.; 1991.
9. Braunstein GD. Diagnosis and treatment of gynecomastia. *Hosp Pract*. 1993;28:37-46.
10. Harris PJ. Understanding pediatric heart sounds. *N Engl J Med*. 1992; 327:741-742.
11. Sailer J. Auscultation in the physical examination of the abdomen. *J Am Med Assoc*. 1923;81;728.
12. Amerson JR. Inguinal canal and hernia examination. In: Walker HK, Hall WD, Hurst JW, eds. *Clinical Methods: The History, Physical, and Laboratory Examinations*. Butterworths; 2011.
13. Adamyan L, Cundiff G. Congenital anomalies of the female reproductive tract. In: Gomel V, Brill A, eds. *Reconstructive and Reproductive Surgery in Gynecology*. Vol 51. CRC Press; 2010:191-199.

14. Smith WG, Metcalfe M, Cormode EJ, Holder N. Approach to evaluation of sexual assault in children. Experience of a secondary-level regional pediatric sexual assault clinic. *Can Fam Physician*. 2005;51:1347-1351.
15. Takada T, Nishiwaki H, Yamamoto Y, et al. The role of digital rectal examination for diagnosis of acute appendicitis: a systematic review and meta-analysis. *PLoS One*. 2015;10:e0136996.
16. Othersen Jr HB, Greenberg L, Morse TS. Rectal examination in children; a diagnostic procedure of major importance. *Clin Pediatr*. 1965;4:391-393.
17. Probasco J, Sahin B, Tran T, et al. The preoperative neurological evaluation. *Neurohospitalist*. 2013;3:209-220.
18. Matics TJ, Sanchez-Pinto LN. Adaptation and validation of a pediatric sequential organ failure assessment score and evaluation of the Sepsis-3 definitions in critically ill children. *JAMA Pediatr*. 2017;171:e172352.
19. Secker DJ, Jeejeebhoy KN. Subjective global nutritional assessment for children. *Am J Clin Nutr*. 2007;85:1083-1089.
20. Zambouri A. Preoperative evaluation and preparation for anesthesia and surgery. *Hippokratia*. 2007;11:13-21.
21. Bratzler DW, Dellinger EP, Olsen KM, et al. Clinical practice guidelines for antimicrobial prophylaxis in surgery. *Am J Health Syst Pharm*. 2013;70:195-283.
22. Grover TR, Brozanski BS, Barry J, et al. High surgical burden for infants with severe chronic lung disease (sCLD). *J Pediatr Surg*. 2014;49:1202-1205.

Chapter 2

Fluids and Electrolytes in Children

Nadine Najjar

ASSESSMENT OF FLUID STATUS

- Intravenous fluids provide daily maintenance requirements of electrolytes and prevent volume depletion or dehydration. This is essential in successful treatment of surgical pediatric patients.
- Fluids must maintain volume requirements, replete electrolyte and fluid deficits, and restore ongoing losses. However, maintenance requirements differ based on age.
- Assessment of fluid status depends on the degree of dehydration:
  - Loss of less than 5% of weight → no clinical manifestations
  - Loss of 5% to 8% of weight → moderate clinical signs
  - Loss of 10% or more of weight → severe signs and poor peripheral circulation
- Signs of moderate fluid loss: irritability, dry mucous membranes, oliguria, increased thirst, depressed fontanelle, decreased tears, cool pale skin, delayed capillary refill (>2), and decreased skin turgor.
- Signs of severe fluid loss: decreased blood pressure, marked tachycardia, cool cyanotic or mottled skin, parched mucous membranes, sunken fontanelle, very delayed capillary refill (>3), and absent tears.

GOALS OF FLUID THERAPY

- The goal of fluid therapy is to preserve normal fluid volume and electrolyte composition of the body.
- Maintenance therapy covers ongoing sensible and insensible losses of volume due to physiologic processes such as respiration, urination, defecation, and sweating. These requirements vary depending on the setting and age of the child.

TABLE 2.1				
Compensation for Fluid Loss				
% Weight Loss	H$_2$O mL/kg	Na mEq/kg	Cl mEq/kg	K mEq/kg
5	50	4	3	3
10	100	8	6	6
15	150	12	9	9

Data from Wesley JR, Adolph V. Chapter 6: Fluids and electrolytes. In: Arensman RM, Bambini D, Almond S, et al, eds. *Pediatric Surgery*. 2nd ed. Austin, TX: Landes Bioscience; 2009.

- Replacement therapy replenishes acute losses of water and/ or electrolytes due to illness.
- Fluid replacement corrects the deficit depending on the degree of loss. These are given in addition to maintenance requirements.
  - For example, if a 5000 g infant exhibits moderate signs of dehydration (ie, decreased urine output), she may have lost 5% to 8% of body mass.
  - Requirement = 5000 × 5% mL = 250 mL to correct deficit.
- Add to maintenance fluids for any losses from dehydration (Table 2.1).
- Although, historically, hospitalized children received hypotonic fluids with electrolyte additives, current literature asserts that isotonic saline solutions are preferred in hospitalized children. Administration of hypotonic fluids increase the risk of inappropriate antidiuretic hormone (ADH) release and hyponatremia compared with administration of isotonic fluids.[3]

CAUSES OF FLUID LOSS

- Fluid losses can occur as a result of normal physiologic processes (such as urination, defecation, sweating, and respiration) or abnormal physiologic processes (examples listed below). Losses are classified as sensible or insensible in nature.
- Sensible water loss are easily measured:
  - Urine—ie, diabetes insipidus, osmotic diuresis
  - Third space—ie, necrotizing enterocolitis, burns
  - Diarrhea—ie, gastroenteritis

TABLE 2.2
Maintenance Daily Fluids for Premature to Term Neonates (mL/kg per day)

Day	Premature, <1250 g	Premature, >1250 g	Term
1	100	75	60-75
2	100-120	75-100	75-85
3+	120+	100+	100

From Wesley JR, Adolph V. Fluids and Electrolytes. In: Arensman RM, et al. eds. *Pediatric Surgery*. 2nd ed. Austin, Tex.: Landes Bioscience; 2009:21. Copyright © 2009 Landes Bioscience. Reproduced by permission of Taylor and Francis Group, LLC, a division of Informa plc.

- Insensible water loss cannot be measured easily. Examples include the following:
  - Respiratory water loss: affected by humidity of inspired air and minute ventilation
  - Transepithelial water loss: affected by surface area, body mass, activity level, body temperature, postural changes, ambient humidity, and ambient temperature

ESTIMATED FLUID NEEDS FOR INFANTS AND CHILDREN

- Maintenance daily fluid needs for premature to term neonates are given in Table 2.2.
- Maintenance daily fluid needs for term infants and older children are given in Table 2.3.

TABLE 2.3
Maintenance Daily Fluids for Term Infants and Older Children (mL/kg per day)[2]

Weight	Daily Fluid Requirements
0-10 kg	100 mL/kg per day
10-20 kg	1000 mL for first 10 kg of body weight +50 mL/kg for every kg over 10
>20 kg	1500 mL for first 20 kg of body weight +20 mL/kg per day for every kg over 20 *Maximum of 2400 mL daily

Source: Holliday MA, Segar WE. The maintenance need for water in parenteral fluid therapy. *Pediatrics*. 1957;19(5):823-832.

MAINTENANCE ELECTROLYTES

- Maintenance electrolyte needs for infants and children up to 20 kg are given in Table 2.4.

TABLE 2.4			
Maintenance Electrolytes for Infants and Children up to 20 kg			
Electrolyte	Supplied as	Amount Required: >30 wk	Comments
Na	NaCl; Na acetate	2-4 mEq/ kg per day (3-5 mEq/ kg per day if <30 wk)	Use the acetate salt if patient is hyperchloremic. Generally not given in first 24 h.
K	KCl; K phosphate, K acetate	2-4 mEq/kg/ per day	Decrease maintenance need with renal dysfunction or extensive tissue breakdown (necrotizing enterocolitis, burns). Increase need with diuretics and nephrotoxic drugs.
Ca	Ca gluconate	0.5-3.0 mEq/ kg per day	Premature infants need more calcium than full-term infants.
PO_4	K phosphate, Na phosphate	0.5-1.5 mM/ kg per day	Each millimole of K phosphate provides 1.5 mEq of K. Each millimole of Na phosphate provides 1.3 mEq of Na.
Mg	$MgSO_4$	0.5-1.0 mEq/ kg per day	

From Wesley JR, Adolph V. Fluids and Electrolytes. In: Arensman RM, et al. eds. *Pediatric Surgery*. 2nd ed. Austin, Tex.: Landes Bioscience; 2009:22. Copyright © 2009 Landes Bioscience. Adapted by permission of Taylor and Francis Group, LLC, a division of Informa plc.

CHANGES IN MAINTENANCE NEEDS

- Fluid requirements change when homeostatic balance of water and electrolytes is altered. These alterations center on changes in water loss and ADH action.
- Examples:
  - Prematurity causes increased insensible transepidermal water loss due to thinner dermis.
  - Patients with burns have increased water and electrolyte loss.
  - Mechanical ventilation with prehumidified air will decrease water loss.
  - Diarrhea will increase fluid loss.
  - Syndrome of inappropriate ADH release, a common comorbidity in hospitalized children, results in decreased fluid loss.
  - Diabetes insipidus (central or nephrogenic) results in increased fluid loss.

PEARLS AND PITFALLS

- Fluid and electrolyte requirements are derived from body weight in children.
- Assessment of fluid status indicates degree of volume depletion.
- Sensible and insensible losses should be considered when assessing sources of fluid loss.
- Isotonic solutions are preferred over hypotonic solutions in hospitalized pediatric patients.

REFERENCES

1. Wesley JR, Adolph V. Fluids and electrolytes. In: Arensman RM, Bambini D, Almond S, et al. *Pediatric Surgery.* 2nd ed. Austin, TX: Landes Bioscience; 2009:20-23.
2. Holliday MA, Segar WE. The maintenance need for water in parenteral fluid therapy. *Pediatrics.* 1957;19(5):823-832.
3. McNab S, Duke T, Choong K, et al. Isotonic versus hypotonic solutions for maintenance intravenous fluid administration in children. In: The Cochrane Collaboration, ed. *Cochrane Database of Systematic Reviews.* 2011. doi:10.1002/14651858.CD009457.

Chapter 3

Surgical Nutrition and TPN in the Pediatric Patient

Nadine Najjar

INTRODUCTION

- Nutritional requirements in a hospitalized or surgical pediatric patient provide a unique challenge. Pediatric patients respond more rapidly to severe illnesses and stress to the body because of decreased energy stores.
- Adequate provision of nutrition requires careful nutritional assessment, determination of energy needs, and appropriate route of administration (eg, enteral or parenteral).
- Although parenteral nutrition (PN) in adult patients has been described in the literature as early as the 1600s, Dr William C Heird and colleagues reported the first successful and safe administration of PN in infants in 1972.[1]
- Energy expenditure increases during periods of stress to the body, but the change is variable. Considerations in feeding route should be made based on the clinical course of the patient, the anticipated length of fasting, the underlying function of the GI (gastrointestinal) tract and nutritional status of the patient, and the degree of nutritional intake at baseline.[2]
- Since then, advances in both enteral and parenteral modes of nutrition have optimized nutrition in the surgical pediatric patient.

PHYSIOLOGY

- Enteral feeds are preferred over parenteral feeds because they most closely resemble the normal physiologic activity of the GI tract.
- PN involves delivery of nutrients intravenously; therefore, it is nonphysiological because nutrients bypass the liver. This can put patients at risk for liver dysfunction and cholestasis.[2]

- Bypassing the GI tract can cause structural and functional changes, such as thinning of the mucosa, blunting of the villi, and increased bacterial translocation.[3]
- Additionally, early initiation of PN may affect infants' development of eating behaviors later in life.[4]
- Not only do enteral feeds decrease risk of complications in pediatric patients but also they are less expensive and easier to administer.[5]
- For these reasons, enteral nutrition is preferred over PN whenever possible. However, oftentimes critically ill and surgical pediatric patients are at risk for malnourishment in the hospital setting, so PN is sometimes necessary.

INDICATIONS FOR PARENTERAL NUTRITION

- PN may be given to complement enteral feeding, or it may substitute enteral feeds, known as total parenteral nutrition (TPN).
- PN is appropriate in children when enteral feeding is either not tolerated or unable to meet the patient's energy needs.
- In neonates, PN can begin within 48 to 72 hours of birth if the enteral route cannot be used.
- In older infants and children, PN should only be used if a fasting period of 5 or more days is anticipated.[6]
- Central venous access is necessary for TPN administration. Umbilical venous access may be used in neonates.[7] Peripheral lines can be considered for partial PN administration (see chapter 5, Central Venous and Arterial Access in the Pediatric Patient).

HOW TO PRESCRIBE PARENTERAL NUTRITION

Administration of a PN solution requires determination of osmolarity of the solution. This can be determined with the following equation[8]:

$$mOsm/L = (grams\ amino\ acids/L \times 10) + \\ (grams\ dextrose \times 5) + ([mEq\ Na + mEq\ K] \times 2)/L + \\ (mEq\ Ca \times 1.4)/L.$$

- Peripheral nutrition must have an osmolarity of 900 Osm or less. PN via central venous access can exceed this amount.

Calorie requirements are based on the patient's energy needs, which can vary based on the patient's age, weight, underlying disease, and many other factors. As an approximate estimate, the following are the energy requirements based on age[9]:

- Preterm neonate: 90 to 120 kcal/kg per day
- <6 months: 85 to 105 kcal/kg per day
- ≥6 to 12 months: 80 to 100 kcal/kg per day
- ≥1 to 7 years: 75 to 90 kcal/kg per day
- ≥7 to 12 years: 50 to 75 kcal/kg per day
- ≥12 to 18 years: 30 to 50 kcal/kg per day

The main macronutrients in PN include lipids, carbohydrates, and protein. Carbohydrates (primarily dextrose) and lipids (in the form of fat emulsion) provide the energy in PN, while proteins (in the form of crystalline amino acids) maintain lean body mass.[2]

- **Dextrose**: Initiate infusion at a rate of 5 mg/kg per minute using 5% to 10% concentration.
- **Lipids**: Initiate infusion at a rate of 1 g/kg per day and increase each day to reach a maximum of 3 g/kg per day.
- **Protein**: Initiate infusion at a rate of 1 g/kg per day in infants and children and 0.5 g/kg per day in preterm newborns. Increase the rate by 1 g/kg per day to reach the goal intake of 2.5 g/kg per day.

Micronutrient requirements encompass fat-soluble and water-soluble vitamins, as well as trace elements and minerals such as zinc, iron, copper, and selenium.

- Multivitamin preparations should be administered in addition to PN, and it should include vitamin C, vitamin A, vitamin D, vitamin B1, vitamin B2, vitamin B6, niacin, dexpanthenol, vitamin E, vitamin K1, folic acid, biotin, and vitamin B12.
- *Zinc* should be supplemented in patients who experience losses via severe diarrhea.
- *Selenium* should be supplemented in patients who must receive PN for 2 or more months.
- *Copper and manganese* may contribute to biliary cholestasis in patients receiving PN, who are already vulnerable to cholestasis, so decreased doses may be necessary depending on the patient's condition.

MONITORING

Routine laboratory test results should be obtained to monitor patients depending on their condition.

- Before beginning PN, obtain laboratory test results including metabolic panel, liver function tests (LFTs), albumin, prealbumin, and C-reactive protein (CRP). Be sure to weigh infants daily and weigh children or adolescents 3 times per week.

- In patients with critical illness, measure magnesium and phosphate daily. Measure LFTs, prealbumin, and CRP 3 times per week and triglycerides weekly.
- In patients who are medically stable, requirements for laboratory work are less stringent. Magnesium and phosphorus should be measured 3 times per week, and LFTs, prealbumin, CRP, and triglycerides should be measured weekly.

COMPLICATIONS

- Catheter-related infection is a common complication of PN, and this can lead to sepsis. Skin flora and GI flora often cause these infections (eg, *Staphylococcus epidermidis*). Sepsis must be considered in such patients.
- Hepatic complications include fatty liver disease, intrahepatic cholestasis, cholecystitis, and cholelithiasis.[10] Pediatric patients are at a particularly increased risk because of their immature biliary system.
- Multiple metabolic derangements have been reported, including electrolyte imbalances, hyper- and hypoglycemia, hyperlipidemia, and trace element deficiencies.

PEARLS AND PITFALLS

- Enteral feeds are always preferable over PN because they resemble normal physiology.
- Indications for PN are based on age, immaturity or dysfunction of GI tract, and inability to tolerate enteral feeds.
- Central venous access is the preferred modality for PN. Peripheral lines may be used if nutritional requirements are less than 900 Osms.
- Catheter-associated infections, fatty liver disease, and cholestasis are the most common complications of PN.

REFERENCES

1. Heird WC, Driscoll JM, Schullinger JN, Grebin B, Winters RW. Intravenous alimentation in pediatric patients. *J Pediatr.* 1972;80(3): 351-372.
2. Mehta N. Chapter 2: Nutritional support of the pediatric patient. In: *Ashcraft's Pediatric Surgery.* N.p.: Elsevier Health Sciences; 2014:8-9 [Print].
3. Kudsk KA. Effect of route and type of nutrition on intestine-derived inflammatory responses. *Am J Surg.* 2003;185(1):16-21.

4. Gahagan S. The development of eating behavior-biology and context. *J Dev Behav Pediatr*. 2012;33(3):261.

5. Arthur LG, Timmapuri SJ. Chapter 4: Enteral nutrition. In: Mattei P, ed. *Fundamentals of Pediatric Surgery*. Berlin: Springer; 2011:27-32 [Print].

6. Garrison AP, Helmrath MA. Chapter 5: Parenteral nutrition. In: Mattei P, ed. *Fundamentals of Pediatric Surgery*. Berlin: Springer; 2011:33-36 [Print].

7. Wesley JR, Adolph V. Chapter 7: Nutrition and metabolism. In: Arensman RM, Bambini DA, Almond S, et al, eds. *Pediatric Surgery*. 2nd ed. Berlin: Springer; 2009:20-23 [Print].

8. Baker RD, Baker SS, David AM. *Pediatric Parenteral Nutrition*. Gaithersburg: Aspen Publishers, Inc.; 2001.

9. Mirtallo J, Canada T, Johnson D, et al. Safe practices for parenteral nutrition. *J Parenter Enteral Nutr*. 2004;28(6):S39-S70.

10. Hartl WH, Jauch KW, Parhofer K, Rittler P, Working group for developing the guidelines for parenteral nutrition of The German association for Nutritional Medicine. Complications and monitoring – guidelines on parenteral nutrition, Chapter 11. *Ger Med Sci*. 2009;7:Doc17. doi:10.3205/000076.

Chapter 4

Pediatric Anesthesia

Arielle D. Henderson

- Pediatric anesthesia is more complex than simply adjusting drug dosages and equipment size.
- Pediatric patients have different anesthetic requirements.
- A detailed understanding of the anatomic, physiologic, and pharmacologic characteristics of pediatric populations is essential (Figure 4.1).
- This chapter will review the anatomy and physiology of pediatric patients, as it pertains to pediatric anesthesia, the pharmacologic differences of pediatric versus adult patients undergoing anesthesia, and various pediatric anesthetic techniques.

RELEVANT ANATOMY AND PHYSIOLOGY

Respiratory System

- A comprehensive understanding of the characteristics that differentiate pediatric respiratory anatomy and physiology from those of adults is essential to the practice of pediatric anesthesia.
- For one, neonates and infants have fewer and smaller alveoli, thus reducing lung compliance and increasing airway resistance.[1]
- This increases the work of breathing, and in combination with weaker intercostal muscles and weaker diaphragms, respiratory muscles fatigue more easily in patients of this age.
- Furthermore, a decreased functional residual capacity (FRC) in neonates and infants results in decreased oxygen reserve during periods of apnea (ie, intubation attempts).[2]
- This puts neonates and infants at an increased risk for atelectasis and hypoxemia.
- It is not until late childhood that the alveoli become fully mature (around 8 y of age) (Figure 4.2).

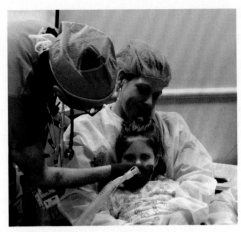

Figure 4.1 Induction of anesthesia. (Reprinted with permission from Holzman RS, Mancuso TJ, Polaner DM. *A Practical Approach to Pediatric Anesthesia*. 2nd ed. Philadelphia, PA: Wolters Kluwer; 2016.)

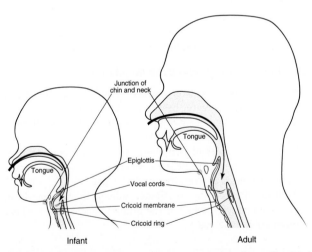

Figure 4.2 Anatomic differences of infant versus adult airway. (Reprinted with permission from Nichols DG, Ackerman AD, Biagas K, Argent AC, Rogers MC, eds. *Rogers' Textbook of Pediatric Intensive Care*. 4th ed. Philadelphia, PA: Lippincott Williams & Wilkins; 2008.)

Cardiovascular System

- Neonatal hearts are relatively noncompliant given an immature left ventricle, and thus stroke volume is relatively fixed.[1]
- In other words, newborns and infants rely almost entirely on heart rate to manage cardiac output.
- This is further complicated by a sympathetic nervous system and baroreceptor reflexes that are not fully mature.[3]
- The immature heart is more susceptible to depression by anesthetics, which can result in intraoperative bradycardia and decreased cardiac output.
- Bradycardia and reductions in cardiac output can lead to hypotension, asystole, and intraoperative death for neonates and infants undergoing extended surgical procedures.[4]

Renal and Gastrointestinal Systems

- Neonates have a relatively decreased glomerular filtration rate, thus, impaired creatinine clearance, sodium retention, bicarbonate reabsorption, and impaired diluting and concentrating ability.[3]
- In neonates and infants, the immature liver conjugates drugs less readily early in life.
- The immature hepatic biotransformation pathways result in an increased risk of systemic toxicity by anesthetic drugs.

Metabolism and Temperature Regulation

- Neonates have a greater surface area relative to weight, which promotes greater heat loss to the environment.[1]
- This becomes significant in operating rooms where temperatures are often kept fairly cold.
- Even mild degrees of hypothermia can cause perioperative problems in pediatric patients, including delayed awakening from anesthesia and respiratory depression.
- Additionally, volatile anesthetics inhibit thermogenesis in brown adipocytes, which is the primary mechanism for heat production in neonates.

PHARMACOLOGIC DIFFERENCES

- Neonates and infants have a proportionately greater total water content than adults. Consequently, the volume of distribution for most intravenous (IV) drugs is disproportionately greater in younger patients.[3]

- Decreased muscle mass in pediatric patients extends the clinical duration of action of anesthetic drugs (such as thiopental and fentanyl) by delaying redistribution of the drugs to muscles.
- Neonates have been found to have decreased protein binding for various drugs (ie, thiopental, bupivacaine). Decreased protein binding increases the concentration of free drugs in circulation, thus enhancing the potency of the drugs and increasing the risk for systemic toxicity.

INDUCTION TECHNIQUES

Intravenous Induction

- IV induction is similar in pediatric patients and adults.
- Typically IV induction is performed with propofol (2-3 mg/kg) followed by a muscle relaxant (ie, succinylcholine).[2]
- The benefits of IV induction include the availability of IV access if emergency drugs need to be administered to the child rapidly.
- The drawback of IV induction is that many children become anxious at the sight of needles; thus, IV access can be difficult to attain while the patient is awake.
- Application of EMLA cream (eutectic mixture of local anesthetic) may help to decrease pain.[3]
- However, the cream needs to be in contact with the skin for at least 30 to 60 minutes before cannulation to have an effect.

Inhalational Induction

- Sevoflurane (or halothane) is typically the drug of choice for inhalational induction in pediatric patients.[2]
- It is less pungent than other anesthetics (ie, desflurane and isoflurane), and thus it can be tolerated better by pediatric patients.
- To speed induction, a single breath induction technique with 7% to 8% sevoflurane in 60% nitrous oxide can be used.[1]
- It is important to recognize anatomic differences between children and adults to ensure proper mask ventilation.
- Compression of submandibular soft tissues ought to be avoided in young children to prevent upper airway obstruction during mask ventilation.
- Following sufficient depth of anesthesia via mask ventilation, IV access can be obtained, and propofol and a muscle relaxant can be administered to facilitate the process of intubation.

TRACHEAL INTUBATION

- Adequate preoxygenation with 100% oxygen is recommended before intubation to prevent hypoxemia during periods of apnea while intubating the patient.
- Straight laryngoscope blades can be useful in aiding intubation of the anterior larynx in pediatric patients (Figure 4.3A).[1]
- The cricoid cartilage is the narrowest portion of the airway in children younger than 5 years (Figure 4.3B).
- It is essential not to try to force the endotracheal tube through the cricoid cartilage, as trauma to the area can cause postoperative edema and airway obstruction (Figure 4.3C).
- The recommended diameter of the endotracheal tube for pediatric patients can be estimated by the following formula:

$$\text{Tube diameter (mm)} = 4 + \text{Age}/4.$$

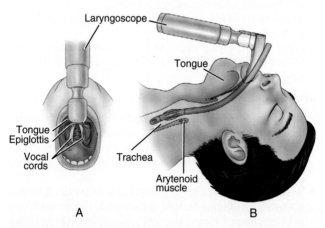

Figure 4.3 Endotracheal intubation in a patient without a cervical spine injury. A, The primary glottis landmarks for tracheal intubation as visualized with proper placement of the laryngoscope. B, Positioning the endotracheal tube. (Reprinted with permission from Honan L. *Focus on Adult Health: Medical-Surgical Nursing.* 2nd ed. Philadelphia, PA: Wolters Kluwer; 2019.)

FURTHER CONSIDERATIONS

- In recent years, there has been increased concern in the possibility that general anesthetic agents are toxic to the brains of young children.[5]
- However, more research studies need to be carried out in this area of concern.
- While the experimental data in animals are worrisome, the clinical data are currently inconclusive with regard to the extent of anesthetic risk in the pediatric population.

PEARLS AND PITFALLS

- A detailed understanding of the anatomic, physiologic, and pharmacologic characteristics of pediatric populations is essential to the practice of pediatric anesthesia.
- The cricoid cartilage is the narrowest portion of the airway in children younger than 5 years.[3]
- A decreased FRC puts neonates and infants at an increased risk for atelectasis and hypoxemia during periods of apnea (ie, intubation attempts).
- Even mild hypothermia can cause perioperative problems in pediatric patients, including delayed awakening from anesthesia and respiratory depression.[1]
- Decreased protein binding in neonates increases the concentration of free drugs in circulation, thus enhancing the potency of the anesthetics and increasing the risk for systemic toxicity.
- IV induction is typically performed with propofol (2-3 mg/kg) followed by a muscle relaxant (ie, succinylcholine).
- Sevoflurane (7%-8%) in nitrous oxide (60%) is well tolerated by pediatric patients for inhalational induction.[2]
- More research studies need to be carried out on the long-term neurologic effects of general anesthetic agents in young children.

REFERENCES

1. Butterworth JF, Mackey DC, Wasnick JD. Pediatric anesthesia. In: *Morgan & Mikhail's Clinical Anesthesiology*. 5th ed. New York, NY: McGraw-Hill; 2013.
2. Cravero JP, Havidich JE. Pediatric sedation—evolution and revolution. *Paediatr Anaesth*. 2011;21:800.
3. Cote CJ. Pediatric anesthesia. In: Miller RD, ed. *Miller's Anesthesia*. 8th ed. Elsevier Inc.; 2015:2757-2798.

4. Morray JP. Cardiac arrest in anesthetized children: recent advances and challenges for the future. *Paediatr Anaesth*. 2011;21:722.
5. Butler MG, Hayes BG, Hathaway MM, Begleiter ML. Specific genetic diseases at risk for sedation/anesthesia complications. *Anesth Analg*. 2000;91:837.

Chapter 5

Central Venous and Arterial Access in the Pediatric Patient

Rennier A. Martinez

- Difficult pediatric vascular access issues arise often and unexpectedly.
- These issues tend to be related to small vessels, intravascular depletion, lack of cooperation, and other unique anatomic and physiologic qualities of the pediatric population.
- There are different indications for obtaining vascular access.[1]
- Most difficult accesses can be obtained percutaneously aided either by ultrasound (US) or fluoroscopy guidance; however, open access may be needed in certain situations.[2]
- As with any surgical procedure, no matter how simple, complications arise and the pediatric surgeon must know how to manage them.

RELEVANT ANATOMY

- Preoperatively the surgeon must decide what type of access to obtain and the size and number of lumens required.
- In neonates the femoral vein lies posterior (rather than medial) to the femoral artery. This requires a different US-guided approach than in older children or adults.[2]
- Common access sites:
  - Blood sampling: heel, antecubital arteries/veins, scalp arteries/veins, femoral veins (last resort)
  - Peripheral venous access: hand veins (dorsum), antecubital veins, cephalic vein at wrist, long greater saphenous at ankle, femoral veins
  - Central venous access: subclavian, internal jugular (IJ) or external jugular, femoral, umbilical vein and artery
  - Intraosseous (IO): anterior tibia, distal femur **(Figure 5.1)**

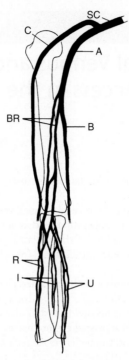

Figure 5.1 Upper extremity veins. The upper extremity veins are paired into deep and superficial drainage. The superficial veins tend to be larger and the dominant system of the upper extremity. The superficial system comprises the cephalic and basilic veins at the forearm. The cephalic vein extends along the lateral forearm. The cephalic vein joins the axillary vein at the humeral head or clavicle. The cephalic vein can be paired. The basilic vein runs through the medial forearm and continues to the upper arm. The basilic vein joins the brachial vein at the mid–upper arm to form the axillary vein. The median antebrachial vein runs on the ventral forearm and drains the palmar venous plexus. The deep veins (radial and ulnar veins) are small and paired, communicate with each other, and accompany the forearm arteries. SC, subclavian; C, cephalic; A, axillary; BR, brachial; B, basilic; R, radial; I, interosseous; U, ulnar. (Reprinted with permission from Dyer R. *Handbook of Basic Vascular and Interventional Radiology.* New York, NY: Churchill Livingstone; 1993:160.)

VENOUS CATHETERS

Peripheral Venous Access

- This type of access is adequate for intravenous (IV) hydration, most medications, and often blood sampling.[2]
- It is the first access obtained in most inpatients.

- It can become quite difficult to obtain in volume depleted, restless, small pediatric patients, ie, emergency situations.
  - In these cases, a surgeon's expertise may be requested.
  - In cases where peripheral intravenous (PIV) access has failed, IO or cutdown techniques become quick and efficient alternatives.
- Common peripheral target veins are in dorsum of hand, forearm, dorsum of foot, medial ankle, and scalp (neonates).
- Scalp veins and external jugular veins are easily accessible but hard to maintain because of patient movements.

Techniques Aiding Peripheral Cannulation

- They include warming extremity, transillumination, and epidermal vasodilators.[1]
- US can be used to cannulate cephalic and basilic veins.

Complications

- They include phlebitis, thrombosis, and extravasation with chemical burns or necrosis of surrounding tissues.[1]
- Recent studies show that US in PIV access increases accuracy and decreases attempts required.
- Other recent technologic advances include infrared-based vein finders.[4-7]

Intraosseous Access

- If PIV access fails, then IO is the fastest and most effective route of administering fluids, drugs, or blood in children <6 years of age.[8]
- Most effective in children <6 years of age because the bone marrow is better perfused.
- For children >6 years of age, venous cutdown should be performed if percutaneous attempts fail.
- Best IO access sites are midline of anterior tibia below tibial tuberosity or distal femur.
  - Angle needle 60° from horizontal and point toward middle of tibia/femur depending on the bone chosen
  - Once cortex is penetrated, aspirate to ensure proper position
  - IO access is faster and safer than emergency central venous catheter (CVC) placement[1]
  - **Contraindications**: diseases of the bone or ipsilateral extremity fractures

- **Complications**: 1% complication rate; subperiosteal or sub-cutaneous infiltration (most common); fracture, growth plate injury, fat embolism, compartment syndrome, and osteomyelitis rare[3]
  - Remove needle as soon as better access obtained

Venous Cutdown

- With increased IO access use, venous cutdown as well as emergency CVC placement has been almost eliminated.[1,2]
- However, this set of skills is still essential for any pediatric surgeon.
- Best target vessel is long saphenous vein near medial malleolus, although cephalic vein at the deltopectoral groove is another good target (Figure 5.2).
  - Ankle cutdown: short transverse incision proximal and anterior to medial malleolus
  - Exposed vein is encircled with a silk suture, and an appropriate angiocatheter is introduced. No need to ligate or transect vein[8]

Central Venous Catheters

- This type of catheter is used less with the advent of peripherally inserted central catheters (PICCs). Indications range from emergent to long-term use.
- Many different types of CVCs are available, and the pediatric surgeon must know each type and indications for each.
- Main determinants of catheter selection are intended duration and frequency of use.[2]
  - CVCs designed for long-term use include the tunneled lines, ie, Broviac and Hickman catheters.
  - These are ideal for continuous infusion of medications or for total parenteral nutrition (TPN).[2]
  - If long-term intermittent use is desired (chemo), then ports are typically used.
    - Both types of catheters allow for more than one lumen is so desired.
  - CVCs designed for acute or emergent use are the nontunneled lines.
    - Tunneling allows for longer duration by reducing chances of infection.
  - Hemodialysis (HD) lines follow similar indications.
- US guidance for insertion is gold standard.

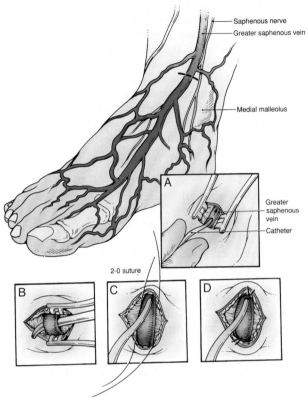

Figure 5.2 Saphenous vein cutdown at the ankle. A, Introduction of catheter into vein without ligation of vein. B, Isolation of vein. C, Insertion of catheter with vascular control of vein. D, Vein ligated distally and catheter tied in proximally. (Reprinted with permission from Scott-Conner CEH, Dawson DL, eds. *Scott-Conner & Dawson Essential Operative Techniques and Anatomy*. 4th ed. Philadelphia, PA: Wolters Kluwer/Lippincott Williams & Wilkins; 2014.)

- Most common access sites include, but are not limited to, IJ, facial, external jugular, subclavian, saphenous, and common femoral veins.
  - Less common sites include gonadal, intercostal, azygous, and hemiazygous veins and the right atrium (RA).[9]
  - These are rarely needed and typically used if common sites are unavailable.
  - Right subclavian access site is associated with 4-fold increased incidence of malposition than left.[9]

- Left has smoother, less angulated course into the innominate vein and right side of the heart.
- In premature neonates the relevant central vein or one of its tributaries such as the common facial vein, external jugular vein, cephalic vein, and saphenous vein are exposed surgically and cannulated directly.[1]
  - Care not to injure surrounding structures such as the carotid artery, vagus, esophagus, and trachea.
  - It is worth remembering that in neonates all these structures are incredibly small and close.

PERCUTANEOUS TECHNIQUE

- US is placed across the table, and patient, supine across radiolucent table.
- Extremities are extended if they contain target vessel otherwise tucked.
- If subclavian or IJ access is desired, then the patient is placed in Trendelenburg position (prevent air embolism) with the neck extended.
- Shoulder roll can be used to aid in neck extension for IJ access (not for subclavian access, as it can decrease the cross-sectional area of the vein).
- Femoral vein exposure can be aided by abduction and external rotation of the leg.[2]
- Seldinger technique is almost universally used to gain access into vessels.
- Most venous access in children can be obtained with a 21 or 22 g needle.
- This allows for a 0.018-inch coaxial wire (straight tip).
- Avoid J or C wires.[2]
- Routine use of micropuncture sets is helpful.
  - It is imperative to confirm proper placement before and after inserting the catheter.
    - When using percutaneous approach, it is important to ensure one is in the vein before dilating the tract and placing the catheter.
    - Dilating a tract in an artery can be disastrous especially in the pediatric population with small vasculature.
    - There are many strategies to ensure IV access.

TECHNIQUES TO CONFIRM VENOUS ACCESS

- Pulsatile flow indicates arterial puncture.
- However, in hypotensive patients this may not be the case.

- Return of deoxygenated color of blood (dark) indicates venous blood.
- However, in very sick patient with poor oxygenation this is not always true.
- Premature atrial contractions on ECG indicate right heart placement of wire.
- An angiocatheter may be placed and pressure transduced, aiding in confirming positioning via proper waveform.
- Fluoroscopic imaging with or without contrast can be used to delineate anatomy.
- Recognition of unintended intra-arterial access before dilation and placement is of utmost importance when accessing the subclavian vein.
  - In this location, it is difficult to hold pressure and the low-pressure system in the thoracic cavity may aid in continued bleeding.
    - Development of hemothorax is a risk, and inadvertent placement into an artery may need operative repair.
- It is also imperative that when inserting the stiff dilators, fluoroscopy is used to ensure wire is not kinking.
  - Kinking of the wire may result in dilator to lacerate vein and cause significant injury depending on the location.[9]
- Proper position:
  - From lower body: The tip of CVC should be at the junction of RA and inferior vena cava (IVC). Proper positioning prevents thrombosis.[1]
  - From upper body: The tip of CVC should be at the junction of RA and superior vena cava (SVC).
  - Same location applies for PICCs. Failure to do this leads to higher complications (Figure 5.3).[9]

Umbilical Vein Central Access

- Typically used in critically ill neonates
- Often possible within a few hours of birth; however, the pediatric surgeon can often dissect umbilical stump and cannulate it after it has undergone early dissection[1]
  - Used for CVP or arterial pressure monitoring, fluids, medications, and TPN
  - Removed after maximum of 14 days to minimize complications; 5 days for umbilical artery

Complications

- Perforation of IVC, extravasation into peritoneal cavity, and portal vein thrombosis

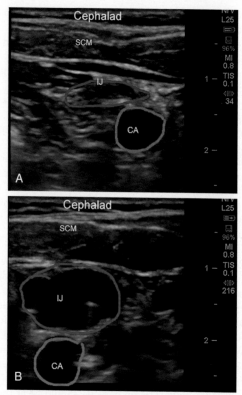

Figure 5.3 A, Noncompressible left internal jugular vein in a patient with a chronic deep venous thrombosis (DVT). Maximal force was being applied, and the vein was still noncompressible. The vein also has the classic heterogeneous appearance of a chronic DVT. B, The right internal jugular vein of the previous patient. Notice how the right internal jugular vein is of normal size and anechoic appearance. CA, carotid artery; IJ, internal jugular vein; SCM, sternocleidomastoid muscle. (Reprinted with permission from Bigeleisen PE, ed. *Ultrasound-Guided Regional Anesthesia and Pain Medicine*. 2nd ed. Philadelphia, PA: Wolters Kluwer Health; 2015.)

Peripherally Inserted Central Catheters

- Suitable for fluids, medications, TPN, and blood products
- Versatile and durable and can be used for long-term (weeks) medication infusion in outpatients
- Often placed by ancillary staff
- Evidence exists that early PICC placement is preferable to treatment through multiple PIV access[1]

Complications

- Infections, occlusion, and dislodgement of catheter
  - Symptomatic upper extremity deep venous thrombosis (DVT) 1% versus 7% if receiving chemotherapy in adults

Totally Implanted Central Venous Catheters (Ports)

- Long-lasting central venous access
- Used often in patients with conditions such as malignancies, renal failure, and hemolytic disorders
- Some can be used for high-flow contrast infusion for imaging
- Best sites are pectoral area, parasternal, and subclavicular

Complications

- Inability to access port, disconnection of catheter from port, flipping of port, embolization of the catheter, and breakdown of overlying skin

Measures to Ensure Durability of Catheter

- Careful placement using US or fluoroscopy to reduce vessel injury
- Sterile technique
- Good stabilization to prevent dislodgement
- Heparin infusion, heparin-coated catheters, and antibiotic-coated catheters to prevent infection

Alternate Routes for Central Venous Access

- Patients with multiple previous CVC placements are at risk for central vein stenosis or thrombosis, which will preclude placement of a new catheter.
- These patients are by far the most difficult vascular access patients.
- Venography should be used to survey available central veins.
  - CT or MRI venogram
  - Venogram in the interventional radiology (IR) suite (allows for treatment if stenosis present)
  - Target vessels include brachiocephalic vein, SVC, and IVC
  - Malpositioned catheters have higher rates of complications
- Possible "last resort" access sites:
  - Percutaneous transhepatic cholangiography (PTC) access via a patent IVC using a translumbar (more durable) or transhepatic (dislodges often because of diaphragmatic excursion) approach
  - PTC access via patent brachiocephalic vein using supra-sternal route

- Other possible sites are the azygous via intercostal veins percutaneously or open (thoracotomy)
- Direct RA access if all else fails

Complications Common to All Vascular Access Procedures

- Pseudoaneurysm (commonly due to unrecognized arterial puncture), infections, thrombosis, extravasation, hematoma, distal embolization
- Arterial puncture: common but usually treated easily with immediate recognition and adequate compression[9]
  - Use techniques explained elsewhere in this chapter to ensure venous access is obtained and prevent unintended placement of catheter into arterial vasculature

Immediate Postprocedural Care and Recovery

- Early complications must be assessed:
  - Any IJ or subclavian access routine chest X-ray (CXR) rules out pneumothorax and confirms proper position of line
  - In general, line can be used immediately after placement
  - Few limitations on activity
  - If patient to be discharged, then proper education on care of the catheter should be given

Removal of Catheters

- Indications for removal of lines depend on type and intended use.
- But generally they are removed because they are no longer needed, they stopped working, or they are infected.
- Complexity of removal also depends on the type of catheter.
  - Nontunneled CVCs and PICCs are generally pulled out while patient is bearing down, and pressure is applied for hemostasis.[2]
  - Tunneled CVCs often require local anesthesia and sedation in children. Ports may require general anesthesia, as the port is sutured to the chest wall.[2]
  - Occasionally, a long-standing catheter is unable to be removed, indicating adherence to the venous endothelium.
    - If catheter is unable to be removed by gentle, constant pulling, the surgeon should place a wire down the catheter into the IVC before proceeding with more aggressive maneuvers.
    - This will facilitate retrieval if the catheter breaks and embolizes to the heart.[2]

- If cuff removal is difficult, it may be best to cut down to it rather than risk catheter rupture and embolization into central vasculature or heart.[9]
- If distal embolization of catheter occurs, then interventional cardiology is best for retrieval followed by IR.
- Line-related procedures are NEVER routine.
- It is when one has become "comfortable" doing these procedures that the "line that would not end" usually occurs.[9]

ARTERIAL CATHETERS

- Intra-arterial catheters allows for continuous hemodynamic monitoring and arterial blood sampling.
- Arteries carry their own set of risks when instrumented, and thus it is paramount to be aware of these to prevent them or lessen their morbidity when they do occur.
- Common access sites:
  - Radial arteries: common target because of dual blood supply to hand (ulnar artery) and good collateralization
    - Use Allen test to evaluate
    - Allows preductal monitoring
    - Often carried out percutaneous with or without US guidance
    - Cutdown can be performed as well
  - Dorsalis pedis or posterior tibial arteries are also sometimes used
  - Femoral arteries: usually for catheter-based interventions; less frequently for monitoring
    - Avoid using main artery to extremity for chronic catheter placement to prevent thromboembolic and ischemic complications

HEMODIALYSIS CATHETERS

- For HD access, autologous arteriovenous fistulas are the gold standard; however, it is common for pediatric patients to require HD emergently and continue to need it long-term, and thus in this setting a temporary or a tunneled dialysis catheter may be necessary until permanent access can be obtained if required (Figure 5.4).
  - Temporary or tunneled HD catheters:
    - Preferentially in right jugular vein either percutaneously or by cutdown

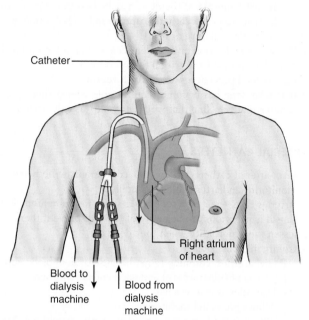

Catheter

Right atrium
of heart

Blood to
dialysis
machine

Blood from
dialysis
machine

Figure 5.4 Hemodialysis access sites. Hemodialysis requires vascular access. The site and type of access depend on expected duration of dialysis, surgeon's preference, and patient's condition. Central venous access using the Seldinger technique: The surgeon inserts an introducer needle into the subclavian vein and then inserts a guide wire through the introducer needle and removes the needle. Using the guide wire, the surgeon threads a 5- to 12-inch (12.5- to 30.5-cm) plastic or Teflon catheter (with a Y-hub) into the patient's vein. Another large vein, such as the femoral vein, also may be used. Central venous access usually is used temporarily when hemodialysis must be started immediately and the patient does not have a functioning arteriovenous (AV) fistula or graft. This access may be used long-term if the patient has problems maintaining an AV fistula or graft. (Reprinted with permission from Lippincott Nursing Advisor 2011. © Wolters Kluwer.)

MANAGEMENT OF COMMON COMPLICATIONS

Infection

- Management is controversial, and approach is surgeon- and institution-dependent.
- Three types of infections exist.
  - Exit-site infection: typically caused by skin pathogen and treated with antibiotics and local wound care

- Tunnel/pocket infection: more serious than exit-site infections and might lead to sepsis. Removal is often indicated, as antibiotics have poor penetration
- Central-line–associated blood stream infection (CLABSI): most serious and can lead to systemic sepsis
  - External signs may be absent
  - Need cultures from central and peripheral sites
- In children it has been shown that chlorhexidine skin preparation and chlorhexidine-impregnated dressing as well as use of heparin and antibiotic-impregnated central catheters prevent CLABSI.[10,11]
- Use of ethanol lock or vancomycin lock therapy has also been useful.
- If suspected infection, then peripheral and central blood cultures should be drawn before starting empiric antibiotics.
- Antibiotics are sometimes sufficient; however, if after 72 hours bacteremia has not cleared, then catheter should be removed.
- Catheter removal is also required if involving resistant organisms.

Failure of Flow

- Algorithmically check position of tip in CXR.
- If tip is in correct position, then do a dye study to evaluate for thrombus at the end of tip and the need for lytic therapy (tPA) versus removal.[9]
  - Occlusion due to lipids or mineral deposits may be cleared with 70% ethanol and hydrochloric acid, respectively.
  - If medical therapy is ineffective, then catheter removal and replacement may be necessary.

Perforation

- Perforation of the SVC or RA by central catheter is extremely rare with incidence ranging from 0.0001% to 1.4%.[2]
- Choice of catheter material (silastic vs polyurethane) does not affect perforation rate.
- Right IJ catheters have the least risk because the course of the catheter is straight and the side tends to contact the vessel wall as opposed to the tip.
- Perforation below the pericardial reflection leads to cardiac tamponade as opposed to that above the reflection, where it leads to hemothorax.
- To avoid this complication, the tip of the catheter should be at the cavoatrial junction.[2]

PEARLS AND PITFALLS

- Vascular access especially in the pediatric population is never routine.
- Use techniques that ensure you are at your target access site—vein versus artery.
- Confirm proper positioning of catheters to increase its life span.
- Always be aware of possible complications, as complications have best outcomes when recognized early.

REFERENCES

1. Holcomb III G, Murphy JP, eds. *Ashcraft's Pediatric Surgery*. 5th ed. Philadelphia: Saunders; 2010.
2. Church JT, Jarboe MD. Vascular access in the pediatric population. *Surg Clin North Am*. 2017;97(1):113-128.
3. Arensman RM, Bambini DA, Almond PS, Adolph V, Radhakrishnan J, eds. *Pediatric Surgery*. 2nd ed. Austin, Texas: Landes Bioscience; 2009.
4. Ishii S, Shime N, Shibasaki M, Sawa T. Ultrasound-guided radial artery catheterization in infants and small children. *Pediatr Crit Care Med*. 2013;14(5):471-473.
5. Tang L, Wang F, Li Y, et al. Ultrasound guidance for radial artery catheterization: an updated meta-analysis of randomized controlled trials. *PLoS One*. 2014;9(11):e111527.
6. Guillon P, Makhloufi M, Baillie S, Roucoulet C, Dolimier E, Masquelier AM. Prospective evaluation of venous access difficulty and a near-infrared vein visualizer at four French haemophilia treatment centres. *Haemophilia*. 2015;21(1):21-26.
7. Chiao FB, Resta-Flarer F, Lesser J, et al. Vein visualization: patient characteristic factors and efficacy of a new infrared vein finder technology. *Br J Anaesth*. 2013;110(6):966-971.
8. Grosfeld JL, O'Neil JAJ, Fonkalsrud EW, Coran AG, eds. *Pediatric Surgery*. 6th ed. Philadelphia: Mosby; 2006 [No. 1].
9. Gaty MG, ed. *Complications in Pediatric Surgery*. New York: Informa Healthcare USA; 2009.
10. Chen IC, Hsu C, Chen YC, et al. Predictors of bloodstream infection associated with permanently implantable venous port in solid cancer patients. *Ann Oncol*. 2013;24(2):463-468.
11. Freeman JJ, Gadepalli SK, Siddiqui SM, Jarboe MD, Hirschl RB. Improving central line infection rates in the neonatal intensive care unit: effect of hospital location, site of insertion, and implementation of catheter-associated bloodstream infection protocols. *J Pediatr Surg*. 2015;50(5):860-863.

Chapter 6

Common Pediatric Drug Dosing

Grace E. Pryor

- Proper drug dosing enables the physician to achieve a desired pharmacologic effect while avoiding unnecessary toxicity.[1]
- There are specific characteristics in the pediatric patient that must be considered to understand adequate drug dosing and pharmacologic mechanism of action.
- The anatomic differences in a neonate versus an infant, child, or adolescent pose a unique challenge in drug therapy, and one that cannot always be investigated through clinical trials as in adults.
- These differences in body composition may affect the volume of distribution of a particular drug and thus the ability of the drug to achieve a desired effect.[1]

PHARMACOKINETICS OF THE PEDIATRIC PATIENT

- Note that total body water makes up 75% to 80% of body weight in the full-term newborn, decreasing to 60% at 5 months of age.[1]
- By 5 months of age, total body fat doubles at the expense of total body water.[1]
- By 2 years of age, protein mass begins to rise at the expense of body fat and is physically noticeable, as infants become toddlers and begin to ambulate.[1]
- Fat-soluble and water-soluble drugs will therefore distribute differently in a child depending on body composition.[1]
- These changes in composition are important to recognize in the pediatric patient and may contribute to inadequate drug concentration or toxicity.
- The GI tract is a common route of absorption in pediatrics.
- Gastric acid is lowest in the newborn and does not reach adult levels until 2 years of age.[1]
- Motility in the GI tract in the infant is also erratic and characterized by peristalsis, corresponding to longer transit times.[1]

- Premature infants may have transit times of anywhere from 8 to 96 hours, as opposed to 4 to 12 hours observed in adults.[1]
- This delayed gastric emptying, also complicated by regurgitation in the infant, may result in delayed absorption in the duodenum.[1]
- Once a child hits school age, however, there are few differences in the absorption of drugs in the GI tract from adults.[1]
- Hepatic and renal functions are decreased in the neonate and develop as the child ages.
- The ability of the liver and kidney to metabolize drugs develops as these organs mature, usually after 1 year of age.
- Rectal administration of drugs is a common route of choice, especially if an infant is vomiting or unable to swallow medicine.[1]
- Note that medicine administered rectally is absorbed through the hemorrhoidal veins and into the systemic circulation, bypassing first-pass metabolism in the liver.[1]

COMMON ANTIBIOTICS

- Prophylactic antibiotic usage accounts for about 75% of prescriptions of antibiotics on a surgical service.[2]
- Antibiotics may also be required either as necessary in the management of the primary disease process or as a result of postoperative infection.
- Antibiotic prophylaxis is indicated during clean-contaminated, contaminated, and dirty cases.[2]
- If used, the first dose of antibiotics should be given 30 minutes to 1 hour before the first incision.[3]
- Additional doses may be indicated if a procedure lasts longer than 2 half-lives of the drug given to maintain appropriate serum levels or if excessive blood loss is encountered during the procedure.[4]
- If prophylaxis is continued postoperatively, antibiotics should not be given for longer than 24 hours.[4]
- Note that data for dosing have been extrapolated from adult dosing and based on expert opinion.[5]
- In general, fluoroquinolones should not be used for surgical prophylaxis in pediatric patients owing to their potential for toxicity.[5]
- Pediatric dosages should not exceed adult dosages.
- If a calculated mg per kg dose exceeds adult dosage, as may be found in adolescent patients, adult dosing should be used instead.[5]

VENOUS THROMBOEMBOLISM PROPHYLAXIS

- The overall risk of venous thromboembolism (VTE) is low in the pediatric patient, estimated to be from 0.02% to 0.33% of injured, hospitalized children.[6]
- Adequate prophylaxis is complicated by the fact that there are very few studies investigating VTE and anticoagulation in children. Most of the recommendations used today are extrapolated from adult data.[6]
- Despite the lack of trial data, low-molecular-weight heparin (LMWH) agents are the most popular anticoagulant of choice in children.[7]
- Benefits of LMWH include reduced need for monitoring and decreased risk of interaction with other medications.[7]
- For both neonates and children, target anti-Xa activity should be 0.5 to 1.0 units/mL in a sample taken 4 to 6 hours after injection.[7]
- Recent consensus indicates that children younger than 12 years who can ambulate may not require chemical VTE prophylaxis.[6]
- Mechanical prophylaxis should be used in all adolescents who are unable to ambulate.[6]
- Anticoagulation should be considered in adolescents with at least 2 risk factors for development of thromboembolism.[8]
- It is essential to remember that with patients of all ages, the risk of thromboembolism versus the risk of acute bleed must be balanced.
- Contraindications to pharmacologic prophylaxis are similar to those of the adult patient. Absolute contraindications include history of a bleeding disorder, evidence or high risk of hemorrhage, and platelet count <50 000/mm.[8]

PAIN MANAGEMENT

- Effective postoperative pain management that achieves pain relief with minimal side effects has been associated with faster recovery and quicker returns to school and play.[2]
- However, studies continue to report undertreatment in both medical and surgical patients.
- In the pediatric patient, poor pain management may be inadequate owing to inability to evaluate the infant's pain level or physician and parental fear of opioid side effects or "addiction."[2]

- Pain scales for the nonverbal neonate to the school-aged child are available and should be used to evaluate pain.
- These include the Face, Legs, Activity, Cry, Consolability Scale (FLACC) for children from 1 month to 4 years of age, the Wong-Baker Faces Pain Rating Scale for those from 5 to 9 years of age and in children who are developmentally appropriate, and a numerical scale for those older than 10 years of age.[2]
- Opioid use in the pediatric patient is common.[2]
- Morphine is the equivalence by which all other opioids are measured.[2]
- Intermittent bolus administration of morphine to opioid-naive children should be started at 0.05 to 0.1 mg/kg every 2 to 4 hours.[2,9]
- Patient-controlled analgesia use may be appropriate in older children and adolescents.
- Hydromorphone is 5 to 7 times more potent than morphine and has a similar duration of action to morphine.[2,9]
- Fentanyl is 100 times more potent than morphine and has a short duration of action owing to high absorption into fat.[2,9]
- Note that this shorter half-life may potentiate tolerance easier than morphine/hydromorphone.[2]
- Side effects of opioids should be closely monitored, the most serious of which is dose-dependent respiratory depression.[2,9]
- Respiratory depression may be more prominent in neonates and young infants.
- Other side effects in pediatric patients are dysphoria, somnolence, nausea and vomiting, pruritus, constipation, and urinary retention.[2]
- Appropriate bowel regimen should be prescribed with all opioid use.[2,9]
- Nonsteroidal anti-inflammatory agents are effective for mild to moderate pain relief.[2]
- Ketorolac is effective and is not associated with nausea, vomiting, or respiratory depression seen with opioids.[2]
- Note that NSAIDs are contraindicated in renal disease, coagulopathy, or a history of gastric ulcers.[2]
- NSAID use is also limited in patients at risk for postoperative bleeding.[2]
- Home pain management offers a number of concerns unique to the pediatric patient.
- As opposed to crying, children may become withdrawn and irritable in response to pain and parents may not able to recognize this.[2]

- Parents may also fail to provide adequate pain medication owing to fear of adverse effects or perceived potential for addiction.[2]
- In the past, codeine was commonly prescribed for pain management at home.
- However, recent studies have shown that some patients have increased CYP2D6 activity.[10]
- These patients, known as ultrarapid metabolizers, have increased plasma levels of morphine in the body.[10]
- This has caused the FDA to issue a strong warning to restrict the use of codeine and tramadol in patients younger than 12 years due to reports of respiratory depression.[10]
- In addition, care should be taken when prescribing opioids to adolescents.
- Surveys of high school seniors in the United States older than 40 years show that the use of prescription opioids is strongly correlated with misuse in adolescents and that misuse typically follows medical use by the patient.[11]
- Alternatives to opioids should always be considered and if opioids are prescribed, the smallest necessary amount should be written.[11]

POSTOPERATIVE NAUSEA AND VOMITING

- Postoperative nausea and vomiting (PONV) is the most common cause of delayed discharge from the postanesthesia care unit and the most common reason for unanticipated hospitalization after outpatient surgery in the pediatric patient.[2]
- Incidence is quite high and has been found to be between 33.2% and 82% of pediatric patients.[12]
- Common risk factors for PONV include previous PONV or positive family history of PONV, anesthesia >30 minutes, and age >3 years.[12,13]
- In addition, the type of surgical procedure may increase the risk of PONV.
- Strabismus and ENT procedures such as tonsillectomy and adenoidectomy may be associated with PONV rates as high as 54% and 82%, respectively.[12]
- New data suggest that pediatric patients undergoing appendectomy and combined herniotomy/orchidopexy are also at an increased risk for PONV.[12]
- Perioperative use of any opioid is associated with a very high incidence of PONV, even when general anesthetic drugs associated with a lower incidence of nausea, such as propofol, are used.[2,12]

- Common approaches to treat or prevent PONV include alteration of the anesthetic technique, perioperative administration of antiemetics (either prophylactically or as treatment), and limitation of postoperative oral intake.[2,12]
- Current recommendations for children older than 3 years include the following[12]:
1. Outpatient (short anesthesia or surgery time less than 30 minutes, rare use of postoperative opioids):
   a. Small pediatric surgery: single prophylaxis
   b. Strabismus or ear-nose-throat surgery or high-risk patients: double prophylaxis
2. Inpatient (longer anesthesia or surgery time greater than 30 minutes, frequent use of postoperative opioids):
   a. Different pediatric surgical procedures: double prophylaxis
   b. Strabismus or ear-nose-throat surgery or high risk: triple prophylaxis
- Rescue therapy is dependent on the agent used.
- Droperidol is an effective dopamine antagonist, whereas dimenhydrinate is an effective histamine antagonist.[12,13]
- When using combination therapy, agents from different drug classes should be used.[12,13]
- Consensus guidelines suggest prophylactic use of a combination of dexamethasone and ondansetron in most pediatric patients at high risk for PONV unless there are contraindications.[12,13]

PEARLS AND PITFALLS

- GI absorption of drugs in the pediatric patient normalizes once the child hits school age.
- In pediatrics, drug dosage is weight-based; if a calculated mg per kg exceeds the adult dosage, the adult dosage should be used instead.
- Children younger than 12 years with no risk factors for VTE development do not require chemical prophylaxis.
- Morphine is the equivalence by which all other opioids are measured; hydromorphone is 5 to 7 times more potent than morphine, whereas fentanyl is 100 times more potent.
- To prevent postoperative nausea and vomiting, single-agent prophylaxis should be used in small, outpatient surgical procedures, whereas longer, inpatient surgical procedures necessitate double prophylaxis.

REFERENCES

1. Yaffe S, Aranda J. *Neonatal and Pediatric Pharmacology Therapeutic Principles in Practice.* 4th ed. Wolters Kluwer Health; 2015.

2. Holcomb G, Murphy J, Ostlie D. *Ashcraft's Pediatric Surgery Expert Consult.* 6th ed. London: Elsevier Health Sciences; 2014.

3. Berrios-Torres SI, Umscheid CA, Bratzler DW, et al. Centers for Disease Control and Prevention guideline for the prevention of surgical site infection, 2017. *JAMA Surg.* 2017. doi:10.1001/jamasurg.2017.090.

4. CHOC Children's Hospital. *Antibiotic Prophylaxis for Surgery Guideline.* 2017. https://www.choc.org/userfiles/AntibioticProphylaxis ForSurgeryGuideline.pdf.

5. Bratzler DW, Dellinger EP, Olsen KM, et al. Clinical practice guidelines for antimicrobial prophylaxis in surgery. *Am J Health Syst Pharm.* 2013;70:195-283.

6. Hanson SJ, Faustino EV, Mahajerin A, et al. Recommendations for venous thromboembolism prophylaxis in pediatric trauma patients: a national, multidisciplinary consensus study. *J Trauma Acute Care Surg.* 2016;80:695-701

7. Monagle P, Chan AKC, Goldenberg NA, et al. Antithrombotic therapy in neonates and children: antithrombotic therapy and prevention of thrombosis, 9th ed: American College of Chest Physicians evidence-based clinical practice guidelines. *Chest.* 2012;141(2 suppl):e737S-e801S. doi:10.1378/chest.11-2308.

8. Multidisciplinary VTE Prophylaxis BESt Team. *Best Evidence Statement Venous Thromboembolism (VTE) Prophylaxis in Children and Adolescents.* Cincinnati Children's Hospital Medical Center; 2014:1-14. http://www.cincinnatichildrens.org/service/j/anderson-center/ evidence-based-care/bests/BESt181.

9. Pain Management and Dosing Guide. *Pain Assessment and Management Initiative.* University of Florida College of Medicine- Jacksonville. Department of Emergency Medicine; 2016. http://americanpainso- ciety.org/uplo ads/education/PAMI_Pain_Mangement_and_Dosing_ Guide_02282017.pdf.

10. U.S. Food and Drug Administration. *FDA Restricts Use of Prescription Codeine Pain and Cough Medicines and Tramadol Pain Medicines in Children; Recommends against Use in Breastfeeding Women.* Drug Safety Communications; 2017. https://www.fda.gov/downloads/ Drugs/DrugSafety/UCM553814.pdf.

11. McCabe SE, West BT, Veliz P, McCabe VV, Stoddard SA, Boyd C. Trends in medical and nonmedical use of prescription opioids among US adolescents: 1976-2015. *Pediatrics.* 2017;139:e2016-e2387.

12. Hohne C. Postoperative nausea and vomiting in pediatric anesthesia. *Curr Opin Anesthesiol.* 2014;27:303-308. doi:10.1097/ ACO.0000000000000073.

13. Gan TJ, Diemunsch P, Habib AS, et al. Consensus guidelines for the management of postoperative nausea and vomiting. *Anesth Analg.* 2014;118(1):85-113. doi:10.1213/ane.0000000000000002.

Pediatric Trauma Surgery

Chapter 7

The Approach to the Pediatric Trauma Patient

Joshua P. Parreco

- Unintentional injury is the leading cause of morbidity and mortality in children in the United States.
- Injuries related to motor vehicles are the leading cause of death in children, whereas injuries from falls are the leading cause of nonfatal injury.[1]
- In high-income countries, the annual rate of physical abuse is 4% to 16% of children,[2] and children with abuse-related fractures are missed by physicians in 20% of first visits.[3]
- In the 1970s and 1980s, J Alex Haller of Johns Hopkins University first developed, implemented, and championed a modern trauma system for pediatric patients.[4]

TRAUMA RESUSCITATION

- The resuscitation of the pediatric trauma patient is guided by fundamental advanced trauma life support (ATLS) principles, including the primary (ABCDE), secondary (AMPLE), and tertiary surveys.
- With acute blood loss, children will maintain a normal central blood pressure longer than adults.
- Shock in children is manifested as tachycardia, delayed capillary refill, altered mental status, decreased urine output, and tachypnea.
- Normal values for heart rate (beats per minute), blood pressure (mm Hg), and respiratory rate (breaths per minute), respectively[5]:
  - <1 year: <160, >60, <60
  - 1 to 2 years: <150, >70, <40

- 3 to 5 years: <140, >75, <35
- 6 to 12 years: <120, >80, <30
- >12 years: <100, >90, <30
- Hypovolemia should be treated with a bolus of 20 mL/kg of an isotonic crystalloid solution. Failure to improve should result in a second bolus. Continued failure should then result in transfusion of packed red blood cells followed by fresh frozen plasma and platelets.[6]
- The Broselow Pediatric Emergency Tape is a widely used color-coded tape measure that relates a child's height to weight and provides instructions regarding medication dosages and other equipment sizes. The colors typically correspond to a colored pouch in a resuscitation kit or colored drawer in the pediatric resuscitation cart.

PRIMARY SURVEY

- Airway
  - Protect airway and stabilize C-spine manually or with a collar.
  - In small children, avoid passive flexion of the neck that can result in anterior buckling of the pharynx owing to a larger occiput.
  - Indications for endotracheal intubation include inadequate ventilation, inability to protect airway, or respiratory failure that is anticipated.
  - Newborns require an uncuffed endotracheal tube to avoid pressure-induced damage. Traditionally an uncuffed tube was recommended for all children younger than 8 years of age; however, modern tubes that support low pressures with high volumes are safe.
  - The diameter of a child's fifth finger can serve as an approximate tube diameter.
  - Surgical cricothyrotomy is contraindicated below the age of 12 years owing to potential laryngeal injury or stenosis. Needle cricothyroidotomy can be safely performed on patients of any age.
- Breathing
  - Identify and treat impairments to adequate ventilation.
  - Hemothorax: Place the chest tube.
  - Pneumothorax: Place the chest tube or perform needle decompression.
  - Open pneumothorax: Place 3-sided occlusive dressing.
- Circulation
  - Check distal pulses first and then central.
  - Start cardiac compressions for absent pulse.

TABLE 7.1			
Pediatric Glasgow Coma Score			
Score	**Motor**	**Verbal**	**Eye Opening**
6	Spontaneous	NA	NA
5	Localizes	Age appropriate	NA
4	Withdrawals	Cries but consolable	Spontaneous
3	Flexion	Irritable	To voice
2	Extension	Restless	To pain
1	None	None	None

Adapted from Mattox KL, Moore EE, Feliciano DV. *Trauma.* 7th ed. McGraw Hill Professional; 2012.

- Emergency department (ED) thoracotomy is indicated after blunt injury with loss of vitals in the ED or after penetrating injury with loss of vitals in the field or ED.
- Control hemorrhage with direct pressure or proximal tourniquet.
- Secure intravenous or intraosseous access and start fluid resuscitation.
- Disability
  - Calculate Glasgow coma score (GCS) (Table 7.1).
  - Assess pupils.
- Exposure
  - Remove clothing and cover with warm blanket.
- Adjuncts to the primary survey
  - Focused assessment with sonography for trauma assesses for free fluid in the following spaces:
    - Hepatorenal
    - Splenorenal
    - Pelvic
    - Pericardial
    - Pleural (extended FAST)
  - Diagnostic peritoneal lavage is rarely used in children but can be useful if FAST or computed tomography (CT) scan is unavailable
  - Chest/pelvis X-rays
  - Foley catheter and oro-/nasogastric tube

SECONDARY SURVEY

- Reassess vital signs.
- Complete a comprehensive history (AMPLE: Allergies, Medications, Past medical history, Last meal, Events, and Environment).

- Complete a comprehensive head-to-toe physical examination.
- Unstable patients with concerns for ongoing intra-abdominal hemorrhage go to the OR.
- Decisions regarding CT scans for stable pediatric patients should consider exposure to ionizing radiation and the need for sedation to remain still.
- Head CT is indicated for altered mental status, loss of consciousness, severe mechanism of injury, or other signs of skull fracture.[7]

TERTIARY SURVEY

- The tertiary survey consists of a repeated comprehensive history and physical examination in a calm setting.
- This is especially important in young children who are unable to communicate injuries that may have been missed during the primary or secondary surveys.
- Communication with caregivers can reveal more details regarding the injury and the treatment plan can be clearly conveyed.

SIGNS OF CHILD ABUSE

- Discrepancies in history and severity of injury
- Multiple visits to different hospitals or delayed presentation
- Different colored bruises or radiographic scars indicating recurrent trauma
- Perioral, perianal, or genital injuries
- Sharp demarcation of burn injuries indicating intentional scald

INJURY PREVENTION

- *The Injury Free Coalition for Kids* is a comprehensive physician-led pediatric injury prevention program operating out of level 1 trauma centers.
  - The Coalition developed a model known as the ABC's of injury prevention[8]:
    - A: Analyze injury data through local injury surveillance.
    - B: Build a local coalition.
    - C: Communicate the problem and raise awareness that injuries are a preventable public health problem.
    - D: Develop interventions and injury prevention activities to create safer environments and activities for children.
    - E: Evaluate the interventions with ongoing surveillance.

PEARLS AND PITFALLS

- Unintentional injury is the leading cause of morbidity and mortality in children in the United States.
- The resuscitation of the pediatric trauma patient is guided by fundamental ATLS principles, including the primary (ABCDE), secondary (AMPLE), and tertiary surveys.
- Unstable patients with concerns for ongoing intra-abdominal hemorrhage go to the OR.
- Consider risks from radiation exposure for CT scans of stable pediatric trauma patients.
- Signs of child abuse include discrepancies in history, multiple visits to different hospitals, delayed presentation, and scarring indicating recurrent trauma.

REFERENCES

1. Borse NN, Julie Gilchrist MS, Dellinger MDAM, Rudd RA, Ballesteros MF, Sleet DA. *Patterns of Unintentional Injuries Among 0-19 Year Olds in the United States, 2000-2006.* 2008. Available from https://www.cdc.gov/safechild/pdf/cdc-childhoodinjury.pdf.
2. Gilbert R, Widom CS, Browne K, Fergusson D, Webb E, Janson S. Burden and consequences of child maltreatment in high-income countries. *Lancet.* 2009;373(9657):68-81.
3. Ravichandiran N, Schuh S, Bejuk M, et al. Delayed identification of pediatric abuse-related fractures. *Pediatrics.* 2010;125(1):60-66.
4. Haller JA Jr. Toward a comprehensive emergency medical system for children. *Pediatrics.* 1990;86(1):120-122.
5. American College of Surgeons Committee on Trauma. *ATLS, Advanced Trauma Life Support for Doctors: Student Course Manual.* American College of Surgeons; 2008.
6. Mattox KL, Moore EE, Feliciano DV. *Trauma.* 7th ed. McGraw Hill Professional; 2012:1472.
7. Kuppermann N, Holmes JF, Dayan PS, et al. Identification of children at very low risk of clinically-important brain injuries after head trauma: a prospective cohort study. *Lancet.* 2009;374(9696):1160-1170.
8. Pressley JC, Barlow B, Durkin M, Jacko SA, Dominguez DR, Johnson L. A national program for injury prevention in children and adolescents: the injury free coalition for kids. *J Urban Health.* 2005;82(3):389-402.

Chapter 8

Abdominal and Pelvic Trauma

Joshua P. Parreco

- The vast majority of children presenting to the emergency department with injuries involve a blunt mechanism and approximately 22% of these patients have an intra-abdominal injury.[1]
- Anatomic considerations that make children more susceptible to abdominal traumatic injury include the following[2]:
  - Compact torso with smaller anterior-posterior diameters with less surface area to dissipate injury force.
  - Liver and spleen that extend below the protective costal margin.
  - Less fat and abdominal musculature to protect intra-abdominal structures.
- Solid organ injury in children typically involves a direct blow to the abdomen such as a bicycle handlebar/sports-related impact or fall from significant height.

INITIAL MANAGEMENT

- Start with advanced trauma life support primary (including adjuncts: X-ray, focused assessment with sonography for trauma [FAST], Foley catheter/gastric tube), secondary, and tertiary surveys.
- Signs of abdominal injury in children:
  - Abdominal distention
  - Rebound tenderness
  - Involuntary guarding
  - Rigidity
  - Pelvic instability
  - Abdominal abrasions
  - Seat belt sign (abdominal bruise) after a motor vehicle collision[3]
- Children who are hemodynamically stable and have signs of abdominal trauma should undergo computed tomography (CT) scan.[4]

- Children who have blunt trauma with hemodynamic stability and no signs of abdominal trauma should undergo laboratory testing including the following:
  - Hemoglobin and hematocrit
  - Urinalysis
  - Aspartate transaminase (AST)/Alanine transaminase (ALT)
  - Pancreatic enzymes
- An abdominal CT scan should be performed for children with[5]
  - Gross or microscopic hematuria
  - Elevated AST/ALT
- Diagnostic peritoneal lavage can be useful if FAST or CT scan is unavailable and considered positive if contains the following[6]:
  - 5 mL of gross blood
  - Enteric contents
  - >100 000 RBCs per cc
  - >500 WBCs per cc
  - Elevated amylase level

INDICATIONS FOR LAPAROTOMY

- Hemodynamic instability
- Replacement of >40 mL/kg blood products[8]
- Hollow viscus injury demonstrated by free intraperitoneal air or extravasated contrast on imaging
- Clinical deterioration[7]

BOWEL INJURY

- Jejunal perforation is the most common small bowel injury (Table 8.1).[9]
- Crush injuries can result in damage to the transverse colon due to compression against the spine (Table 8.2).
- Rapid deceleration can result in bowel injuries at fixed points such as the ligament of treitz, the ileocecal valve, and the rectosigmoid junction.
- Delayed ischemic necrosis and perforation can result from mesenteric injuries.[10]

SPLENIC INJURY

- The need for operative management in children with splenic injury is usually apparent within 24 hours of admission.[12]

TABLE 8.1		
Small Bowel Injury Scale		
Grade[a]	**Type of Injury**	**Description of Injury**
I	Hematoma	Contusion or hematoma without devascularization
	Laceration	Partial thickness, no perforation
II	Laceration	Laceration <50% of circumference
III	Laceration	Laceration >50% of circumference without transection
IV	Laceration	Transection of the small bowel
V	Laceration	Transection of the small bowel with segmental tissue loss
	Vascular	Devascularized segment

Reprinted with permission from Moore EE, Cogbill TH, Malangoni MA, et al. Organ injury scaling II: pancreas duodenum small bowel, colon, and rectum. *J Trauma*. 1990;30(11):1427-1429.
[a]Advance one grade for multiple injuries up to grade III.

- Direct repair or partial splenectomy should be favored in children, but splenectomy may be required for ongoing instability or multiple other injuries.[13]
- Asplenic children are at increased risk for overwhelming postsplenectomy sepsis compared with adults and should receive vaccinations and antibiotic prophylaxis.[14]

TABLE 8.2		
Colon Injury Scale		
Grade[a]	**Type of Injury**	**Description of Injury**
I	Hematoma	Contusion or hematoma without devascularization
	Laceration	Partial thickness, no perforation
II	Laceration	Laceration <50% of circumference
III	Laceration	Laceration >50% of circumference without transection
IV	Laceration	Transection of the colon
V	Laceration	Transection of the colon with segmental tissue loss
	Vascular	Devascularized segment

Reprinted with permission from Moore EE, Cogbill TH, Malangoni MA, et al. Organ injury scaling II: pancreas duodenum small bowel, colon, and rectum. *J Trauma*. 1990;30(11):1427-1429.
[a]Advance one grade for multiple injuries up to grade III.

TABLE 8.3		
Liver Injury Scale		
Grade[a]	**Type of Injury**	**Description of Injury**
I	Hematoma	Subcapsular, <10% surface area
	Laceration	Capsular tear, <1 cm parenchymal depth
II	Hematoma	Subcapsular, 10%-50% surface area, intraparenchymal <10 cm in diameter
	Laceration	Capsular tear, 1-3 cm parenchymal depth, <10 cm in length
III	Hematoma	Subcapsular, >50% surface area of ruptured subcapsular or parenchymal hematoma; intraparenchymal hematoma >10 cm or expanding
	Laceration	>3 cm parenchymal depth
IV	Laceration	Parenchymal disruption involving 25%-75% hepatic lobe or 1-3 Couinaud segments
V	Laceration	Parenchymal disruption involving >75% of hepatic lobe or >3 Couinaud segments within a single lobe
	Vascular	Juxtahepatic venous injuries; ie, retrohepatic vena cava/central major hepatic veins
VI	Vascular	Hepatic avulsion

Reprinted with permission from Moore EE, Cogbill TH, Jurkovich GJ, Shackford SR, Malangoni MA, Champion HRF. Organ Injury Scaling: Spleen and Liver (1994 Revision). *J Trauma.* 1995;38(3):323-324.
[a]Advance one grade for multiple injuries up to grade III.

LIVER INJURY

- Only 5% to 10% of children with liver injuries will require surgery.[15]
- Operative liver trauma may require damage control measures including abdominal packing with temporary abdominal closure (Table 8.3).
- After temporary closure, resuscitation in the intensive care unit should continue with rewarming and correction of coagulopathy with definitive repair within 12 to 24 hours.[16]

TABLE 8.4		
Bladder Injury Scale		
Grade[a]	Injury Type	Description of Injury
I	Hematoma	Contusion, intramural hematoma
	Laceration	Partial thickness
II	Laceration	Extraperitoneal bladder wall laceration <2 cm
III	Laceration	Extraperitoneal (>2 cm) or intraperitoneal (<2 cm) bladder wall laceration
IV	Laceration	Intraperitoneal bladder wall laceration >2 cm
V	Laceration	Intraperitoneal or extraperitoneal bladder wall laceration extending into the bladder neck or ureteral orifice (trigone)

Reprinted with permission from Moore EE, Cogbill TH, Jurkovich GJ, et al. Organ injury scaling. III: Chest wall, abdominal vascular, ureter, bladder, and urethra. *J Trauma*. 1992;33(3):337-339.
[a]Advance one grade for multiple lesions up to grade III.

BLADDER INJURY

- The bladder in children resides above the pelvis, and this presents an increased risk for injury from blunt mechanisms such as seat belts (Table 8.4).
- Diagnosis of bladder injury can be performed by conventional or CT cystography.
- Intraperitoneal injury requires operative repair in multiple layers with absorbable suture because permanent suture could be a nidus for bladder stone formation.
- Extraperitoneal injury can be treated with antibiotics and foley drainage for 1 week.[16]

PANCREATIC INJURY

- Pancreatic injuries are rare and are usually diagnosed by CT scan; however, magnetic resonance cholangiopancreatography or endoscopic retrograde cholangiopancreatography can identify ductal involvement.
- Distal pancreatic ductal disruption may require distal pancreatectomy (Table 8.5).
- Pancreatic injury without ductal disruption or with proximal duct disruption can usually be treated conservatively with bowel rest.[13]

TABLE 8.5

Pancreatic Injury Scale

Grade[a]	Type of Injury	Description of Injury
I	Hematoma	Minor contusion without duct injury
	Laceration	Superficial laceration without duct injury
II	Hematoma	Major contusion without duct injury or tissue loss
	Laceration	Major laceration without duct injury or tissue loss
III	Laceration	Distal transection or parenchymal injury with duct injury
IV	Laceration	Proximal transection or parenchymal injury involving ampulla
V	Laceration	Massive disruption of pancreatic head

Reprinted with permission from Moore EE, Cogbill TH, Malangoni MA, et al. Organ injury scaling II: pancreas duodenum small bowel, colon, and rectum. *J Trauma.* 1990;30(11):1427-1429.
[a]Advance one grade for multiple injuries up to grade III.

PEARLS AND PITFALLS

- Children are more susceptible to abdominal traumatic injury than adults.
- An abdominal CT scan should be performed for children with hematuria or an elevated AST/ALT.
- Jejunal perforation is the most common small bowel injury.
- The bladder in children resides above the pelvis and this presents an increased risk for injury from blunt mechanisms such as seat belts.
- Splenic preservation is preferred since asplenic children are at increased risk for overwhelming postsplenectomy sepsis compared with adults.

REFERENCES

1. Bixby SD, Callahan MJ, Taylor GA. Imaging in pediatric blunt abdominal trauma. *Semin Roentgenol.* 2008;43(1):72-82.
2. Mendez DR. *Overview of blunt abdominal trauma in children.* In: Bachur RG, Woodward GA, Wiley JF, eds. *UpToDate.* Waltham, MA: UpToDate; 2017.
3. Lutz N, Nance ML, Kallan MJ, Arbogast KB, Durbin DR, Winston FK. Incidence and clinical significance of abdominal wall bruising in restrained children involved in motor vehicle crashes. *J Pediatr Surg.* 2004;39(6):972-975.

4. Holmes JF, Sokolove PE, Brant WE, et al. Identification of children with intra-abdominal injuries after blunt trauma. *Ann Emerg Med.* 2002;39(5):500-509.

5. Isaacman DJ, Scarfone RJ, Kost SI, et al. Utility of routine laboratory testing for detecting intra-abdominal injury in the pediatric trauma patient. *Pediatrics.* 1993;92(5):691-694.

6. American College of Surgeons Committee on Trauma. *ATLS, Advanced Trauma Life Support for Doctors: Student Course Manual.* American College of Surgeons; 2008.

7. Haley G, William M. *Hollow viscus blunt abdominal trauma in children.* In: Torrey SB, Wiley JF, eds. *UpToDate.* Waltham, MA: UpToDate; 2017.

8. Wesson DE, Filler RM, Ein SH, Shandling B, Simpson JS, Stephens CA. Ruptured spleen—when to operate? *J Pediatr Surg.* 1981;16(3):324-326.

9. Grosfeld JL, Rescorla FJ, West KW, Vane DW. Gastrointestinal injuries in childhood: analysis of 53 patients. *J Pediatr Surg.* 1989;24(6):580-583.

10. Holland AJ, Cass DT, Glasson MJ, Pitkin J. Small bowel injuries in children. *J Paediatr Child Health.* 2000;36(3):265-269.

11. Mattox KL, Moore EE, Feliciano DV. *Trauma.* 7th ed. McGraw Hill Professional; 2012:1472.

12. Nance ML, Holmes JH IV, Wiebe DJ. Timeline to operative intervention for solid organ injuries in children. *J Trauma.* 2006;61(6):1389-1392.

13. Wesson DE. *Liver, spleen, and pancreas injury in children with blunt abdominal trauma.* In: Torrey SB, Wiley JF, eds. *UpToDate.* Waltham, MA: UpToDate; 2016.

14. Pasternack MS. *Prevention of sepsis in the asplenic patient.* In: Weller PF, Thorner AR, eds. *UpToDate.* Waltham, MA: UpToDate; 2017.

15. Landau A, van As AB, Numanoglu A, Millar AJW, Rode H. Liver injuries in children: the role of selective non-operative management. *Injury.* 2006;37(1):66-71.

16. Mattei P, ed. *Fundamentals of Pediatric Surgery.* New York: Springer; 2011.

Chapter 9

Thoracic Trauma

Kenneth F. Newcomer

- Trauma is a leading cause of death in children and young adults.
- It has been estimated that almost 25% of deaths are attributed to some type of chest trauma and the vast majority are from blunt injury.[1]
- Most frequent causes of chest trauma include motor vehicle crashes, falls, and pedestrian and sports injuries.[1]

RELEVANT ANATOMY AND PHYSIOLOGY

- Compared with adults, the chest wall of children has a greatly increased compliance, transmitting more force to internal structures.
- Occurrence of rare but deadly injuries such as commotio cordis and traumatic asphyxia is also attributed to increased chest wall compliance.[2]
- A mobile mediastinum in children makes them particularly susceptible to shift, notably in tension pneumothorax.
- **Physiology**: A higher rate of tissue O_2 consumption in children makes children prone to hypoxia.
- Increased heart rate is able to maintain arterial pressure, despite severe intravascular volume loss, but can rapidly decompensate.
- Hypothermia is a concern because the body volume to surface area ratio is smaller than adults.

EPIDEMIOLOGY AND ETIOLOGY

- **Incidence**: It varies from approximately 4% to 25% in trauma patients.[3]
- Thoracic trauma is a marker of severe injury in pediatric patients and has increased mortality when combined with head and abdominal trauma (25%) and central nervous system trauma (40%).[3,4]
- Blunt mechanisms account for 80% to 95% of pediatric thoracic trauma.

- **Etiology**: Motor vehicle accidents are the most common etiology for blunt trauma. Gunshots cause most penetrating trauma.
- **Most common injuries**: They include pulmonary contusion, rib fracture, and pneumothorax.

COMMON INJURY PATTERNS

Chest Wall Injury

- Rib fractures, especially first rib fractures, are suggestive of high-energy trauma and should prompt an investigation for intrathoracic injury (Figure 9.1).
- Rib fracture in children aged 0 to 3 years is suspicious for nonaccidental trauma (especially posterior rib fractures).
- Open pneumothoraxes (sucking wounds) can cause rapid mediastinal shift and are treated with chest tube and occlusive dressing.
- Pain management and breathing exercises are the mainstay of treatment for all rib fractures.

Pulmonary Injury

- Contusion is a common injury and may occur in the absence of rib fractures.
- Severe contusion can lead to respiratory failure or acute respiratory distress syndrome.

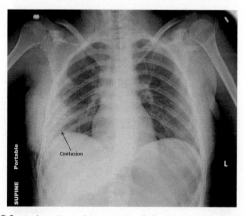

Figure 9.1   A chest X-ray demonstrates rib fractures in a pediatric patient that are associated with soft tissue swelling, subcutaneous emphysema, and intrathoracic injury (contusion). (Reprinted with permission from Shaw KN, Bachur RG, eds. *Fleisher & Ludwig's Textbook of Pediatric Emergency Medicine.* 7th ed. Philadelphia: Wolters Kluwer; 2016.)

- Traumatic pneumothorax is typically managed with a chest tube.
- Hemothorax and hemopneumothorax are associated with higher mortality but are also typically managed with chest tube.
- Thoracotomy is indicated for high-volume hemothorax (15-20 cc/kg initially or 2-4 cc/kg per hour over 4 h).[3,5]
- Pulmonary parenchymal injury can lead to air embolism, especially in the setting of positive pressure ventilation.
- Suspected tension pneumothorax necessitates immediate needle decompression and definitive management with chest tube.

Mediastinal Injury

- Damage to the great vessels, tracheobronchial tree, esophagus, and heart can occur in the absence of obvious external injury.
- Although rare, these injuries are often life-threatening.

IMAGING FINDINGS

Supine Anteroposterior Chest X-ray

- **It remains the most common initial imaging tool.**
- Nonanatomic consolidation near the site of injury suggests pulmonary contusion (Figure 9.2).

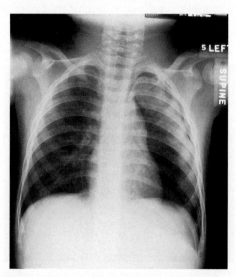

Figure 9.2 A 3-year-old who was an unrestrained passenger in an motor vehicle collision has chest X-ray findings of left-sided pulmonary contusion and small pneumothorax. (Reprinted with permission from Kline-Tilford AM, Haut C. *Lippincott Certification Review: Pediatric Acute Care Nurse Practitioner.* Philadelphia: Wolters Kluwer; 2016.)

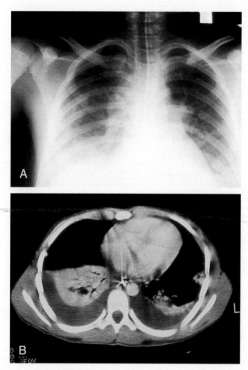

Figure 9.3 A 15-year-old who was involved in an autopedestrian accident has bilateral pleural fluid collections, suggestive of hemothorax (A). The finding is well demonstrated on the computed tomography scan (B). (Reprinted with permission from Shah K, Egan D, Quaas J. *Essential Emergency Trauma.* Philadelphia: Lippincott Williams & Wilkins; 2011.)

- Layering hemothorax can have a similar appearance.
- Careful attention should be paid to small pneumothoraxes.
- Apical pleural cap or dependent fluid collection is seen in hemothorax, often obscuring the costophrenic angles (Figure 9.3).
- Mediastinal widening may be concealed by thymic tissue.

Bedside Ultrasound

- Bedside technique is becoming increasingly common in trauma.
- Ultrasound has a high specificity for pneumothorax and can quickly reveal the presence of pericardial fluid.

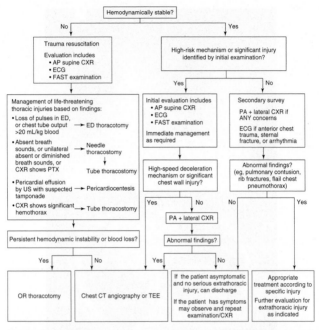

Figure 9.4 Algorithm showing an approach to blunt thoracic trauma. (Reproduced with permission from: Eisenberg M. *Thoracic trauma in children: Initial stabilization and evaluation trauma.* In: UpToDate, Post TW (Ed), UpToDate, Waltham, MA. (Accessed on 6/27/2018.) Copyright © 2018 UpToDate, Inc. For more information visit www.uptodate.com.)

Computed tomography-Angiogram

- Computed tomography angiography is pursued in patients with known or suspected intrathoracic injury and in stable patients if they have a high-risk injury mechanism.
- Hemo- and pneumothorax are readily visualized.
- It is more accurate for studying injuries to blood vessels and mediastinum.

SURGICAL MANAGEMENT

- 90% of pediatric thoracic trauma can be managed noninvasively or with tube thoracostomy[3] (Figure 9.4).
- Indications for emergent thoracotomy include rapid decompensation and witnessed arrest.
- After placement of a chest tube, thoracotomy is indicated for a massive hemothorax.

- Fiber-optic bronchoscopy is often used to address persistent air leak and/or suspected tracheobronchial injury.
- Severe tracheobronchial injuries may require operative repair such as pulmonary resection (Figure 9.5).

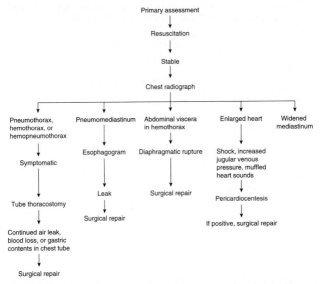

Figure 9.5   Indications for surgery in thoracic trauma. (Reprinted with permission from Fleisher GR, Ludwig S. *Textbook of Pediatric Emergency Medicine.* 6th ed. Philadelphia: Lippincott, Williams & Wilkins; 2010.)

PEARLS AND PITFALLS

- Blunt thoracic trauma is commonly associated with other injuries.
- Associated abdominal and head injuries are associated with worse outcomes.
- Pulmonary contusion, rib fracture, and pneumothorax are the most common traumatic thoracic injuries.
- Intrathoracic injuries can occur in the absence of rib fractures.
- Many injuries will be recognized on initial anteroposterior chest X-ray.
- The majority can be managed noninvasively or with chest tube.
- Prophylactic antibiotics are generally reserved for cases of extensive soft tissue disruption, pulmonary contusion with hemoptysis, or recognized need for operative intervention.[6]

REFERENCES

1. Pauze DR, Pauze DK. Emergency management of blunt chest trauma in children: an evidence-based approach. *Pediatr Emerg Med Pract.* 2013:1-24.
2. Santorellia KH, Vanea WV. The diagnosis and management of children with blunt injury of the chest. *Semin Pediatr Surg.* 2004;13:98-105.
3. Puapong DP, Tuggle DW. *Thoracic trauma.* In: Holcomb GW, Murphy JP, eds. *Ashcraft's Pediatric Surgery.* 5th ed. Philadelphia: Elsevier; 2010:183-189.
4. Peclet MH, Newman KD, Eichelberger MR, et al. Thoracic trauma in children: an indicator of increased mortality. *J Pediatr Surg.* 1990;25:961-966.
5. Cullen ML. Pulmonary and respiratory complications of pediatric trauma. *Respir Clin North Am.* 2001;7:59-77.
6. Mandal AK, Montano J, Thadepalli H. Prophylactic antibiotics and no antibiotics compared in penetrating chest trauma. *J Trauma.* 1985;25:639-643.

SUGGESTED READINGS

Bliss D, Silen M. Pediatric thoracic trauma. *Crit Care Med.* 2002;30:409-415.
Riley JP, Brandt ML, Mattox KL, et al. Thoracic trauma in children. *J Trauma.* 1993;34:329-333.

Chapter 10

Common Fractures in Children

Blaze D. Emerson and Bijan J. Ameri

- Pediatric fractures are a very common reason for physician visits with 17.6% to 20% of pediatric injuries associated with fractures.[1,2] Furthermore, it is estimated that 42% of boys and 27% of girls will sustain a fracture of some form before the age of 16 years.[2]
- Fracture incidence increases linearly with age, peaking at approximately 12 years, then decreasing until 16 years of age. This is possibly related to a decline in female fractures with more advanced skeletal maturity.[2]
- Most commonly, fractures are due to low-energy trauma and occur in the upper extremity, especially the distal radius.[2,3]
  - The incidence of specific fractures, in descending order, is distal radius 23.3%, hand 20.1%, elbow area 12.0%, clavicle 6.4%, radius shaft 6.4%, tibia shaft 6.2%, foot 5.9%, distal tibia 4.4%, femur 2.3%, humerus 1.4%, and other 11.6%.[2]

BONE PHYSIOLOGY

- Pediatric fractures in children are challenging, as they often involve regions of growing bone. The unique anatomy of the immature skeleton includes the epiphysis, metaphysis, and diaphysis (Figure 10.1).
- The epiphysis is a secondary ossification center and is separated from the metaphysis by the cartilaginous physis.
- The epiphysis and physis are primary growth centers, and damage may lead to growth derangements including angular deformity, limb-length discrepancy, and/or epiphyseal distortion.[2]
- Physeal injuries in children are common and may account for up to 30% of all pediatric fractures.[2]
- The age of ossification of the epiphysis is variable, which makes fracture identification difficult. X-rays of the unaffected side may be needed for comparison.

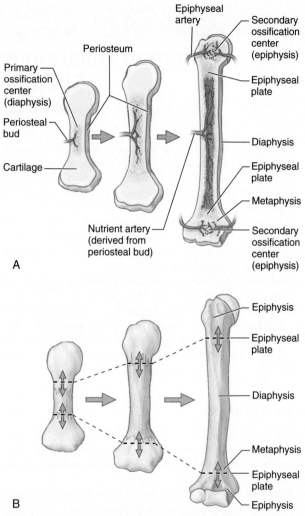

Figure 10.1 Development and growth of a long bone. A, The formation of primary and secondary ossification centers is shown. B, Growth in length occurs on both sides of the cartilaginous epiphyseal plates (double-headed arrows). The bone formed from the primary center in the diaphysis does not fuse with that formed from the secondary centers in the epiphyses until the bone reaches its adult size. When growth ceases, the depleted epiphyseal plate is replaced by a synostosis (bone-to-bone fusion), observed as an epiphyseal line in radiographs and sectioned bone. (Reprinted with permission from Moore KL, Dalley AF, Agur AMR. *Clinically Oriented Anatomy.* 7th ed. Philadelphia, PA: Wolters Kluwer Health/Lippincott Williams & Wilkins; 2014.)

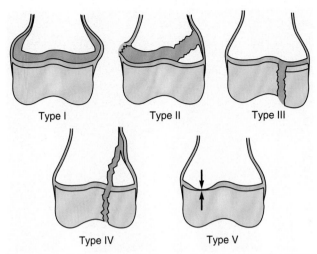

Type I   Type II   Type III

Type IV   Type V

Figure 10.2   Salter-Harris classification of epiphyseal injuries. Type I injury is an epiphysiolysis of the involved growth plate without associated fracture. Type II has an additional metaphyseal fracture fragment; type I and II injuries have a good prognosis and are usually treated with closed reduction and casting. Type III injury results in a fracture through the growth plate and epiphysis. Type IV fracture crosses the epiphysis, growth plate (physis), and metaphysis. Type III and IV injuries require careful open reduction and internal fixation if displaced. Type V injury involves a crush of the growth plate without a fracture and is usually detected late by asymmetric or premature closure of the growth plate. (Reprinted with permission from Fiser SM. *The ABSITE Review*. 4th ed. Philadelphia, PA: Wolters Kluwer Health/Lippincott Williams & Wilkins; 2013.)

- The unique physiology of immature bone gives rise to several unique fracture patterns. As discussed previously, physeal fractures are common.
- The Salter-Harris classification system stratifies injuries based on their likelihood of growth derangement, with higher numbers being severe (Figure 10.2).
- Also, children have thicker periosteum with a greater osteogenic potential than that of an adult's.[4] This unique periosteal profile within children's bones leads to a greater propensity to bend rather than break when exposed to stress.
- A torus fracture (buckle fracture) occurs when a longitudinal force causes the periosteum to fail in compression rather than breaking completely (Figure 10.3).
- Greenstick fractures occur when the bone fails on the tension side of the cortex as the result of a lateral force being applied to a long bone (Figure 10.4). Both torus and greenstick fractures are incomplete.

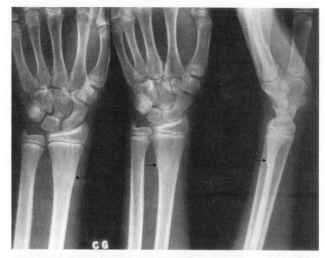

Figure 10.3 Left wrist PA, oblique, and lateral radiographs. Torus fracture (arrows) or a nondisplaced fracture of the distal left radius. (Reprinted with permission from Smith WL. *Radiology 101*. 4th ed. Philadelphia, PA: Wolters Kluwer Health/Lippincott Williams & Wilkins; 2014.)

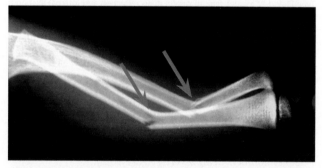

Figure 10.4 Greenstick fracture (arrows) of the forearm. Greenstick fractures are common in the forearm, as the bone bends before it fractures and the periosteal sleeve maintains apposition. (Reprinted with permission from Staheli LT. *Fundamentals of Pediatric Orthopedics*. 5th ed. Philadelphia, PA: Wolters Kluwer; 2015.)

HEALING AND REMODELING

- Anatomic reduction in a pediatric patient is not as crucial as in an adult because of the bone remodeling potential of children. Remodeling in the diaphysis and metaphysis may realign previously maligned fragments; however, anatomic reduction should always be the goal owing to the unpredictability of the remodeling process.

- The potential for complete remodeling of the fracture is greater with younger age, fractures closer to the physis, and alignment of angulation in the normal plane of motion.[2]
- Furthermore, children are better able to withstand prolonged immobilization and usually do not suffer from postimmobilization stiffness and decreased range of motion, which can be a debilitating problem in adults.
- Children's bones remodel and grow at an accelerated rate. As a result, pediatric fractures often exhibit an increased rate of longitudinal growth after a fracture. Therefore, it is sometime recommended that during realignment there exists some shortening or overlap of the fragments to account for this expected longitudinal growth.[1]
- In general, pediatric patients have an excellent prognosis after a fracture. It is recommended to consult an orthopedic surgeon when the fractures are displaced, especially with Salter-Harris type classifications above III.[1]
- If the clinician decides to manage the fracture, it is suggested that X-ray views are obtained monthly for 3 to 6 months to ensure optimal healing response.[1]

DISTAL RADIUS

Epidemiology

- Distal radius fractures are the most common pediatric fracture with an incidence of 23.3% and are 3 times more common in boys than girls.[2]
  - Fracture incidence is increased around the adolescent growth spurt phase and is usually secondary to a sporting event.

Mechanism

- A direct fall on an outstretched hand is the usual mechanism of injury (Figure 10.5).

Presentation

- Generally, patients present with dorsal displacement/angulation of the carpus relative to the forearm (Figures 10.6 and 10.7). However, patients may present with volar displacement when the mechanism is a fall on a flexed wrist (Figure 10.8).
- Patients will complain of pain, swelling, and limited motion of the wrist and hand.

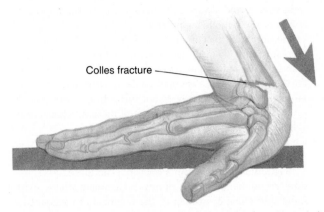

Figure 10.5 Colles fracture. (Reprinted with permission from Anatomical Chart Company. *Hand and Wrist Anatomical Chart.* Lippincott Williams & Wilkins; 2000.)

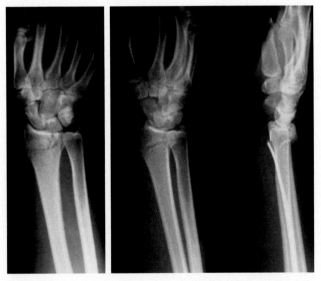

Figure 10.6 X-ray of Colles fracture. (Reprinted with permission from Silverberg M. Colles' and Smith's fractures. In: Greenberg MI, ed. *Greenberg's Text-Atlas of Emergency Medicine.* Philadelphia, PA: Lippincott Williams & Wilkins; 2005:483.)

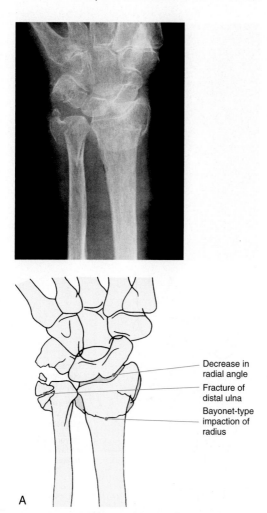

Decrease in
radial angle

Fracture of
distal ulna

Bayonet-type
impaction of
radius

A

Figure 10.7 Posteroanterior (A) and lateral (B) radiographs of the distal forearm demonstrate the features of Colles fracture. On the posteroanterior projection, a decrease in the radial angle and an associated fracture of the distal ulna are evident. The lateral view reveals the dorsal angulation of the distal radius as well as a reversal of the palmar inclination. On both views, the radius is foreshortened secondary to bayonet-type displacement. The fracture line does not extend to the joint (Frykman type II). (Reprinted with permission from Greenspan A. *Orthopedic Imaging*. 6th ed. Philadelphia, PA: Wolters Kluwer Health; 2014.)

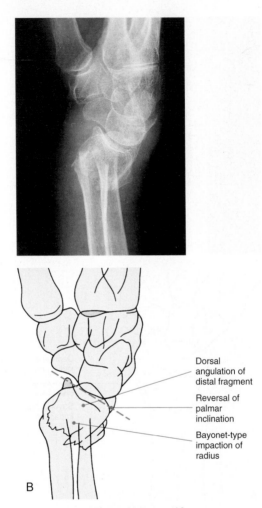

Dorsal angulation of distal fragment

Reversal of palmar inclination

Bayonet-type impaction of radius

B

Figure 10.7—cont'd

- Deformity will depend on the degree of fracture displacement; however, a "dinner fork" deformity may be noted with dorsally displaced fractures (Figure 10.9).

Management

- Standard anteroposterior (AP) and lateral X-ray views should be ordered if a fracture is suspected. Neurovascular examination includes the median, radial, and ulnar nerves.

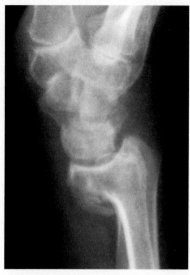

Figure 10.8 Smith fracture. A fracture of the distal radius with volar angulation such as this is called a Smith fracture. This is a much less common injury than the Colles fracture. (Reprinted with permission from Brant WE, Helms C. *Fundamentals of Diagnostic Radiology.* 4th ed. Philadelphia: Wolters Kluwer Health/Lippincott Williams & Wilkins; 2012.)

- The physician should also rule out compartment syndrome.
- Always inspect the joints above and below the injury to detect associated injuries.
- Nondisplaced and minimally displaced Salter-Harris types I and II fractures may be treated with closed reduction and cast immobilization.

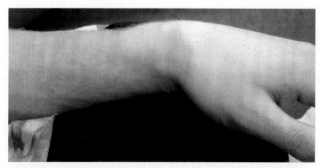

Figure 10.9 "Dinner fork" deformity of the Colles fracture. (Reprinted with permission from Silverberg M. Colles' and Smith's fractures. In: Greenberg MI, ed. *Greenberg's Text-Atlas of Emergency Medicine.* Philadelphia, PA: Lippincott Williams & Wilkins; 2005:483.)

- Of note, Salter-Harris type I fractures of the distal radius are easily missed. Presence of the pronator fat pad on lateral radiograph is an indication of an occult Salter-Harris type I fracture (Figure 10.10).[5]
- Closed reduction and percutaneous pinning is indicated for neurovascular compromise and physeal fracture involvement. Open reduction is reserved for irreducible fractures, displaced Salter-Harris types III, IV, V, and open fractures.[2]

DIGITS

Epidemiology

- Injuries to the hand and wrist are the second leading fracture location in children. These injuries account for nearly 25% of pediatric fractures, and the annual incidence is 26.4 fractures per 10 000 children.[2]
- Hand fractures in children occur in a bimodal distribution with most of the fractures occurring in toddlers and adolescents.
- The index and small finger are the most commonly injured.

Mechanism

- Toddler hand fractures are usually crush injuries of the distal phalanges.
- Adolescent hand injuries tend to be Salter-Harris type II fractures of proximal phalangeal base and are often related to sporting activities.

Presentation

- Swelling, deformity, ecchymosis, and/or limited motion are indicators of a hand fracture. Fractures may rotate during active grasp or passive tenodesis (Figure 10.11) and cause a scissoring motion of the phalanges (Figure 10.12).

Management

- AP, lateral, and oblique radiographic views should be obtained. The normal ossification patterns of the pediatric hand may complicate interpretation of fractures or ligamentous injuries.
- For this reason, contralateral imaging of the uninjured hand is desirable.

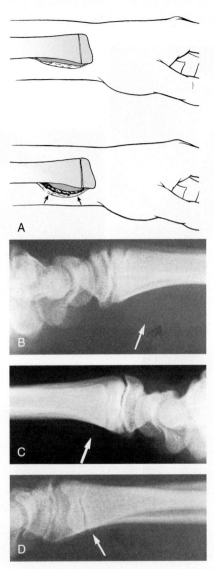

Figure 10.10 A, Subperiosteal hemorrhage from an occult fracture of the distal radius causes an anterior displacement of the normal pronator quadratus fat pad (arrows). B, Radiograph of a 13-year-old girl with tenderness over the distal radius after a fall. The only radiographic finding is an anterior displacement of the normal pronator quadratus fat pad (arrow). C, The opposite normal side (arrow indicates normal fat pad). D, 2 weeks later, there is a small area of periosteal new bone formation (arrow) anteriorly, substantiating that bony injury has occurred. (Reprinted with permission from Flynn JM, Waters PM, Skaggs DL. *Rockwood and Wilkins' Fractures in Children*. 8th ed. Philadelphia, PA: Wolters Kluwer Health; 2014.)

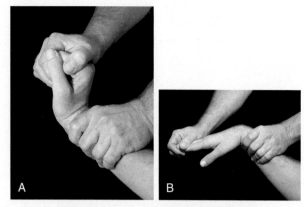

Figure 10.11 Ranging to facilitate tenodesis grasp. A, When the wrist is extended, the fingers are flexed. B, When the wrist is flexed, the fingers are extended. (Reprinted with permission from Radomski MV, Latham CAT. *Occupational Therapy for Physical Dysfunction.* 7th ed. Philadelphia: Wolters Kluwer Health/Lippincott Williams & Wilkins; 2013.)

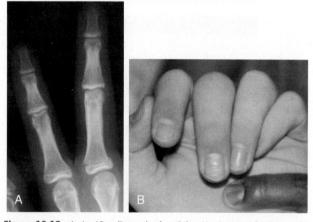

Figure 10.12 A, An AP radiograph of an Salter-Harris type II fracture at the long finger proximal phalanx. The radiograph reveals slight angulation and can appear benign. Clinical examination must be carried out to assess the digital cascade for malrotation. B, Tenodesis of the wrist with passive extension reveals unacceptable malrotation as evident by the degree of overlap of the middle finger on the ring finger. (Reprinted with permission from Flynn JM, Waters PM, Skaggs DL. *Rockwood and Wilkins' Fractures in Children.* 8th ed. Philadelphia: Wolters Kluwer Health; 2014.)

- Neurovascular examination may be complicated by pain or young age of the patient. However, excessive bleeding may indicate a digital nerve laceration; this is due to the proper digital artery that runs dorsal to the proper digital nerve (Figure 10.13).
- If there is question as to whether a nerve has been injured, the wrinkle test may be performed. This consists of immersion of the digit in warm water for 5 minutes. Wrinkling should be noted on the volar surface. The absence of wrinkling indicated nerve damage.[2]
- Most children's hand fractures are treated conservatively. Remodeling will take place in digits with moderate sagittal or coronal deformity. However, it will not properly occur in a malrotated digit. Reduction and stabilization are required with these injuries to prevent scissoring defects.
- Nondisplaced fractures may be immobilized and then reevaluated in 3 to 4 weeks. Fractures that required reduction should be checked weekly to ensure proper alignment and rotation. Immobilization of the injured digit with at least one of the uninjured digits is recommended. Short arm immobilization with the metacarpal phalangeal joints flexed and the interphalangeal joints extended is the standard of care.
- Unstable or maligned fractures should be treated with closed reduction and internal fixation to maintain alignment.

SUPRACONDYLAR FRACTURES

Epidemiology

- The distal humerus is the most common site for elbow fractures, accounting for approximately 86% of the fractures in this region, and of these 55% to 75% are supracondylar fractures.[2]
- The peak age for supracondylar fractures is between 5 and 7 years. This age period coincides with the time when there is a natural hyperextension of the elbow joint in children.[2]

Mechanism

- A fall on an outstretched hand is the usual mechanism for supracondylar fractures.
- When a child falls on an extended extremity, the laxity of the elbow ligaments causes the elbow to lock into hyperextension.
- The hyperextension converts a linear force into an anterior tension force because of the olecranon being compressed into the olecranon fossa.

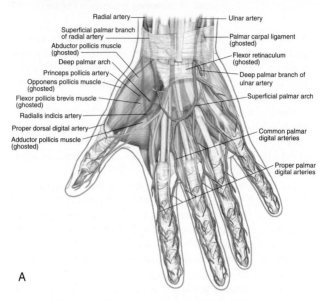

Superficial view

Radial artery

Ulnar artery

Superficial palmar branch of radial artery

Palmar carpal ligament (ghosted)

Abductor pollicis muscle (ghosted)

Flexor retinaculum (ghosted)

Deep palmar arch

Princeps pollicis artery

Deep palmar branch of ulnar artery

Opponens pollicis muscle (ghosted)

Flexor pollicis brevis muscle (ghosted)

Superficial palmar arch

Radialis indicis artery

Proper dorsal digital artery

Common palmar digital arteries

Adductor pollicis muscle (ghosted)

Proper palmar digital arteries

A

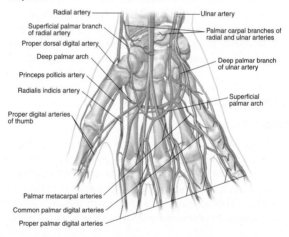

Deep view

Radial artery

Ulnar artery

Superficial palmar branch of radial artery

Palmar carpal branches of radial and ulnar arteries

Proper dorsal digital artery

Deep palmar arch

Deep palmar branch of ulnar artery

Princeps pollicis artery

Radialis indicis artery

Superficial palmar arch

Proper digital arteries of thumb

Palmar metacarpal arteries

Common palmar digital arteries

Proper palmar digital arteries

B

Figure 10.13 A, Three common palmar digital arteries find their origin from the convexity of the superficial palmar arch and proceed distally on the second, third, and fourth lumbrical muscles to give off the proper palmar digital arteries, which course along the sides of the index, middle, ring, and little fingers. B, The proper palmar digital arteries lie just below their corresponding digital nerves, each artery lying just dorsal to its respective digital nerve. The proper palmar digital arteries interconnect and anastamose with the smaller arteries that supply the interphalangeal joints and pulp of the fingertips. (Reprinted with permission from Tank PW, Gest TR. The upper limb. In: *Lippincott Williams & Wilkins Atlas of Anatomy*. Philadelphia, PA: Lippincott Williams & Wilkins; 2009:66.)

- If the force applied is great enough, the humerus will fail anteriorly and the distal fracture fragment will be pulled proximally owing to the pull of the triceps muscle.

Presentation

- Pain, swelling, and sometimes obvious deformity of the joint are apparent. Often pain is the only presenting symptom, and the child may report only minor trauma.
- Care should be taken to rule out infection, occult fracture, nursemaid's elbow, or other associated fractures.

Management

- All patients with suspected elbow injury should be initially managed with comfortable splint immobilization of the region in a 90° elbow flexion if permissable.
- Aggressive positioning or splinting may result in neurovascular compromise.
- The antecubital fossa should not be overpacked with cast padding, and a robust elbow pad should be applied.
- Patients must undergo a full radiographic examination of the upper extremity in addition to standard elbow X-rays. Imaging should include an AP view and a lateral view with the elbow flexed to 90° and the forearm neutral.
- There are several ossification centers of the elbow that may be confused with a fracture. The mnemonic, "Come Read My Tale of Love" may be helpful and refers to the order and location of ossification centers of the elbow (Figures 10.14 and 10. 15). Otherwise, an X-ray of the uninjured extremity may be helpful to characterize an ossifying epiphysis.[6]
- Supracondylar fractures and displaced nonossified portions of the elbow may be difficult to detect on X-ray, but several radiographic features may indicate a fracture:
  - The anterior humeral line is a line drawn down the anterior cortex of the humerus and should bisect the capitellum (Figures 10.16 and 10.17).
  - The radiocapitellar line is drawn down the shaft of the radius and should intersect the capitellum in all views (Figures 10.16 and 10.18). Disruption of the anterior humeral or radiocapitellar lines indicates a fracture.
  - A fat pad sign may be detected when there is an occult fracture. This is due to the effusion causing the anterior or posterior fat pad to lift off the capsule (Figures 10.17 and 10.19).

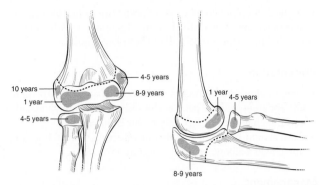

Figure 10.14 Secondary ossification centers of the elbow, with a range of ages of appearance. (Reprinted with permission from Skaggs DL, Flynn JM. *Staying Out of Trouble in Pediatric Orthopaedics.* Philadelphia, PA: Lippincott Williams & Wilkins; 2006.)

- Fracture lines may not be apparent in type I fractures, and a fat pad sign may be your only clue to pathology.[7] The anterior fat pad is more sensitive for fracture, while the posterior is more specific.
- Owing to the intimate anatomic relationship of the elbow's neurovascular structure, nerve injury occurs in approximately 7% of elbow fractures, while vascular injury occurs

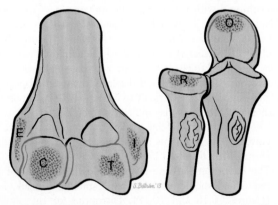

Figure 10.15 CRITOE—the order and age of appearance of ossification centers around the elbow joint. C, capitellum (1 year); R, radius (3 years); I, internal (medial) epicondyle (5 years); T, trochlea (7 years); O, olecranon (9 years); E, external (lateral) epicondyle (11 years). (Reprinted with permission from Greenspan A. *Orthopedic Imaging.* 6th ed. Philadelphia, PA: Wolters Kluwer Health; 2014.)

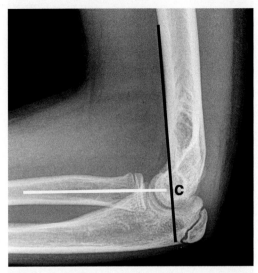

Figure 10.16   Anterior humeral and radiocapitellar lines. Lateral radiograph of the elbow shows the anterior humeral line (black line) paralleling the anterior cortex of the humerus and bisecting the capitellum (C). The radiocapitellar line (white line), drawn along the long axis of the radius, intersects the capitellum. (Reprinted with permission from Siegel MJ, Coley BD. *Pediatric Imaging*. Philadelphia, PA: Lippincott Williams & Wilkins; 2005.)

in 1%.[2] On physical examination, injury to the brachial artery can be ruled out by testing radial and ulnar pulses, capillary refill, Allen test, and the color of the hand. Sensation should be tested in the dorsal first web space (radial), palmar index finger (median), and palmar little finger (ulnar).

- Motor testing is appreciated by extending the wrist, finger, and thumb (radial), thenar strength (median), interosseous function (ulnar), and thumb interphalangeal flexion (anterior interosseous nerve [AIN]). Of note, the median nerve, especially the AIN branch is the most commonly injured.
- The Gartland classification system is the most commonly used guideline for communicating the pattern of supracondylar fractures (Figure 10.20).
  - Type I fractures are nondisplaced, type II are minimally displaced with an intact posterior cortex, type III are displaced with loss of cortical contact, and type IV fractures occur with periosteal stripping:

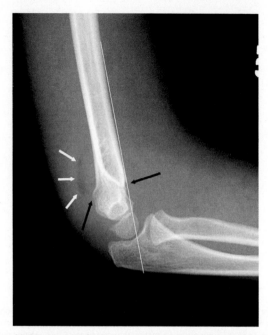

Figure 10.17 Lateral radiograph of an elbow with a supracondylar humerus fracture (black arrows) and an elevated posterior fat pad (white arrows). The anterior humeral line (thin white line) passes through the capitellum but not through the middle third, so some posterior angulation is present. This fracture may be considered borderline between a type II fracture (as there is some posterior angulation) and a type I fracture, as the anterior humeral line touches the capitellum. (Reproduced with permission from Children's Orthopaedic Center, Los Angeles, CA.)

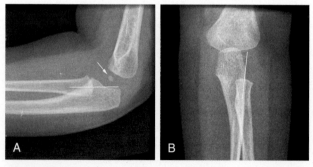

Figure 10.18 Small child with pulled elbow. A and B, Lateral and AP radiographs show that the radiocapitellar line (white line) does not intersect the middle of the ossification center (arrow) of the capitellum. (Reprinted with permission from Chew FS. *Skeletal Radiology*. 3rd ed. Philadelphia, PA: Wolters Kluwer/Lippincott Williams & Wilkins; 2010.)

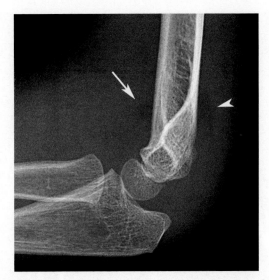

Figure 10.19 When there is an elbow joint effusion, the anterior fat pad (white arrow) looks bulbous or saillike ("sail sign") and the posterior fat pad becomes visible (arrowhead). (Reprinted with permission from Iyer RS, Chapman T. *Pediatric Radiology: The Essentials*. Philadelphia, PA: Wolters Kluwer; 2015.)

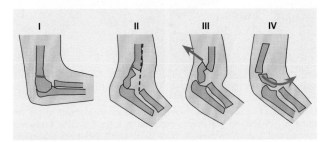

Figure 10.20 Classification of supracondylar humerus fractures. Gartland type I is non- or minimally displaced. Type II is displaced posterior to a line drawn along the anterior cortex of the distal humerus (blue dashed line), with intact posterior cortex. In type III, the posterior cortex is disrupted as the distal fragment is displaced posterior to the humerus. Flexion of the distal fragment has been designated type IV. (Reprinted with permission from Diab M, Staheli LT. *Practice of Pediatric Orthopedics*. Philadelphia, PA: Wolters Kluwer; 2015.)

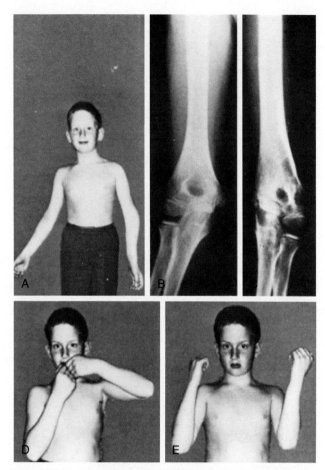

Figure 10.21 Cubitus varus (reversal of the carrying angle) of the left elbow of a 9-year-old boy due to malunion of a supracondylar fracture of the humerus 1 year previously. A, Note the unsightly deformity (sometimes referred to as a "gunstock" deformity). B and C, Radiographs of this boy's upper limbs. Unfortunately the supracondylar fracture of the left humerus had been allowed to unite in a position of varus. D, Because of the altered plane of the elbow joint, the boy cannot put the left hand to his mouth without abducting his shoulder. E, For the same reason his hand and forearm are deviated laterally when he keeps his elbow to his side (which could create problems for a dinner partner seated on his left side during the soup course). The appearance and function of this boy's arm can be improved by a supracondylar osteotomy of the humerus. (Reprinted with permission from Salter RB. *Textbook of Disorders and Injuries of the Musculoskeletal System: An Introduction to Orthopedics, Fractures, and Joint Injuries, Rheumatology, Metabolic Bone Disease, and Rehabilitation.* 3rd ed. Baltimore, MD: Williams & Wilkins; 1999.)

- Management of type I fractures consists of a posterior splint with the elbow flexed and the forearm in the neutral position. Type I fractures are inherently stable because of intact periosteum. Repeat X-rays should be taken in 3 to 7 days to confirm maintenance of alignment. A cast may be applied at the first follow-up but should be supported with a sling to prevent fracture displacement from the weight of the cast.
- Type II supracondylar fractures are inherently stable, and cast immobilization is sufficient if adequate reduction is maintained. However, if medial column collapse, significant swelling, neurovascular injuries, excessive angulation, or other injuries are present, closed reduction internal fixation is recommended. Pin stabilization is the procedure of choice, and the pins may be removed at 3 to 4 weeks.
- In completely displaced type III fractures, neurovascular and soft tissue injury is common. A careful inspection is required to rule out compartment syndrome or circulatory compromise, which if found requires emergent reduction and stabilization. Most type III fractures are initially managed with closed reduction and pinning. If closed reduction is not possible, there is a risk that neurovascular structures are impeding the correction and open reduction is required.
- Type IV fractures are diagnosed during surgery and should be suspected with more significant fractures.

CLAVICLE

Epidemiology

- Owing to the unique function and location of the clavicle, it is one of the most commonly fractured bones in the body with an estimated rate of 8% to 15% of all pediatric fractures.[2]
- Fractures are described by their anatomic location with 76% to 85% of clavicular fractures occurring in the middle third, 10% to 21% in the distal third, and 3% to 5% involving the medial third of the clavicle (Figure 10.22).[1,2]
- The clavicle is the most common site of all obstetric fractures with an occurrence rate of 1% to 13% of all births.[2]

Mechanism

- Because the clavicle is the only bony attachment site of the upper extremity to the trunk, nearly all the forces transmitted through the upper extremity travel through the clavicle.

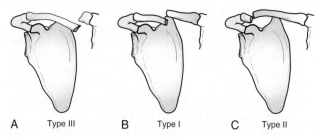

Figure 10.22 A, Fracture of the medial third of the clavicle. B, Fracture of the middle third of the clavicle. C, Fracture of the lateral third of the clavicle. (Reprinted with permission from Flynn JM, Waters PM, Skaggs DL. *Rockwood and Wilkins' Fractures in Children.* 8th ed. Philadelphia, PA: Wolters Kluwer Health; 2014.)

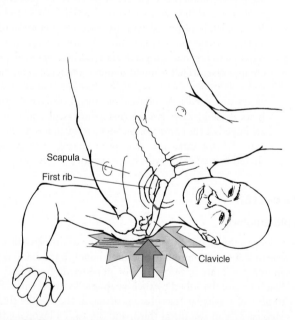

Figure 10.23 A typical way to fracture the clavicle. A fall on the top of the shoulder produces a downward force on the clavicle pushing it down onto the first rib. The first rib prevents depression of the medial aspect of the clavicle, but the force of the fall continues to depress the lateral portion of the clavicle resulting in a fracture in the middle third of the clavicle. (Reprinted with permission from Oatis CA. *Kinesiology - The Mechanics and Pathomechanics of Human Movement.* Baltimore: Lippincott Williams & Wilkins; 2004.)

- Therefore, a fall onto the shoulder is the most common mechanism of injury in children (Figure 10.23).
- Trauma directly over the clavicle may also result in an open fracture because the clavicle runs subcutaneously for most of its course and has little soft tissue protection.

Presentation

- Children with clavicular fractures usually present with pain, tenderness, and refusal to move the extremity. Children may also turn their head toward the fracture to relax the sterno-cleidomastoid muscle (SCM).
- Bony prominence or deformity is common in fractures associated with a significant displacement because of the superior pull of the SCM on the proximal fragment and weight of the arm on the distal segment.
- If sternoclavicular (SC) or acromioclavicular (AC) joints are injured, crepitus and instability are likely.
- Associated injuries to the neck, upper arm, or forearm are common in clavicle fractures. Special attention should be given to posterior clavicular dislocations or posteriorly displaced physeal separations, as the clavicle may impinge on the trachea, esophagus, or great vessels.
- Consider posterior displacement when a child presents with a clavicle injury and has difficulty speaking, breathing, or swallowing or has diminished pulses in the ipsilateral arm.

Management

- AP radiography is typically the only study needed to diagnose a clavicle fracture. However, several views may be helpful depending on the fracture site:
  - X-rays taken with the beam directed 20° to 40° cephalad to the clavicle may be necessary to illustrate the degree of fracture displacement.
  - The serendipity view is a broad X-ray beam with 40° of cephalic tilt. This view is advantageous because it allows comparison of both clavicles and an enhanced view of the medial end of the clavicle.
  - If a medial third clavicle fracture is suspected, a CT is warranted. CT imaging provides information about the medial physis and the degree of displacement and will help determine if there is injury to the intrathoracic structures.

- Treatment options for clavicular fractures are based on their anatomic location:
  - Middle third fractures are most commonly treated with a sling or figure-of-eight splint. Only fractures that violate the integrity of the skin, open fractures, or fractures that compromise neurovascular structures are treated surgically. Surgical options include plating or intramedullary nail fixation.
  - Distal third fractures are also most often treated conservatively. Frequently, these fractures occur through the metaphysis or physis and have an excellent ability to remodel. Surgical fixation is only recommended for grossly unstable fractures.
  - Medial third fractures are most often through the physis and have a great potential for remodeling. Because of this, conservative management is usually the treatment of choice.
  - Closed reduction, and if unsuccessful, open reduction is indicated for posteriorly dislocated fractures that impinge on the airway or great vessels.

TIBIA

Epidemiology

- Roughly 10.8% of all pediatric fractures involve the tibia.[2] Most tibial fractures are isolated, but it is estimated that up to 30% of tibial fractures involve the ipsilateral fibula.[2]
- In decreasing occurrence, the most commonly involved areas for fracture are the distal, middle, and proximal thirds of the tibial shaft.
- Most tibial/fibular fractures are secondary to a motor vehicle accident. The tibia is the second most common fracture sight in cases of child abuse.

Mechanism

- Approximately 81% of isolated tibia fractures are oblique or spiral in nature.[2] Oblique/spiral fractures are generally low force and are secondary to the body rotating around a planted foot.
- In children younger than 4 years, the fractures tend to be located at the distal or middle third of the tibia. In older children and adolescents, most tibial fractures are located near the ankle.

- Tibial fractures may be nondisplaced (greenstick or torus) or complete. Most tibial fractures are isolated, and the intact fibula usually prevents significant displacement.

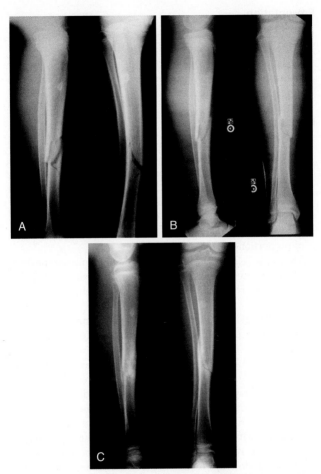

Figure 10.24 A, Anteroposterior and lateral radiograph of the lower leg in a 12-year-old child showing a comminuted tibial fracture with a concomitant plastic deformation of the fibula. Note the valgus alignment of the tibia. B, This patient had a closed manipulation and casting correcting the valgus alignment in the tibia and partially correcting the plastic deformation of the fibula. C, At union, there is an anatomic alignment of the tibia with a mild residual plastic deformation of the fibula. (Reprinted with permission from Flynn JM, Waters PM, Skaggs DL. *Rockwood and Wilkins' Fractures in Children.* 8th ed. Philadelphia, PA: Wolters Kluwer Health; 2014.)

- However, 30% of pediatric tibial shaft fractures also involve the fibula. Loss of fibular support may cause tibial shaft fractures to fall into coronal plane malalignment (Figure 10.24).

Presentation

- Children with tibial shaft fractures present with inability to bear weight, pain, tenderness, and deformity.
- 9% of tibial fractures are open, and compartment syndrome occurs in up to 5% of open fractures.[2] Associated injuries to the ankle and foot are common.

Management

- A careful neurovascular examination should be completed to rule out compartment syndrome. Arterial pulses are not reliable to definitively rule out compartment syndrome, as compartment pressures may rise enough to cause ischemia but not to the level of occluding blood supply.
- Be on the lookout for tense compartments, nerve dysfunction, burning/throbbing pain, and the complaint of pain out of proportion to the injury.
- The most sensitive indicators for compartment syndrome are pain out of proportion, increased analgesia requirement, grossly tense compartments, and pain with passive stretch.
- If pulses are no longer present, then compartment syndrome was likely missed, as this is a late event in the sequence.
- AP and lateral X-rays of the tibia as well as the knee and ankle should be ordered. If suspected fractures are not found on initial X-ray but a fracture is still suspected, then the child should be casted with follow-up X-rays planned.
- New bone formation on follow-up x-ray confirms the diagnosis.
- Children with uncomplicated fractures can be managed with closed reduction and a long leg cast for 6 to 8 weeks. Weekly follow-up X-rays are recommended to confirm alignment.[1]
- Operative treatment is considered for open fractures, those accompanied by compartment syndrome, and unstable fractures that fail closed manipulation and casting.

PEARLS AND PITFALLS

- Tibial shaft fractures with concomitant fibular shaft fractures are extremely common. Ipsilateral fibular fractures will compromise stability of the tibial fracture and should be followed up closely.
- Compartment syndrome is a surgical emergency and should be ruled out if a tibial fracture is suspected.
- Obtain a CT for medial third clavicle fractures to determine if there is an injury to the medial physis or if posterior dislocation has occurred.
- Of note, medial column collapse in supracondylar fractures may lead to nonunion and a varus angulation of the elbow. Untreated varus deformity may result in loss of full extension and a "gunstock" deformity (Figure 10.21).
- Malrotated digit fractures, as evidenced by scissoring defects, should be closely followed up, and if reduction is unsuccessful, the patient should be referred for internal fixation.
- If wrist fracture is suspected, look for pronator fat pad on lateral X-ray; new bone formation on follow-up X-ray confirms the occurrence of a fracture.

REFERENCES

1. Patrice ME, Hatch RL. Boning up on common pediatric fractures. *Contemp Pediatr*. 2003;20:30.
2. Rockwood CA, Wilkins KE, Beaty JH, Kasser JR, eds. *Rockwood and Wilkins' Fractures in Children*. 6th ed. Philadelphia: Lippincott Williams & Wilkins; 2006.
3. Valerio G, Gallè F, Mancusi C, et al. Pattern of fractures across pediatric age groups: analysis of individual and lifestyle factors. *BMC Publ Health*. 2010;10:656.
4. Ogden JA. Chondro-Osseus development and growth. In: Urist MR, ed. *Fundamental and Clinical Bone Physiology*. Philadelphia: JB Lippincott; 1980.
5. Musharafieh RS, Macari G. Salter-Harris I fractures of the distal radius misdiagnosed as a wrist sprain. *J Emerg Med*. 2000;19:265.
6. Chacon D, Kissoon N, Brown T, et al. Use of comparison radiographs in the diagnosis of traumatic injuries of the elbow. *Ann Emerg Med*. 1992;21:895.
7. Skaggs DL, Mirzayan R. The posterior fat pad sign in association with occult fracture of the elbow in children. *J Bone Joint Surg Am*. 1999; 81:1429.

Chapter 11

Management of the Pediatric Burn Patient

Stephanie Scurci

- For centuries, physicians have searched for treatments for burn victims; however, survival has improved dramatically in the last 50 years with advancements and better understanding of the pathophysiology.
- Ancient burn care consisted primarily of topical treatments including honey, rendered pig fat, wine, and myrrh.
- The discovery of penicillin by Sir Alexander Fleming in 1928 played a large part in burn treatments with systemic antibiotics.[2]
- In the 1940s, Underhill studied the importance of fluid resuscitation in burn patients. In 1952, body weight and body surface area burned were combined to create a formula for resuscitation, which underwent substitution of normal saline for lactated ringers and is now known as the Parkland formula.[2]

RELEVANT ANATOMY

- Children have thinner skin and less developed thermoregulation systems compared with adults, so they tend to get deeper burns, lose heat more rapidly, and have greater insensible fluid loss.
- Pediatric patients also differ in the larger body surface area of their heads and smaller legs.
- The traditional classification for burns (first, second, third) has been adjusted to reflect the need for surgical therapy, which now includes superficial (first), superficial partial-thickness (second), deep partial-thickness (second), full-thickness (third), and fourth degree burns (Figure 11.1).
- Second degree burns are divided into superficial partial and deep partial because of the difference in treatment. Deep partial may require surgical excision, whereas superficial partial can often be treated topically.

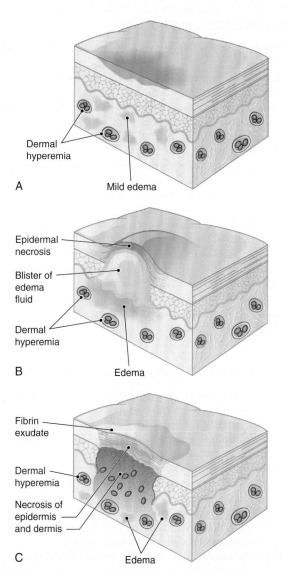

Figure 11.1 Skin burns are classified as superficial, partial thickness, or full thickness. A, Superficial burns affect only the outer layer of epidermis. B, Partial-thickness burns affect the lower layers of epidermis. C, Full-thickness burns destroy the entire layer of epidermis. (Reprinted with permission from Shaw KN, Bachur RG, eds. *Fleisher & Ludwig's Textbook of Pediatric Emergency Medicine.* 7th ed. Philadelphia, PA: Wolters Kluwer; 2016.)

EPIDEMIOLOGY AND ETIOLOGY

- One-fourth of burn injuries occur in children under the age of 16 years.
- Burns are the third leading cause of accidental deaths after vehicle and drowning deaths.
- Overall mortality rates are <3%; however, rates are higher for children <4 years of age.
- These 2 defects vary in etiology, epidemiology, and genetic predisposition.
- History and physical examination findings concerning for child abuse include delayed presentation for care, conflicting histories, previous injuries, sharply demarcated margins, uniform depth, absence of splash marks, stocking or glove patterns, flexor sparing, dorsal location on hands, and very deep localized contract injury.
- Common accidental mechanisms for burn injuries in children include biting electrical cords, exposure to hot bathwater, and spilling of hot liquids (Figure 11.2).
- Risk factors for scalding include age, crowded homes, unsupervised play, low socioeconomic status, younger unmarried mothers, and lack of maternal education.

CLINICAL PRESENTATION AND INITIAL EVALUATION

- Initial evaluation of the pediatric burn patient should follow ABCs like other trauma. Any sign of altered mental status, hypoxia, stridor, drooling, oropharyngeal edema, singed facial hair, and carbonaceous sputum should prompt intubation.
- Once airway is assessed, breathing should be evaluated. Specific to burn, circumferential chest burns may constrict respirations and require escharotomy.
- Circulation should be evaluated by checking pulses and capillary refill. Again, escharotomy may be required to restore flow to extremities with circumferential burns.
- Exposure should always include removal of all clothes.

FLUID MANAGEMENT

- Burn injuries affect not only the integumentary system but also all organ systems.

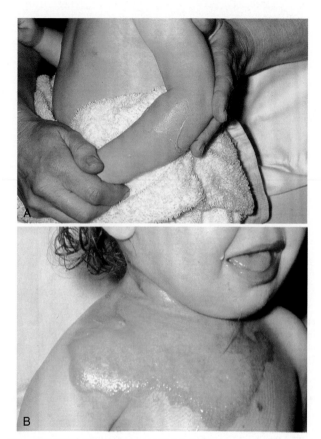

Figure 11.2 Partial-thickness burns. A, Infant with first-degree burn on arm and chest caused by scalding. B, Toddler with second-degree burn caused by scalding. (Reprinted with permission from Hatfield NT. *Broadribb's Introductory Pediatric Nursing.* 7th ed. Philadelphia, PA: Wolters Kluwer Health/Lippincott Williams & Wilkins; 2008.)

- Systemic inflammatory response syndrome results from both local and systemic inflammatory mediators including vasoactives and catecholamines, resulting in capillary leak, loss of protein, interstitial edema, and intravascular volume depletion. Additionally, the loss of the integument barrier causes evaporative fluid losses.
- Rapid fluid resuscitation significantly reduces morbidity.

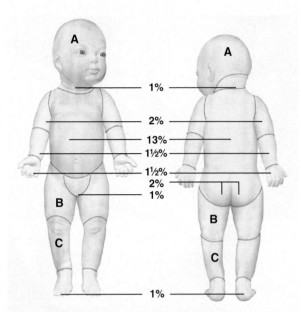

Figure 11.3 The Lund & Browder burn estimation chart. This chart and method for assigning percentage of burns are commonly used in pediatric populations. (Reprinted with permission from Jenson S. *Nursing Health Assessment.* Philadelphia, PA: Wolters Kluwer Health/Lippincott Williams & Wilkins; 2011.)

- Obtaining access with large-bore IVs is paramount. If venous access if difficult, interosseous and central accesses are alternative options.
- The Parkland formula is a good guide for initial resuscitation:
  - 4 cc × weight (kg) × % body surface area burned (Figure 11.3)
  - Half should be given in the first 8 hours and the rest over the next 16 hours
- The Parkland formula may underestimate resuscitation, especially in children because of their larger body surface area to volume ratios.[1]
- It's important to monitor urine output and hemodynamics to adjust resuscitation as required. Urine output goals should be 1 to 2 cc/kg per hour for kids <30 kg and 0.5 to 1 cc/kg per hour for kids >30 kg.
- Children may also need dextrose added to their fluids earlier than adults because of their lower hepatic glycogen reserves.

MEDICAL AND SURGICAL TREATMENT

- The principles of burn management include cleansing, debridement, and topical antimicrobials and dressing changes.
- Superficial burns do not require topical agents or debridements.
- Deeper burns require several steps—first cleansing with saline with mild soap.
- Early mechanical debridement using brushing and gentle scraping techniques clears away necrotic tissue.
- Various topical agents exist, which reduce the incidence of wound infections; no specific one has been found to be superior to others.
- Frequent dressing changes also reduce the risk of infection and promote healing. Dressings range from standard gauze to hydrocolloid and silver impregnated ones. Once again, no specific dressing type has been shown to be superior.

Operative Intervention

- Surgical principles include early excision, grafting, and reconstruction.
- Early excision and grafting allow coverage of large areas, restoring skin barrier function and preserving esthetics.
- When compared with late excision and grafting, early surgical intervention has been found to reduce hospital stay, cost, and mortality.

Skin Grafting

- Skin grafts may be split or of full thickness depending on the characteristics of the burn.
- Split-thickness skin grafts can cover large areas, with less donor skin morbidity, but also poorer cosmesis.
- Full-thickness grafts have improved cosmesis and less contraction allowing their use across joints and cosmetically sensitive areas.
- Skin substitutes (Integra, Matriderm) may supplement thin split-thickness skin grafts when limited donor sites exist.

Escharotomy

- Full-thickness, circumferential burns may require escharotomy.
- Vascular compromise in the case of extremity burns and ventilator impairment in chest and torso burns should be emergently released by escharotomy.

- In children, the chest wall and lungs are more compliant, so circumferential burns can significantly affect respiratory mechanics.
- Briefly, extremity escharotomy should extend down to subcutaneous tissue beginning and ending beyond the burned area.
- Chest wall escharotomy includes incisions along the anterior midaxillary line anteriorly with bridging incisions across the chest.

POSTOPERATIVE CARE

- Pain management postoperatively is a difficult and often overlooked portion of burn care.
- Morphine is the most commonly used opiate for burn patients; however, more recently a multimodal approach has been strongly supported. The inclusion of ketamine and benzodiazepines with careful monitoring can avoid the tolerance, withdrawal, and hyperalgesia associated with high-dose opiates.
- For procedures and extensive dressing changes, conscious sedation with opiates and benzodiazepines should be considered.

PEARLS AND PITFALLS

- Burn patients should be approached with ABCs as with other trauma patients, with careful attention to inhalational injury.
- Patterns of child abuse should be recognized.
- Fluid resuscitation in children can be underestimated by formulas commonly used for adults, so urine output should be closely monitored and resuscitation titrated.
- Early burn wound debridement and grafting reduce morbidity.

REFERENCES

1. Carvajal H. Fluid therapy for the acutely burned child. *Compr Ther.* 1977;3(3):17-24.
2. Kwang C, Joory K, Moiemen N. History of burns: the past, present, and the future. *Burns Trauma.* 2014;2(4):169-180.

SUGGESTED READINGS

Krishnamoorthy V, Ramalah R, Bhananker S. Pediatric burn injuries. *Int J Crit Illn Inj Sci*. 2012;2(3):128-134.

Merrell S, Saffle J, Sullivan J. Fluid resuscitation in thermally injured children. *Am J Surg*. 1986;152(6):664-669.

O'Neill J. Fluid resuscitation in the burned child – a reappraisal. *J Pediatr Surg*. 1982;17(5):605-607.

Chapter 12

Head Trauma in Children

Nicholas Cortolillo, John H. Kimball, Caroline R. Deyoe, and Jessica L. Buicko

- Head injuries account for a significant number of injuries in the pediatric population, resulting in over 300 000 pediatric hospitalizations annually.[1]
- Almost 90% of injury-related deaths in children are associated with head trauma.
- Falls and motor vehicle crashes are the two most common mechanisms for injury.[2]
- The American Association of Neurological Surgeons defines traumatic brain injury (TBI) as a blow or jolt to the head or penetrating head injury that disrupts the normal function of the brain.[1]

RELEVANT ANATOMY AND PHYSIOLOGY

- Primary brain injury refers to immediate physical damage as a result of shear forces.
- Secondary brain injury refers to delayed endogenous cytotoxic injury to brain tissue.
- Inflammatory cytokines released after structural damage induce harmful changes on the cellular level, manifesting with microvascular dysfunction leading to both cerebral edema and ischemia.
- Systemic factors, such as hypotension and hypoxia, can potentiate this cascade and cause neurons to necrose.
- Several anatomical factors exacerbate the severity of TBI in children.
  - Pediatric patients have thinner bones, larger head-to-toe ratio, less myelinated tissue, and late development of air sinuses.[2]
  - Skull fractures in a pediatric patient suggest massive transfer of energy, and TBI should be suspected.[3]

- The brain reaches 80% of adult brain size by age 2 years; this reduces the subarachnoid space and leads to less of a fluid cushion for the brain to be suspended and protected in the skull.[3]
- Underdeveloped neck musculature and higher relative head weight translates to increased head velocity and momentum in children.[3]

EPIDEMIOLOGY AND ETIOLOGY

- Head injury in children occurs in a bimodal distribution; most frequent hospitalizations for TBI are in age groups 0 to 4 and 15 to 19 years, according to Centers for Disease Control and Prevention (CDC) data.[4]
- For ages 0 to 4 years, falls represent the most common mechanism (more than 40%), followed by motor vehicle accidents (MVAs) and assault.[4]
- This trend continues into early teen years, when MVA replaces falls as the most common mechanism of TBI, followed by assault.[4]

INITIAL EVALUATION: HISTORY

- Includes both timing and mechanism: fall, drop, collision, blow to head, MVA.
- *Any delay in presentation is cause for concern and warrants evaluation to exclude nonaccidental cause of injury.*
- Also, discrepancies between the story and extent of injury are suspicious for abuse.
- Condition immediately after injury: loss of consciousness vs immediate cry.
- Condition since the injury: alertness, eating, vomiting, seizures, neurologic deficits (**motor exam most crucial**).

CLINICAL PRESENTATION

- Patients may present with loss of consciousness or vomiting.
- Younger children may show signs of irritability or lethargy.
- Patients may complain of worsening headache or amnesia.
- Impact seizures after injury are seen more frequently in children, and although usually self-limited, require a computed tomography (CT) of the head.

DIAGNOSTIC IMAGING

- CT scan is the imaging modality of choice when imaging is indicated.
- Patients with a skull fracture or other high-risk clinical findings should receive a head CT.[8]
- High-risk clinical findings:
  - Focal neurologic findings; motor examination is the best indicator of prognosis
  - Seizure
  - Persistent altered mental status
  - Prolonged loss of consciousness
- Long-term radiation risk of cranial CT scan in the pediatric population necessitates careful consideration of patient's risk of having an intracranial injury.

MEDICAL AND SURGICAL MANAGEMENT

- Rapid assessment of airway, breathing, circulation, disability, exposure (ABCDE)
- Early endotracheal intubation through rapid sequence in patients who have a Glasgow coma score (GCS) of <8 (see Table 7.1), respiratory failure, or hemodynamic instability
- Neurosurgical evaluation when warranted. Indications include
  - GCS 8 or less
  - Motor score 1 or 2
  - Multiple injuries associated with brain injuries such as major abdominal or thoracic injury and those needing major volume resuscitation
  - Imaging findings showing brain hemorrhage, cerebral swelling, transtentorial or cerebellar herniation[3]
- Hyperventilation with $PaCO_2$ <35 can induce cerebral ischemia, useful in setting of impending herniation
- IV access to ensure adequate cerebral perfusion; use isotonic fluid to avoid cerebral edema[9]

COMMON INJURIES

Scalp injuries

- The human **SCALP** consists of 5 layers. The **S**kin is the outer layer, followed by the **C**onnective tissue, galea **A**poneurotica, **L**oose areolar tissue, and **P**eriosteum.[5]
- The scalp is highly vascular and could be a source of substantial blood loss.

- However, *shock in a child secondary to blood loss from a scalp injury is a diagnosis of exclusion.*
- Subgaleal hemorrhage may produce up to 50% of blood volume loss in children and occurs due to rupture of emissary veins traversing the subgaleal space, allowing blood to dissect within the areolar plane and across cranial suture lines.[5]
- Cephalohematoma forms **beneath** the periosteum of the skull, in the so-called subperiosteal space.
- It is limited to the surface of a cranial bone and the cranial sutures.[5]
- A caput succedaneum, seen in newborns usually after vertex delivery, is a self-limited collection of serosanguinous fluid **above** the galea aponeurotica.[5]
- In the emergent setting, any brisk bleeding should be ligated or clamped.
- Local anesthesia, followed by thorough cleansing with saline and examination under bright lighting, is required to exclude skull fracture or intracranial communication of the wound.[6]
- Lacerations through dermis alone are appropriately closed with skin staples or suture after cleaning the wound.
- Any galea laceration >0.5 cm should be repaired with absorbable suture.[6]

Skull Fractures

- Can be seen in 2% to 20% of children with head trauma.[7]
- Nearly two-thirds of skull fractures have concomitant TBI.[7]
- May involve flat bones (frontal, temporal, occipital, parietal) or the base of the skull (basilar).[8]
- Noncontrast CT is the preferred confirmatory test. Temporal bone CT protocol (with thinner CT slices) is indicated for children with signs of basilar skull fracture.[9]
- Basilar skull fractures may present with Raccoon eyes (periorbital ecchymosis) (Figure 12.1), Battle sign (retroauricular or mastoid ecchymosis), or hemotympanum.
- Most skull fractures are located in the parietal bone and are simple linear fractures without underlying brain injury.
- However, the presence of a skull fracture increases the likelihood of TBI 6-fold.[8]
- All open and/or depressed skull fractures require a neurosurgical opinion.[9]
- General indications for a neurosurgical elevation of a depressed fracture include depression of 5 mm or more, dural injury, underlying hematoma, or gross contamination.[10]

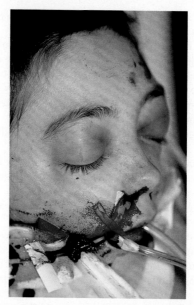

Figure 12.1 "Raccoon eyes" secondary to severe closed head injury with basilar skull fracture. (Reprinted with permission from Fleisher GR, Ludwig S, Baskin MN. *Atlas of Pediatric Emergency Medicine.* Philadelphia: Lippincott Williams & Wilkins; 2004.)

- Open fractures will require exploration with washout, wound coverage, and antibiotic prophylaxis.
- Basilar skull fractures are usually treated conservatively unless there is cerebrospinal fluid (CSF) leakage.
- A CSF leak that is prolonged has been shown to increase the risk of meningitis; however, routine antibiotic prophylaxis against meningitis for CSF leak is not indicated.[11]

Concussion

- Concussion is a form of mild TBI caused by a direct blow to the head or elsewhere on the body with an impulsive force transmitted to the head.[12]
- This leads to a rapid onset of impaired neurologic function that resolves spontaneously.
- Functional deficits, rather than structural brain damage, is the hallmark of this injury.[13]
- Management: supportive care, monitor for resolution, and rest from physical activities including sports.

- A small minority of patients will develop long-term impairment.[14]
- Repetitive concussions are currently theorized but not proven to cause chronic traumatic encephalopathy.

Epidural Hematoma

- Trauma to middle meningeal artery or dural sinus produces hemorrhage between the calvarium and dura, producing the classical lens shape on CT imaging.[15]
- Classic presentation: loss of consciousness, followed by lucid interval, followed by neurologic deterioration.
- Rapid evaluation and care by a neurosurgeon are key for patient outcome; surgical treatment consists of hematoma evacuation.
- Craniotomy may be performed by experienced providers for patients with substantial delays to definitive care in the setting of neurologic deterioration.[16]
- Radiographic factors that suggest the need for hematoma evacuation: Extradural hemorrhage >10 mm, midline shift, or temporal hematoma increases the likelihood of requiring an intervention.[17]
- Clinical factors that suggest the need for hematoma evacuation: pupillary abnormalities, altered mental status, signs of increased ICP, cerebellar signs.[18]

Subdural Hematoma

- Tearing occurs to bridging cortical veins, classically concave on CT imaging (Figure 12.2).
- More severe than epidural hematoma.
- Usually associated with shaken baby syndrome and less commonly with falls.[2]
- If suspect abuse, need to perform skeletal survey and examine for retinal hemorrhage.[15]

Penetrating Head Trauma

- Only accounts for small fraction of total head injuries but are often the most lethal (Figure 12.3).
- Most commonly secondary to gunshot wounds.
- Complications for survivors can include CSF leaks, diabetes insipidus, intracerebral abscess, and hydrocephalus.[2]

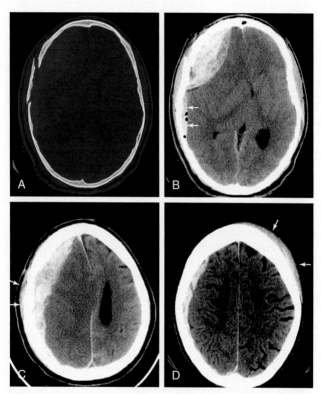

Figure 12.2 Examples of epidural (extradural) hemorrhage/hematoma (A and B) and subdural hematoma/hemorrhage (C and D) resultant to trauma to the head; all are CT and all are in the axial plane. Arrows signify site of trauma. (Reprinted with permission from Haines DE. *Neuroanatomy in Clinical Context.* 9th ed. Philadelphia: Wolters Kluwer Health; 2014.)

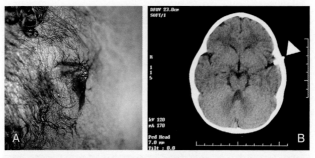

Figure 12.3 A, This 1-year-old child fell on the floor just after his mother dropped and broke a glass. The glass appears superficial but seemed unusually solidly implanted. B, The computed tomography scan shows the piece of glass (arrowhead) penetrating through the skull into sylvian fissure. (Reprinted with permission from Fleisher GR, Ludwig S, Baskin MN. *Atlas of Pediatric Emergency Medicine.* Philadelphia: Lippincott Williams & Wilkins; 2004.)

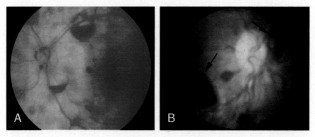

Figure 12.4 Shaken baby syndrome. A, Multiple intraretinal and preretinal hemorrhages in the posterior pole. B, Note the globular nature (arrows) of the preretinal hemorrhage in shaken baby syndrome. (A, Courtesy of Dr Richard Spaide. B, Reprinted with permission from Fineman MS, Ho AC. *Color Atlas and Synopsis of Clinical Ophthalmology – Wills Eye Institute – Retina.* 2nd ed. Philadelphia, PA: Lippincott Williams & Wilkins; 2012.)

Shaken Baby Syndrome/Nonaccidental Trauma

- Subdural hemorrhage caused by shearing of cortical veins from the child being shaken[2] (Figure 12.4).
- Can occur in children of all ages, with 0 to 3 years at greatest risk for death.[15]
- Associated signs and symptoms are altered state of consciousness, seizures, vomiting, developmental delay, and retinal hemorrhages.[15]
- Nonaccidental trauma required more surgical treatment than accidental trauma, with worse outcomes.[15]
- Some of these patients were not immediately identified on first presentation and suffered repeated abuse.[15]

PEARLS AND PITFALLS

- Head injuries are common in the pediatric population and cause significant morbidity.
- Quick evaluation and determination of acuity is of utmost importance, using clinical judgment and head CT.
- Abuse and nonaccidental trauma should be suspected when there is a delay in seeking treatment and when the symptoms do not match the story.
- Obtain neurosurgical evaluation when GCS <9, signs of increased ICP, and signs of herniation.

REFERENCES

1. Atabaki SM. Pediatric head injury. *Pediatr Rev*. 2007;28(6).
2. Alexiou GA, Sfakianos G, Prodromou N. Pediatric head trauma. *J Emerg Trauma Shock*. 2001;4(3):403-408.
3. Adapted from Advanced trauma life support, 9th edition. *J Trauma Acute Care Surg*. 2013;74(5):1363-1366.
4. Percent Distributions of TBI-related Hospitalizations by Age Group and Injury Mechanism — United States, 2006–2010. Concussion. Traumatic Brain Injury. CDC Injury Center. Available at: https://www.cdc.gov/traumaticbraininjury/data/dist_hosp.html.
5. Chen C-E, Liao ZZ, Lee YH, et al. Subgaleal hematoma at the contralateral side of scalp trauma in an adult. *J Emerg Med*. 2017;53:e85-e88.
6. Hollander JE, Singer AJ. Laceration management. *Ann Emerg Med*. 1999;34:356-367.
7. Carson HJ. Brain trauma in head injuries presenting with and without concurrent skull fractures. *J Forensic Leg Med*. 2009;16;115-120.
8. Rabinowitz RP, Caplan ES. Management of infections in the trauma patient. *Surg Clin North Am*. 1999;79:1373-1383 [x].
9. Orman G, Wagner MW, Seeburg D, et al. Pediatric skull fracture diagnosis: should 3D CT reconstructions be added as routine imaging? *J Neurosurg Pediatr*. 2015;16:426-431.
10. Ersahin Y, Mutluer S, Mirzai H, Palali I. Pediatric depressed skull fractures: analysis of 530 cases. *Childs Nerv Syst*. 1996;12(6):323-331.
11. Ratilal BO, Costa J, Pappamikail L, Sampaio C. Antibiotic prophylaxis for preventing meningitis in patients with basilar skull fractures. *Cochrane Database Syst Rev*. 2015 [CD004884].
12. Faul M, Wald MM, Wu L, Coronado VG [National Center for Injury Prevention and Control (U.S.). Division of Injury Response], Traumatic brain injury in the United States: emergency department visits, hospitalizations, and deaths, 2002–2006 (Centers for Disease Control and Prevention, 2010). doi:10.15620/cdc.5571.
13. Eapen BC, Cifu DX. *Rehabilitation After Traumatic Brain Injury*. Elsevier Health Sciences; 2018.
14. Deakin ND, Cronin T, Trafford P, et al. Concussion in motor sport: A medical literature review and engineering perspective. *J Concussion*. 2017;1:2059700217733916.

15. Paul AR, Adamo MA. Non-accidental trauma in pediatric patients: a review of epidemiology, pathophysiology, diagnosis and treatment. *Transl Pediatr*. 2014;3(3):195-207.doi:10.3978/j.issn.2224-4336.2014.06.01.
16. Bullock MR, Chesnut R, Ghajar J, et al. Surgical management of acute epidural hematomas. *Neurosurgery*. 2006;58:S7-S15 [discussion Si-Siv].
17. Schutzman SA, Barnes PD, Mantello M, Scott RM. Epidural hematomas in children. *Ann Emerg Med*. 1993;22:535-541.
18. Paşaoglu A, Orhon C, Koç K, et al. Traumatic extradural haematomas in pediatric age group. *Acta Neurochir*. 1990;106:136-139.

Chapter 13

Diagnosis and Management of Child Abuse Injuries

Lacey P. MenkinSmith and Ashley B. Hink

- Child abuse or nonaccidental trauma (NAT) has always existed, but its recognition by the medical community as a major cause of morbidity and mortality to children was in 1860 by Dr Ambroise Tardieu, a French forensic pathologist who published an article on 32 cases of pediatric physical abuse and raised the attention of physicians to report suspected cases to legal authorities.[1]

- Drs John Caffey and Frederic Silverman, both pediatric radiologists, further defined NAT injuries by publishing multiple articles throughout their careers from the 1940s to 1970s, describing patterns of fractures and head trauma suspicious of abuse.[2-4]

- In 1962, "The Battered Child Syndrome," widely considered a sentinel paper in child abuse published in JAMA, outlined the clinical features of physical abuse and maltreatment in children and provided the framework that led to the creation of child protection and mandatory reporting laws in the United States.[5]

- The Federal Child Abuse Prevention and Treatment Act amended in 2003 provides minimum standards to the states for defining maltreatment as "Any recent act or failure to act on the part of a parent or caretaker, which results in death, serious physical or emotional harm, sexual abuse, or exploitation, or an act or failure to act which presents an imminent risk of serious harm."[6]

- State laws defining physical abuse vary widely, but medical providers are mandated to report all cases of suspected abuse and neglect to child protective services (CPS).

RELEVANT ANATOMY

- Child abuse should be considered in any traumatic injury in a child, especially if the mechanism of trauma described does not match the injury pattern or the child's developmental milestones.

EPIDEMIOLOGY AND ETIOLOGY

- There were 683 000 victims of child abuse and neglect identified by CPS in 2015.[7]
- About 1670 children died from abuse or neglect in 2015 with head trauma being the primary cause of death, and 75% of fatalities were under the age of 3 years.[7]
- Child abuse remains significantly underreported and underrecognized by the medical profession.[8,9]
  - Nearly 20% of child victims of NAT are seen by a medical professional in the month before their death.[10]
- Although the immediate impact of NAT includes acute injuries, children who experience abuse and neglect are more likely to have a number of poor health and social outcomes, including poor school performance, perpetration and victimization of violence, substance abuse, mental illness, and chronic illnesses.[11,12]
- The etiology of child abuse is multifactorial at the individual, family, and community level. Studies show that the following family and social factors are associated with an increased risk of abuse[7,13-19]:
  - Abusers are more likely to be young parents and women, but men are more likely to commit fatal abuse
  - Caregiver history of experiencing child abuse
  - Caregiver history of mental illness and substance abuse
  - Caregiver history of criminal activity
  - Short intervals between pregnancies and high number of unplanned pregnancies
  - Economic stress within the family/household
  - Intimate partner violence
  - Living in households with unrelated adults
  - Perceived poor community and social support
- Children at a higher risk of abuse are under the age of 3 years, born preterm, or with significant perinatal illness and have special needs (chronic illness, mental retardation, and disabilities).[20,21]
  - There is no conclusive evidence that race is associated with abuse, but African American children are more likely to experience fatalities secondary to abuse.[22,23]

CLINICAL PRESENTATION

History Red Flags

- No history available or denial of trauma despite severe injury
- Inconsistent history and stories from witnesses present

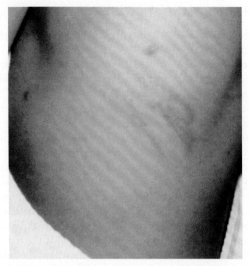

Figure 13.1 Imprint marks from beating with a looped electrical cord. (Reprinted from Carrasco MM, Wolford JE. Child Abuse and Neglect. In: Zitelli BJ, McIntire S, Nowalk AJ, eds. *Atlas of Pediatric Physical Diagnosis.* 7th ed. Elsevier; 2018. Copyright © 2018 Elsevier. With permission.)

- Mechanism and history do not support the injury pattern or severity
- Mechanism and injury pattern are not consistent with development
- Injury blamed on other children or pets, or reported as self-inflicted
- Significant delay in seeking care
- History of previous evaluations for suspicious injuries

Physical Examination Red Flags

- **General appearance and behavior:**
  - Evidence of poor caretaking and neglect
  - Caregiver appearing distant or nervous
  - Inappropriate or concerning interactions between the child and caregiver
- **Skin:**
  - Superficial injury patterns of objects such as loop-of-cord marks, hangers, slap marks, and bites (Figure 13.1)
  - Bruising patterns inconsistent with developmental stage— "those who don't cruise rarely bruise"[24]

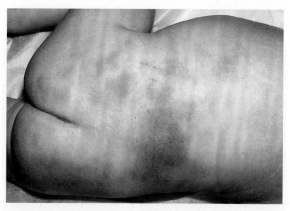

Figure 13.2 Large bruises on a child's body. With this type of injury, carefully assessing the history of the accident would be essential. (Copyright Biophoto Associates. Supplied by SCIENCE SOURCE.)

- Accidental bruising typically occurs over bony prominences (Figure 13.2)
- **TEN4:** Concerning locations for bruising include the following[24,25]:
  - T—Torso
  - E—Ear
  - N—Neck
  - 4—Bruising in these areas in children <4 years of age or ANY bruising in children <4 months of age
- Bruising to the cheek, buttock, back, and genitals should be regarded as suspicious
- **Fractures:**
  - Fractures in nonambulatory infants and toddlers especially in the long bones such as the femur and humerus
  - Multiple fractures and fractures in variable stages of healing
  - Rib fractures (especially posterior)
  - Metaphyseal corner fractures of long bones ("bucket handle fracture" or "corner fracture") have high specificity for NAT[26] (Figure 13.3)
  - Spiral fracture patterns of long bones are suspicious but may be seen with rotational forces (ie, "toddler's fracture" of tibia)
  - Fractures of sternum, scapula, and skull

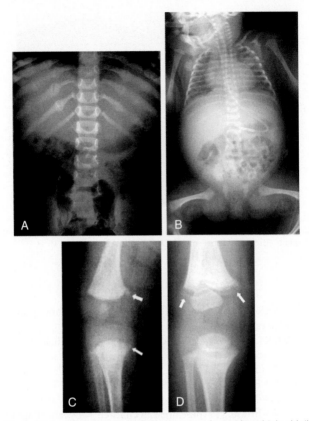

Figure 13.3 Skeletal survey in child abuse. A, Infant with multiple old rib injuries and gastric distension. B, "Babygram": a single frontal radiograph of the long bones and axial skeleton may mask subtle injuries because of geometric distortion and exposure variation. C, Frontal radiograph of the knee showing a characteristic metaphyseal "corner" fracture of the distal femur (arrows). D, Another infant's knee demonstrating the typical and highly specific "bucket-handle" fracture of the distal femur (arrows). (A, Reprinted with permission from Reece RM, Christian C, eds. *Child Abuse Medical Diagnosis & Management.* 3rd ed. Elk Grove Village, IL: American Academy of Pediatrics; 2008. B-D, Courtesy of Evan Geller. Reprinted with permission from Greenberg MI, Hendrickson RG, Silverberg M, et al. *Greenberg's Text-Atlas of Emergency Medicine.* Philadelphia, PA: Lippincott Williams & Wilkins; 2004.)

- **Abdominal injury:**
  - Older toddlers and young children are most susceptible to blunt abdominal injures.[27]
  - Solid organ injuries to the spleen, liver, and pancreas occur with both accidental trauma and NAT, but hollow viscous injuries are more likely associated with abuse, especially in children under the age of 4 years.[28]
  - Many of these injuries may be easily missed because of vague symptoms of abdominal pain, poor appetite, nausea, and emesis.
    - There are high rates of occult abdominal injuries in the setting of abusive head trauma.
    - Bruising rarely occurs, but if noted on examination, this should heighten suspicion for abuse.
- **Head trauma**
  - It is the leading cause of death in pediatric NAT, typically in the first year of life.[29]
    - Head injuries sustained from NAT tend to be more severe requiring operative intervention and result in death compared with accidental head injuries.[30,31]
  - Intracranial injuries, including epidural, subdural, and intraventricular hemorrhage, diffuse axonal injury (DAI), cortical contusions, skull fractures, and retinal hemorrhage may accompany head trauma.[32]
  - Infants are susceptible to shaken baby syndrome that causes a classic triad of subdural hematomas, retinal hemorrhage, and encephalopathy, while infants, toddlers, and older children are all susceptible to direct blunt force trauma.[32]
  - Presentation can be variable based on the acuity and severity of the injury.
    - Severe or acute head injuries may present with altered mental status, apnea, seizures, and emesis.[33]
    - Delayed or chronic symptoms from head injury may include nonspecific symptoms such as failure to thrive, poor feeding, irritability, lethargy, and developmental delays—making it challenging to diagnose if a history of head trauma is not provided.[34]
- **Burns**
  - About 10% of pediatric admissions for burns are secondary to abuse, but upward of 40% of all burns are from abuse. Most are scald (from hot liquids) and thermal (from hot objects) burns.
  - Suspicious burns include the following:
    - Burns to the dorsum of the hands, legs, feet, and buttock
    - In the shape of a hot object

- Forced immersion (stocking-and-glove pattern)
- Cigarette burns
- Spill/splash patterns not consistent with developmental history
- **Injury Patterns**
  - Although patients experiencing NAT may present with an isolated injury, multiple studies have identified injuries that frequently co-occur with abusive head trauma and should raise suspicion for NAT.
    - Injuries including rib fractures, seizures, long bone fractures, retinal hemorrhage, apnea, and head and neck bruising increase the likelihood that a head injury is secondary to NAT, especially if multiple injuries are present.[35,36]

SCREENING

- There is no gold standard in screening for pediatric child abuse, and there is poor evidence on the accuracy of many developed screening instruments.[37]
  - The U.S. States Preventive Task Force found insufficient evidence to universally screen children for NAT; however, there are studies demonstrating improved detection with universal screening in the ED.[38]
- There should be a low threshold for suspecting abuse, and any aforementioned clinical or history "red flags" detected by members of the clinical team (including nurses) should trigger a workup for the diagnosis of child abuse.
- If sexual assault is suspected within the last 72 hours, defer interview and examination to specialized multidisciplinary team; a single comprehensive child sexual abuse evaluation should be conducted by professionals trained and experienced in sexual abuse.

DIAGNOSIS

History and Physical Examination

- A thorough and complete family, social, medical, surgical, and event history is absolutely necessary, including details surrounding the injury (setting, who was present, time, and circumstances).
  - It is important to assess the medical history and a review of systems to identify underlying diseases that may increase the risk of bruising, bleeding, and fractures such as hematologic disorders and pathologic bone disease.

- Physical examination is the key for the initial workup and diagnosis of NAT, which includes exposure and full examination including the skin, extremities, and genitalia when appropriate.

Laboratory Studies

- A complete blood count, comprehensive metabolic panel (including electrolytes, liver function tests [LFTs], lipase), urinalysis, and coagulation studies should be obtained for all children with suspected abuse.
- If an intracranial hemorrhage is identified, additional coagulation studies should be ordered to work up underlying coagulopathies and hematologic disorders.

Skeletal Survey

- Series of X-rays of the axial skeleton and large cortical bones should be obtained in all children <2 years of age with any suspicion for abuse and in children >2 years of age with suspicious fractures (Figure 13.4).
- Other indications:
  - Infants and toddlers with unexplained intracranial injury
  - Infants and siblings <2 years of age who are household contacts of an abused child

Neuroimaging

- Noncontrasted CT of the head should be obtained for all symptomatic patients with concern of intracranial trauma.
  - It is preferred for diagnosis of pathology requiring immediate surgical intervention such as intracranial hemorrhage, as well as skull fractures and scalp injuries.
- MRI is more sensitive for injuries that may be missed on CT, such as hypoxic injury and DAI, and is sometimes used for children with negative CT scans.

Abdominal Imaging

- Children with LFTs twice above normal limits, an elevated lipase, or concerning abdominal examination findings and symptoms (such as pain, nausea, and emesis) should undergo a CT scan with IV contrast of the abdomen and pelvis.
  - Oral contrast should be considered if suspicious of duodenal or other hollow viscous injury.

Ophthalmologic Examination

- Funduscopic examination should occur within 24 to 72 hours by an ophthalmologist to evaluate for the presence and severity of retinal hemorrhages in the setting of suspected or identified head trauma.

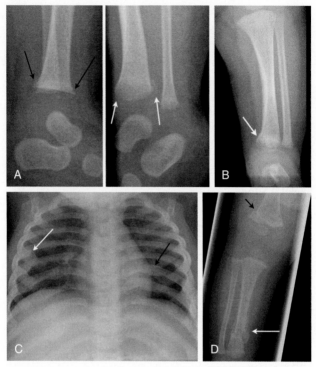

Figure 13.4   A, Classic metaphyseal fracture of the distal tibia seen in 2 projections showing "chip-fracture" (black arrows) and "bucket-handle" (white arrows) appearances. B, Classic metaphyseal lesion with more developed periosteal calcification (arrow). C, AP chest X-ray from skeletal survey showing more than a dozen rib fractures with evidence of healing. One representative posterior (black arrow) and anterior (white arrow) have been labeled. D, Child with multiple fractures at different stages of healing. Although the fracture of the distal femur (black arrow) shows very minor, if any, periosteal reaction or calcification, the fracture of the distal tibia (white arrow) shows robust calcification and periosteal reaction. (Courtesy of Cincinnati Children's Hospital Medical Center, Cincinnati, OH. Reprinted with permission from Lewiss RE, Saul T, Shah K. *Essential Emergency Imaging.* Philadelphia, PA: Lippincott Williams & Wilkins; 2012.)

MANAGEMENT

- Appropriate medical and surgical management of all injuries should be ensured with consultation to appropriate subspecialties for specific injuries (neurosurgery, orthopedic surgery, etc).
- Consult a child abuse multidisciplinary team for further workup and management of the patient.
  - Many hospitals have established child abuse teams (eg, social worker, nurse, child life specialist, child abuse pediatrician).

- Admission may be warranted for the care of injuries and is often necessary for further workup of NAT and to protect the child pending further investigation.
- All aspects of the provided history, events surrounding the injury, and physical findings must be thoroughly documented; body maps and photos of injuries are often useful.
  - Medical records can be used in criminal cases, so it's incredibly important to provide detailed documentation.
- CPS referral must be made whenever child abuse and neglect are suspected. Health care professionals are mandated reporters and do not need to prove abuse; suspicion alone is the minimum requirement for reporting. Law enforcement most likely will need to be notified.
  - Identify and report other children at risk in household.
  - Reporting phone numbers can be obtained from the Child Welfare Information Gateway (www.childwelfare.gov/) or by calling Childhelp (1-800-4-A-CHILD, 1-800-422-4453).
  - The responding CPS worker should evaluate the child and circumstances before the patient is discharged from the health care setting, so an appropriate disposition plan is in place.
- Appropriate referral for counseling should be made.

PEARLS AND PITFALLS

- Child abuse must be considered in the differential diagnosis of any traumatic injury to a child especially if the mechanism of trauma described does not match the injury pattern or developmental milestones, especially in young children.
- Pathology that may be mistaken for child abuse include osteogenesis imperfecta, Mongolian spots, cultural practices such as cupping or coining, bleeding disorders, hemangiomas, or vasculitis.
- Careful documentation of reported and suspected history with mechanism of injury as well as physical examination findings (including drawings or pictures of injury) is important.
- Report! All health care providers are required by law to report any *suspicion* of child abuse to CPS.

REFERENCES

1. Roche AJ, Fortin G, Labbé J, et al. The work of Ambroise Tardieu: the first definitive description of child abuse. *Child Abuse Negl.* 2005;29:325-334.

2. Caffey J. Multiple fractures in the long bones of infants suffering from chronic subdural hematoma. *Am J Roentgenol Radium Ther.* 1946;56:163-173.

3. Silverman FN. The roentgen manifestations of unrecognized skeletal trauma in infants. *Am J Roentgenol Radium Ther Nucl Med.* 1953;69:413-427.

4. Caffey J. The whiplash shaken infant syndrome: manual shaking by the extremities with whiplash-induced intracranial and intraocular bleedings, linked with residual permanent brain damage and mental retardation. *Pediatrics.* 1974;54:396-403.

5. Kempe CH, Silverman FN, Steele BF, Droegemueller W, Silver HK. The battered-child syndrome. *J Am Med Assoc.* 1962;181(1):17-24. doi:10.1001/jama.1962.03050270019004.

6. U.S. Department of Health & Human Services, Administration for Children and Families, Administration on Children, Youth and Families, Children's Bureau. *Child Abuse Prevention and Treatment Act as Amended by P.L. 111–320, the CAPTA Reauthorization Act of 2010.* 2010. Available from https://www.acf.hhs.gov/sites/default/files/cb/capta2010.pdf.

7. U.S. Department of Health & Human Services, Administration for Children and Families, Administration on Children, Youth and Families, Children's Bureau. *Child Maltreatment 2015.* 2017. Available from http://www.acf.hhs.gov/programs/cb/research-data-technology/statistics-research/child-maltreatment [PMID:10201724].

8. Flaherty EG, Sege RD, Griffith J, et al. From suspicion of physical child abuse to reporting: primary care clinician decision-making. *Pediatrics.* 2008;122:611-619.

9. Jenny C, Hymel KP, Ritzen A, Reinert SE, Hay TC. Analysis of missed cases of abusive head trauma [published correction appears in *JAMA.* 1999;282:29]. *J Am Med Assoc.* 1999;281:621-626.

10. Smith JA, Adler RG. Children hospitalized with child abuse and neglect: a case control study. *Child Abuse Negl.* 1991;15:437-456.

11. Altemeier WA, O'Connor S, Vietze PM, et al. Antecedents of child abuse. *J Pediatr.* 1982;100:823-829.

12. Garbarino J, Crouter A. Defining the community context for parent-child relations: the correlates of child maltreatment. *Child Dev.* 1978;49:604-629.

13. Smith SM, Hanson R. Interpersonal relationships and child-rearing practices in 214 parents of battered children. *Br J Psychiatry.* 1975;127:513-520.

14. Oliver JE. Successive generations of child maltreatment: social and medical disorders in the parents. *Br J Psychiatry.* 1985;147:484-490.

15. Rumm PD, Cummings P, Krauss MR, Bell MA, Rivara FP. Identified spouse abuse as a risk factor for child abuse. *Child Abuse Negl.* 2000;24:1375-1381.

16. Schnitzer PG, Ewigman BG. Child deaths resulting from inflicted injuries: household risk factors and perpetrator characteristics. *Pediatrics.* 2005;116(5).

17. Benedict MI, White RB, Cornley DA. Maternal perinatal risk factors and child abuse. *Child Abuse Negl.* 1985;9:217-224.

18. Huang MI, O'Riordan MA, Fitzenrider E, et al. Increased incidence of nonaccidental head trauma in infants associated with the economic recession. *J Neurosurg Pediatr.* 2011;8:171-176.

19. Leventhal JM, Thomas SA, Roseneld NS, et al. Fractures in young children: distinguishing child abuse from unintentional injuries. *Am J Dis Child.* 1993;147:87-92.

20. Wu SS, Ma CX, Carter RL, et al. Risk factors for infant maltreatment: a population-based study. *Child Abuse Negl.* 2004;28:1253-1264.

21. Vinchon M, Defoort-Dhellemmes S, Desurmont M, et al. Accidental and nonaccidental head injuries in infants: a prospective study. *J Neurosurg.* 2005;102:380-384.

22. Falcone RA Jr, Brown RL, Garcia VF. The epidemiology of infant injuries and alarming health disparities. *J Pediatr Surg.* 2007;42: 172-176.

23. Lyman JM, McGwin G, Malone DE, et al. Epidemiology of child homicide in Jefferson county, Alabama. *Child Abuse Negl.* 2003;27:1063-1073.

24. Pierce MC, Kaczor K, Aldridge S, O'Flynn J, Lorenz DJ. Bruising characteristics discriminating physical child abuse from accidental trauma. *Pediatrics.* 2010;125(1):67-74. Epub December 7, 2009. Erratum in *Pediatrics.* 2010;125(4):861.

25. Christain CW, Committee on Child Abuse and Neglect. The evaluation of suspected child physical abuse. *Pediatrics.* 2015;135(5):e1337 -e1354. doi:10.1542/peds.2015-0356.

26. Kleinman PK. Problems in the diagnosis of metaphyseal fractures. *Pediatr Radiol.* 2008;38(suppl 3):S388-S394.

27. Trokel M, Discala C, Terrin NC, Sege RD. Patient and injury characteristics in abusive abdominal injuries. *Pediatr Emerg Care.* 2006;22:700-704.

28. Wood J, Rubin DM, Nance ML, Christian CW. Distinguishing inflicted versus accidental abdominal injuries in young children. *J Trauma.* 2005;59:1203-1208.

29. Alexander RC, Levitt CJ, Smith W. *Abusive head trauma.* In: Reece RM, Ludwig S, eds. *Child Abuse: Medical Management and Diagnosis.* 2nd ed. Philadelphia, PA: Lippincott, Williams & Wilkins; 2001:47-80.

30. Reece RM, Sege R. Childhood head injuries: accidental or inflicted. *Arch Pediatr Adolesc Med.* 2000;154:11-15.

31. Feldman KW, Bethel R, Shugeman RP, Grossman DC, Grady MS, Ellenbogen RG. The cause of infant and toddler subdural hemorrhage: a prospective study. *Pediatrics.* 2001;108:636-646.

32. Greely CS. Abusive head trauma: a review of the evidence base. *Am J Radiol.* 2014;204:967-973.

33. Sieswerda-Hoogendoorn T, Boos S, Spivack B, et al. Educational paper: abusive head trauma part I: Clinical aspects. *Eur J Pediatr.* 2012;171: 415-423.

34. Ferriero DM. Neonatal brain injury. *N Engl J Med.* 2004;351:1985-1995.

35. Hymel KP, Willson DF, Boos SC, et al. Pediatric brain injury research network (PediBIRN) investigators: derivation of a clinical prediction rule for pediatric abusive head trauma. *Pediatr Crit Care Med.* 2013;14:210-220.

36. Cowley LE, Morris CB, Maguire SA et al. Validation of a prediction Tool for abusive head trauma. *Pediatrics*. 2015;136(2):290-298.
37. Bailhache M, Leroy V, Pillet P, Salmi L. Is early detection of abused children possible?: a systematic review of the diagnostic accuracy of the identification of abused children. *BMC Pediatr*. 2013,13:202-213.
38. Louwers E, Korfage I, Affourtit MJ, et al. Effects of systematic screening and detection of child. *Pediatrics*. 2012;130:457-464.

Common Pediatric Surgical Problems

Chapter 14

Hypertrophic Pyloric Stenosis

Jessica L. Buicko

HISTORICAL BACKGROUND

- Although reports date back to the early 1600s, Harald Hirschsprung is credited as the first person to describe hypertrophic pyloric stenosis (HPS) in 1887.
- Hirschsprung reported on 2 cases of term infants who suddenly began vomiting and losing significant amounts of weight. He found at autopsy that both of his young patients had hypertrophied and elongated pyloric channels.[1]
- As the pathology became better understood, a variety of surgical treatments emerged as attempts to correct this disease process.
- In 1912, German surgeon Conrad Ramstedt developed the pyloromyotomy, which is the foundation of surgical treatment today.[2]

RELEVANT ANATOMY (FIGURE 14.1)

- The pyloric channel is the distal portion of the stomach that connects to the first portion of the duodenum.
- At the distal portion of the pyloric channel, there is a circular layer of smooth muscle, which comprises the pyloric sphincter.
- The pyloric sphincter controls the rate of stomach emptying and prevents regurgitation of chyme from the duodenum back into the stomach.
- The normal pyloric muscle thickness is ≤2 mm.

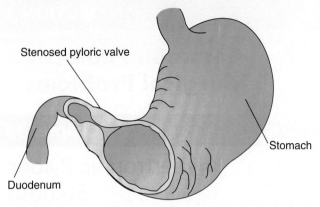

Stenosed pyloric valve

Stomach

Duodenum

Figure 14.1 Fluid is unable to pass easily through the stenosed and hypertrophied pyloric valve. (Reprinted with permission from Pillitteri A. *Maternal and Child Nursing*. 4th ed. Philadelphia, PA: Lippincott Williams & Wilkins; 2003.)

EPIDEMIOLOGY AND ETIOLOGY

Incidence: It varies depending on ethnic and geographic locations although pyloric stenosis occurs in approximately 1 in 300 live births and is more common in Caucasians.

- Males are affected approximately 4 times more frequently than females.
- There is also evidence of a genetic predisposition, as siblings of children with HPS are at approximately 15 times greater risk of also developing the condition.[3]

Etiology: Many theories as to the exact etiology exist, but it is likely multifactorial.

- Some environmental causes have been linked to development of HPS.
- Erythromycin is associated with HPS with a postulated mechanism that its promotility effects can lead to hypertrophy of the sphincter muscle.

CLINICAL PRESENTATION

Classic presentation: an otherwise healthy baby who presents with projectile, nonbilious, nonbloody emesis.

- It is paramount to distinguish this from infants with bilious emesis, which can suggest a multitude of other pathologies that will be discussed in other chapters.
- Unlike other etiologies, patients with HPS are typically hungry and eager to feed after episodes of emesis.

- The average age of patients presenting with HPS is between third and sixth week of life.
- The classic physical examination finding is a palpable "olive-like" mass, although oftentimes this is hard to elicit unless the baby is resting comfortably.

DIAGNOSIS

Laboratory Findings

- If pyloric stenosis is on the differential diagnosis, it is essential to obtain intravenous access and check basic electrolytes.
- Patients with vomiting secondary to HPS usually have a **hypokalemic, hypochloremic, metabolic alkalosis**.

Imaging Findings

- Imaging modality of choice for the diagnosis of HPS is abdominal ultrasound.
- The ultrasound allows for direct visualization of the thickened smooth muscle.
- **Key ultrasound findings** that are suggestive of HPS include a pyloric channel >15 mm long with a pyloric muscle thickness >3.5 mm.
- The channel length can be variable, and the measurement of the muscle thickness is often more reliable.
- On transverse view, the "target sign" can be seen secondary to hypertrophied hypoechoic muscle surrounding echogenic mucosa. Of note, ultrasounds are user-dependent.
- If there is question of the diagnosis and the ultrasound is not feasible, one can obtain an upper gastrointestinal study (UGIS).
- A UGIS suggestive of HPS would demonstrate the **classic "string sign"** caused by the hypertrophied pylorus in addition to showing slowed gastric emptying (Figures 14.2-14.4).

SURGICAL MANAGEMENT

- Surgery for HPS is not an emergency, and it is **paramount to correct the electrolyte imbalances before operative intervention**.
- There are many different algorithms for correction of the metabolic derangement.
- Our practice is to correct electrolyte disturbances with **normal saline boluses at 20 mL/kg**.

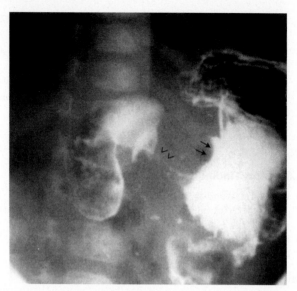

Figure 14.2 The upper GI in this 6-week-old baby shows elongation and narrowing of the pyloric channel (arrowheads). On the stomach side, notice the rounded indentation (arrows) caused by the very hypertrophied pyloric muscle. This is called the shoulder sign. Together this combination of signs is diagnostic for pyloric stenosis. (Reprinted with permission from Erkonen WE, Smith WL. *Radiology 101: The Basics and Fundamentals of Imaging.* 2nd ed. Philadelphia, PA: Lippincott Williams & Wilkins; 2005.)

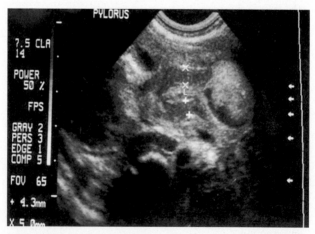

Figure 14.3 Abdominal ultrasound demonstrating pyloric stenosis. Note the thin pyloric lumen (L) and the thickened pyloric musculature (defined by the region between ×'s and +'s). (Reprinted with permission from Daffner RH. *Clinical Radiology: The Essentials.* 4th ed. Philadelphia, PA: Lippincott Williams & Wilkins; 1999.)

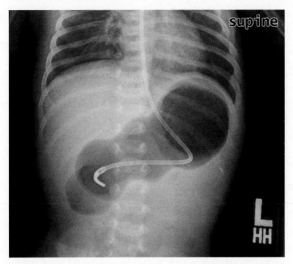

Figure 14.4   Hypertrophic pyloric stenosis on abdominal radiograph. Supine abdominal radiograph in a 1-month-old infant shows marked gastric distention and an undulating contour of the stomach, referred to as the "caterpillar" sign, reflecting peristaltic waves against the obstruction. (Reprinted with permission from Iyer RS, Chapman T. *Pediatric Imaging: The Essentials*. Philadelphia, PA: Wolters Kluwer; 2016.)

- We then recheck the laboratory test results, and if the derangements are improved, patients are then placed on 1.5 times maintenance fluids.
- A nasogastric tube should also be placed to keep the stomach empty before surgical intervention.

OPERATIVE INTERVENTION

- The classic surgical procedure for HPS is **Ramstedt pyloromyotomy**.
- This can be performed either laparoscopically or with an open approach depending on the surgeon's preference.

Open Approach

- The open approach is typically made through a right upper quadrant incision lateral to the rectus muscle.
- The stomach is identified and grasped proximally to the thickened area of the pylorus.

- A longitudinal seromuscular incision is made over the pylorus extending up toward the gastric antrum.
- The vein of Mayo, when seen, is helpful to identify the distal extent of the myotomy.
- The muscle is then carefully split down to the submucosal layer.
- Protrusion of the intact gastric mucosa confirms an appropriate myotomy.
- Of note, occasionally mucosal perforation does occur.
- If this happens, the perforation is repaired and the pylorus is rotated approximately 90° and the myotomy is redone.

Laparoscopic Approach (Figure 14.5)

- For the laparoscopic approach, the patient is placed supine.
- It is the surgeon's preference to enter the abdominal cavity through the umbilicus.
- Two small stab incisions are made in the right and left upper quadrants through which an atraumatic grasper and a myotomy knife or electrocautery device are placed.
- The myotomy is performed in a similar fashion to the open procedure.
- Afterward, air is insufflated into the stomach to assess the integrity of the mucosa.
- Similar to many laparoscopic procedures, laparoscopic pyloromyotomy has been found to have shorter lengths of stay, a lower total complication rate, and a shorter time to full feeding.[4]

POSTOPERATIVE CARE

- Postoperative care is similar after both open and laparoscopic approaches with some surgeons starting feeds sooner after laparoscopic repair.
- It is not uncommon for patients to have episodes of vomiting postoperatively, but this is usually self-limited.
- A recent prospective randomized trial comparing ad lib feeding with protocol feeding postpyloromyotomy concluded that patients with ad lib feeds reached goal feeds faster, yet this did not translate into a significant difference in the length of stay.[5]
- Pain is usually well controlled with acetaminophen, and patients are usually discharged within a few days of surgical intervention.

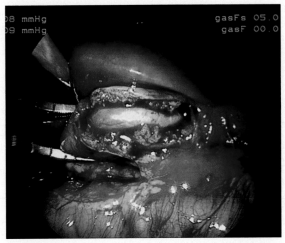

Figure 14.5   Laparoscopic repair of pyloric stenosis. In this image, the surgical cleft created in the hypertrophic muscles of the pylorus can be seen. (Courtesy of Timothy Lautz, MD. Reprinted with permission from Barash PG. *Clinical Anesthesia.* 8th ed. Philadelphia, PA: Wolters Kluwer; 2017.)

Complications

- The major complications after surgery for HPS include mucosal perforation, incomplete myotomy, prolonged postoperative emesis, duodenal injury, and wound infection.
- In regard to long-term outcomes, historically HPS had a mortality of more than 50%, but today with significant advances the mortality rate is almost 0 with an overall complication rate of 1% to 2%.[6]

PEARLS AND PITFALLS

- Always consider pyloric stenosis in patients aged 3 to 6 weeks of life who present with projectile nonbilious vomiting.
- The classic palpable **"olive mass"** may be absent on physical examination.
- Ultrasound is the best imaging modality for diagnosis in these patients.
- Pyloric stenosis is **NOT A SURGICAL EMERGENCY**; the first concern should always be correcting the patient's metabolic derangement.

REFERENCES

1. Georgoula C, Gardiner M. Pyloric stenosis a 100 years after Ramstedt. *Arch Dis Child*. 2012;97:741-745.
2. Stringer MD, Brereton RJ. Current management of infantile hypertrophic pyloric stenosis. *Br J Hosp Med*. 1990;43:266-272.
3. Fujimoto T. Chapter 18: Hypertrophic pyloric stenosis. In: Hollwarth ME, ed. *Pediatric Surgery: Diagnosis and Management*. Berlin: Springer; 2009:171-180 [Print].
4. Sola JE, Neville HL. Laparoscopic vs open pyloromyotomy: a systematic review and meta-analysis. *J Pediatr Surg*. 2009;44(8):1631-1637.
5. Adibe OO, Igbal CW, Sharp SW, et al. Protocol versus ad libitum feeds after laparoscopic pyloromyotomy: a prospective randomized trial. *J Pediatr Surg*. 2014;49(1):129-132.
6. Koontz KS, Wulkan ML. Chapter 29: Lesions of the stomach. In: *Ashcraft's Pediatric Surgery*. N.p.: Elsevier Health Sciences; 2014:403-413 [Print].

SUGGESTED READINGS

Dalton BG, Gonzalez KW, Boda SR, et al. Optimizing fluid resuscitation in hypertrophic pyloric stenosis. *J Pediatr Surg*. 2016;51(8):1279-1282.
Pandya S, Heiss K. Pyloric stenosis in pediatric surgery: an evidence-based review. *Surg Clin North Am*. 2012;92(3):527-539.

Chapter 15

Omphalocele and Gastroschisis

Junyan Gu

- Omphalocele and gastroschisis are congenital abdominal wall defects and were first described in the 16th century by Ambrose Paré and Lycosthenes, respectively.
- The first successful repair of omphalocele was reported by Hey in 1802, and the first successful repair of gastroschisis, by Visick in 1873.[1]
- Coverage of the defect with skin flap was used for the repair of omphalocele before, but the problem was that closure of the resultant hernia could be difficult because of failure of the abdominal cavity to grow without the impetus of the intestines within it and because of intestinal adhesions to the skin flaps.
- Current surgical treatment to the omphalocele, which is unable to be closed primarily, is staged reduction, attaching silastic silo to the abdominal wall, progressively tightening over days to weeks to stretch abdominal wall and make room for intestine to achieve the goal of final primary closure.
- Most of the patients with gastroschisis can be primarily closed. If not, a silastic silo can be applied as well.

RELEVANT ANATOMY AND TERMINOLOGY

Omphalocele

- Omphalocele is a large defect (>4 cm) covered by amniotic membrane that contains midgut and other abdominal organs including the liver and often the spleen and gonad (Figure 15.1).
- Omphalocele with cephalic fold defect (pentalogy of Cantrell) is where the abdominal wall defect is supraumbilical and the heart is in the sac through a defect in the pericardium and the central tendon of the diaphragm (Figure 15.2).
- Ectopia cordis thoracis (when the heart is outside the chest with no pericardial covering as opposed to being inside the omphalocele sac) might be considered a form of a cephalic fold defect as well (Figure 15.3).

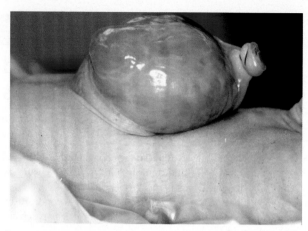

Figure 15.1 Omphalocele in a newborn. (Reprinted with permission from Ricci S. *Essentials of Maternity, Newborn, and Women's Health Nursing.* 4th ed. Philadelphia, PA: Wolters Kluwer; 2016.)

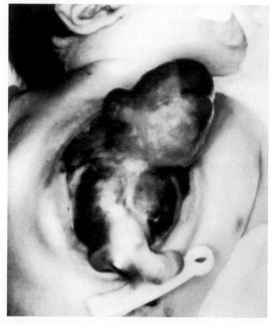

Figure 15.2 Pentalogy of Cantrell. (Reprinted with permission from Mulholland MW, Lillemoe KD, Doherty GM, Maier RV, Upchurch GR, eds. *Greenfield's Surgery: Scientific Principles and Practice.* 4th ed. Philadelphia, PA: Lippincott Williams & Wilkins; 2006.)

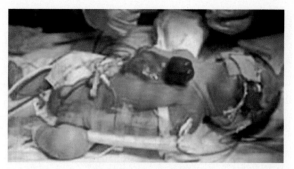

Figure 15.3 Ectopia cordis thoracis. (Reprinted with permission from Kline-Fath BM, Bulas DI, Bahado-Singh R, eds. *Fundamental and Advanced Fetal Imaging*. Philadelphia, PA: Wolters Kluwer Health; 2015.)

- Omphalocele with caudal fold defect is cloacal exstrophy, in which the defect is infraumbilical and accompanied by exstrophy of the bladder, epispadias with ileum prolapsed between the 2 halves of the exstrophied bladder, diastasis of the pubic rami, and imperforate anus.

Gastroschisis

- Gastroschisis is usually less than 4 cm in diameter, has no covering membrane, and usually contains only the midgut with the stomach and possibly a gonad and is almost always to the right of the umbilical cord (Figure 15.4)
- The extruded intestine may be thickened and covered with fibrinous exudate.
- Complicated gastroschisis means the association with other gastrointestinal conditions such as atresia, perforation, necrosis, or volvulus as a separate entity.
- Complicated gastroschisis is usually associated with a poorer outcome (Table 15.1).

ETIOLOGY AND EPIDEMIOLOGY

Omphalocele

- Omphalocele represents a failure of the body folds to grow, migrate, and fuse.
- The risk factors include both advanced and very young maternal age, maternal obesity, vitamin deficiency (especially vitamin B12 or folic acid), and poor glycemic control.[2]

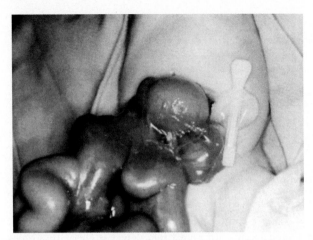

Figure 15.4   Gastroschisis. (Courtesy of Robert J Izant Jr, MD, Case Western Reserve University, Cleveland, Ohio. Reprinted with permission from Stocker JT, Dehner LP, Husain AN. *Stocker and Dehner's Pediatric Pathology*. 3rd ed. Philadelphia, PA: Wolters Kluwer Health/Lippincott Williams & Wilkins; 2010.)

- Omphalocele exists in families and is associated with chromosomal anomalies (especially trisomy 18).[3]
- Omphalocele is included in many syndromes as well.
- For instance, Beckwith-Wiedemann syndrome is the most common.[4]
- However, no specific genes or chromosomal anomalies have been identified with gastroschisis.
- Omphalocele is the second most common abdominal wall defect.
- The overall incidence is 1 out of 6000 to 1 out of 10 000 live births with a male preponderance.
- Up to 45% of patients with omphalocele have been reported to have a cardiac abnormality.[6]

Gastroschisis

- Gastroschisis is caused by failure of the umbilical coelom to develop.
- The elongating intestine then has no space to expand and ruptures out the body wall just to the right of the umbilicus, possibly because the right side of the umbilicus is relatively unsupported as a result of resorption of the right umbilical vein.

TABLE 15.1

Comparison of Gastroschisis and Omphalocele

Defect	Site	Sac	Content	Frequency	Associated Anomalies	Outcome
Omphalocele	Umbilicus	Yes	Liver, intestine, spleen, gonad	Common	Chromosomal, cardiac	Good (depending on associated anomalies)
Omphalocele-cephalic fold (pentalogy of Cantrell)	Superior umbilicus	Yes	Liver, intestine	Rare	Cardiac, sternal cleft, pericardial defect, central tendon diaphragm defect	Poor
Omphalocele-caudal fold (cloacal exstrophy)	Inferior umbilicus	Yes	Intestine	Rare	Bladder exstrophy, imperforate anus, epispadias	Fair
Ectopia cordis thoracis	Midline sternum	No	Heart	Rare	Cardiac	Poor
Gastroschisis	Right umbilicus	No	Intestine	Common	Intestine atresia	Good

Adapted from Coran AG, Adzick NS, Krummel TM, et al, eds. *Pediatric Surgery.* 7th ed. Philadelphia, PA: Saunders; 2012. Copyright © 2012 Elsevier. With permission.

- The risk factors include young maternal age, low socioeconomic status, poor maternal prenatal care, vitamin deficiency, low levels of glutathione and α-carotene, and high levels of nitrosamines, vasoconstrictive agents, and illicit drugs.[2]
- Gastroschisis is the most common of the abdominal wall defects.
- The incidence is about 1 per 2000 to 4000 live births with a male preponderance.
- The intestinal atresia is the most common anomaly associated with gastroschisis.[5]

DIAGNOSIS

- Imaging modality of choice for the diagnosis of omphalocele and gastroschisis is an antenatal ultrasound.
- Omphalocele can be distinguished from gastroschisis by the presence of a sac.
- The sensitivity for detecting omphalocele was 75% (range, 25%-100%), and that for gastroschisis was 83% (18%-100%).
- The first age at which omphalocele was detected was 18 ± 6 weeks, and gastroschisis, 20 ± 7 weeks.[7]
- Routine use of antenatal ultrasound has not been definitively shown to improve perinatal morbidity or maternal outcome.

PREOPERATIVE MANAGEMENT

- Infants with gastroschisis can be safely delivered vaginally.
- Studies did not show significant difference in outcome between vaginal delivery and cesarean section.
- However, cesarean section is preferable for prenatally diagnosed infants with giant omphalocele to prevent birth-related hepatic injury.[8,9]
- it is important to maintain an adequate airway, to keep the infant well humidified, and to use an orogastric (OG) tube for intestinal decompression.
- Intravenous dextrose is administered.
- Infants with gastroschisis will have higher intravenous fluid requirements to maintain euvolemia than infants with omphalocele.
- In gastroschisis, the mesentery should be checked to make certain it is not twisted.
- The tightness of the opening of the abdominal wall should be assessed to ensure that there is sufficient perfusion of the bowel.

- The viscera should be covered with gauze to prevent further contamination, hypothermia, and volume depletion.
- Alternatively the infant's entire lower torso can be placed inside a plastic bowel bag.

SURGICAL APPROACH

- Based on the whether the abdomen can be closed without causing abdominal compartment syndrome, the surgical options for omphalocele include primary closure, reduction of abdominal contents, and closure with skin flap or prosthetic silo (Figure 15.5) to cover viscera with slow reduction over 7 to 10 days.
- The use of tissue expander to either expand the abdominal cavity or obtain more skin in older infants is also an option.

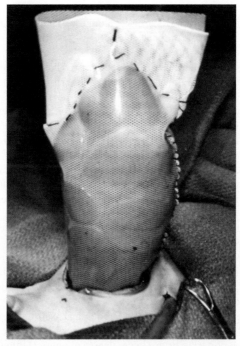

Figure 15.5 Reduction of intestine contained in a preformed silastic silo for omphalocele. (Reprinted with permission from Mulholland MW, Lillemoe KD, Doherty GM, Maier RV, Upchurch GR, eds. *Greenfield's Surgery: Scientific Principles and Practice*. 4th ed. Philadelphia, PA: Lippincott Williams & Wilkins; 2006.)

- A cosmetic closure with preservation of umbilicus can be achieved immediately after birth for gastroschisis.
- It is helpful to evacuate meconium from the rectum by anal dilatation before the procedure.
- Even though patients with gastroschisis usually have a volume deficit, limiting preoperative fluid resuscitation will improve outcomes.
- Compared with bedside placement of the silo, there was a trend to fewer days on the ventilator for the primary closure but no difference in days on total parenteral nutrition (TPN), length of stay, incidence of sepsis, or incidence of necrotizing enterocolitis.
- If there is intestinal atresia, it can simply be placed in the abdominal cavity with stoma creation and repaired 6 weeks after the abdomen has been closed.

POSTOPERATIVE CARE

- Respiratory distress, cardiac failure, or oliguria can develop after repair of omphalocele because of tight closure of abdomen.
- The solution is to return the patient to the operating room to remove the fascial sutures and perform skin closure only.
- Delayed return of bowel function is seen more often after repair of gastroschisis than the repair of omphalocele.
- It is not unusual for the infants with gastroschisis repair to have normalized bowel function up to 4 weeks.[10]
- Particularly, infants with gastroschisis and associated intestinal atresia may have pronounced intestinal dysmotility and may require long-term, sometimes lifelong, dependence on TPN for caloric intake.[11]
- About 15% of infants with gastroschisis develop necrotizing enterocolitis.[12]
- Long-term outcome of infants operated on for gastroschisis or omphalocele is usually dependent on the morbidity and mortality of associated conditions rather than the abdominal wall defect itself.
- Most children with repaired abdominal wall defects enjoy satisfactory health and quality of life, although they have been reported to have a lower degree of physical fitness measured by exercise time and maximal oxygen consumption.[13]

PEARLS AND PITFALLS

- Omphalocele is a large abdominal wall defect covered by amniotic membrane that contains midgut and other abdominal organs.
- Omphalocele represents a failure of the body folds to grow, migrate, and fuse.
- It is usually associated with chromosomal anomalies (especially trisomy 18).
- Gastroschisis is the most common abdominal wall defect.
- Gastroschisis has no covering membrane and is almost always to the right of the umbilical cord.
- Gastroschisis is caused by failure of the umbilical coelom to develop, causing rupture of body wall by elongating intestine.
- Intestinal atresia is the most common anomaly associated with gastroschisis, whereas omphalocele is usually associated with cardiac abnormalities.
- Both omphalocele and gastroschisis can be diagnosed by antenatal ultrasound.
- There is no difference in days on TPN, length of stay, incidence of sepsis, or incidence of necrotizing enterocolitis between primary closure and silo placement.
- Long-term outcomes of gastroschisis or omphalocele are usually dependent on the morbidity and mortality of associated conditions rather than the abdominal wall defect itself.

REFERENCES

1. Coran AG, Adzick NS. *Pediatric Surgery*. 7th ed. Philadelphia, USA: Saunders; 2012.
2. Stoll C, Alembik Y, Dott B, Roth MP. Risk factors in congenital abdominal wall defects (omphalocele and gastroschisi): a study in a series of 265,858 consecutive births. *Ann Genet*. 2001;44(4):201-208.
3. Ardinger HH, Williamson RA, Grant S. Association of neural tube defects with omphalocele in chromosomally normal fetuses. *Am J Med Genet*. 1987;27(1):135-142
4. Wilkins-Haug L, Porter A, Hawley P, Benson CB. Isolated fetal omphalocele, Beckwith-Wiedemann syndrome, and assisted reproductive technologies. *Birth Defects Res A Clin Mol Teratol*. 2009;85(1):58-62.
5. Friedman AM, Ananth CV, Siddiq Z, D'Alton ME, Wright JD. Gastroschisis: epidemiology and mode of delivery, 2005-2013. *Am J Obstet Gynecol*. 2016;215(3):348.e1-348.e9.
6. Salemi JL, Tanner JP, Ramakrishnan R, et al. Prevalence, correlates, and outcomes of omphalocele in the United States, 1995-2005. *Obstet Gynecol*. 2015;126(2):284.

7. Barisic I, Clementi M, Häusler M, Gjergja R, Kern J, Stoll C. Evaluation of prenatal ultrasound diagnosis of fetal abdominal wall defects by 19 European registries. *Ultrasound Obstet Gynecol*. 2001;18(4):309-316.

8. How HY, Harris BJ, Pietrantoni M, et al. Is vaginal delivery preferable to elective cesarean delivery in fetuses with a known ventral wall defect? *Am J Obstet Gynecol*. 2000;182(6):1527.

9. Biard JM, Wilson RD, Johnson MP, et al. Prenatally diagnosed giant omphaloceles: short- and long-term outcomes. *Prenat Diagn*. 2004;24(6):434.

10. Curry JJ, Lander AD, Stringer MD, et al. A multicenter, randomized, double-blind, placebo-controlled trial of the prokinetic agent erythromycin in the postoperative recovery of infants with gastroschisis. *J Pediatr Surg*. 2004;39:565-569.

11. Phillips JD, Raval MV, Redden C, et al. Gastroschisis, atresia, dysmotility: surgical treatment strategies for a distinct clinical entity. *J Pediatr Surg*. 2008;43:2208-2212.

12. Jayanthi S, Seymour P, Puntis JW, et al. Necrotizing enterocolitis after gastroschisis repair: a preventable complication? *J Pediatr Surg*. 1998;33:705-707.

13. Zaccara A, Iacobelli BD, Calzolari A, et al. Cardiopulmonary performances in young children and adolescents born with large abdominal wall defects. *J Pediatr Surg*. 2003;38:478-481.

Chapter 16

Mesenteric, Omental, and Duplication Cysts

Ann Alyssa Kurian

Duplication Cysts

- Duodenal duplication was first described by Calder in 1773.[1,2]
- William Ladd coined the term duplication of the alimentary tract in 1937 and described them as sharing the following features:[1,2]
  - A well-developed coat of smooth muscle
  - An epithelial lining consistent with some portion of the intestinal tract mucosa
  - Attachment to the alimentary tract

EPIDEMIOLOGY AND ETIOLOGY

- Incidence: 1 in 4500 live births[1-3]
- Location of cysts:[3]
  - Gastric—3% to 4% of all duplication cysts
  - Intestinal—45% to 55% of all duplication cysts
  - Duodenal—5% to 6% of all duplication cysts
  - Colon—15% of all duplication cysts
  - Rectal—8% of all duplication cysts
- Multiple cysts present in 10% to 20% of cases[2]
- GI duplication cysts associated with vertebral, spinal cord, or genitourinary anomaly in 30% to 50% of cases[1]
- Etiology—4 theories exist
  - Partial twinning: may lead to long duplicated segments[2,3]
  - Split notochord: endoderm separates from the notochord to form the GI tract; herniations or abnormal deposits of endodermal cells can occur during this process leading to duplications[2,3]
  - Incomplete recanalization: error in creation of gut lumen; duplication may arise from abnormal diverticula[2,3]
  - Environmental factors[2]

CLINICAL PRESENTATION

- They are often asymptomatic and discovered as an incidental finding.[2]
- Duplications can be cystic or tubular.
- Symptoms at presentation can vary depending on location, size, and mucosal features.
  - Duplication in the chest can present with wheezing, pneumonia, and dysphagia.
  - Duplication in the abdomen can present as abdominal pain, vomiting, and abdominal mass. Large cysts can cause extrinsic compression of adjacent bowel and present with obstructive symptoms.
  - Cysts containing gastric mucosa can present with bleeding (melena), ulceration, or perforation.
  - Large gastric duplications can present like hypertrophic pyloric stenosis with symptoms of gastric outlet obstruction.
  - Duodenal duplication cysts can lead to recurrent pancreatitis.
  - Duplications arising from the ileum can present like appendicitis, difficult to differentiate preoperatively.
  - Small intestine duplications can act as a lead point and cause intussusceptions.
  - Colon and hindgut duplication can present as a second opening in the perineum and can cause symptoms of constipation and urinary obstruction from mass effect.[2]

DIAGNOSIS

- Imaging
- CXR and CT scan can show mediastinal mass
- Ultrasound: most common imaging modality for abdominal duplications. Shows inner hyperechoic layer of mucosal/submucosal tissue with an outer hypoechoic muscle layer. May be apparent and monitored with prenatal ultrasound
- Meckel scan: positive for cysts containing gastric mucosa; present in location other than that of Meckel diverticulum[1]
- CT scan shows cystic lesion surrounded by enhancing rim, and may look similar to abscess; however, in the absence of infectious symptoms (fever, leukocytosis), duplication cyst should be suspected[2]

SURGICAL MANAGEMENT

Oropharyngeal

- Most common location is the floor of the mouth
- Treatment: resection of cyst, reapproximation of the oral mucosa

Esophageal

- Often cystic; on right side of thorax
- Most do not share a muscular wall or communicate with esophageal lumen
- Treatment: resection via right thoracotomy or thoracoscopy[1]

Thoracoabdominal

- Tubular duplication from thoracic esophagus, which extends past the diaphragmatic hiatus
- Usually contain gastric mucosa
- Present with dyspnea; can present with bleeding
- 88% have vertebral anomaly
- Treatment: resection. May require staged procedure. May also need to incise the muscular layer of esophageal duplication and denude the epithelium of the cyst without entering the esophageal mucosa, if resection not feasible[1-3]

Gastric

- Often cystic and located along the greater curvature
- Treatment: resection. May require partial gastrectomy. Complex cysts may be treated by resection/stripping of the common wall

Duodenal

- Most are cystic and located on the mesenteric side of the first or second portion of the duodenum
- Treatment: simple excision if possible and blood supply to duodenum not compromised. May alternatively require Roux-en-Y cystojejunostomy or duodenal resection, especially if gastric mucosa present in cyst[1]

Pancreatic

- Most commonly present in the head of pancreas
- Presence of muscle layer differentiates pancreatic duplication cyst from pseudocyst
- Requires resection, or cystojejunostomy, pancreaticoduodenectomy, or partial pancreatectomy depending on location[1]

Small Intestine

- Usually cystic, occur on mesenteric side of small bowel, and may or may not share a wall with true small bowel
- Most common site is ileum
- Treatment: small bowel resection with primary anastomosis; enucleation of cyst (possible for small cysts); mucosal stripping of long, tubular duplications or anastomosis to stomach for long tubular duplication containing gastric mucosa[1]

Colonic

- Most common site is cecum; most are cystic
- Type I are limited to GI tract duplications
- Type II are associated with genital or urinary tract duplication
- Treatment: resection and primary anastomosis if possible; enucleation; for long tubular duplications, they may be treated with creation of distal communication with the true lumen to relieve obstructive symptoms, if resection not feasible[1]

Rectal

- Can present with perianal abscess or fistula
- Usually in presacral area, posterior to rectum
- Treatment: marsupialization through transanal approach, division of septum between cyst and rectum, or excision using posterior sagittal approach[1]

Mesenteric and Omental Cysts

- The mesenteric cyst was first described in an autopsy in 1507.
- First successful surgery for a cystic mesenteric mass was performed by Tillaux in 1880.
- The first marsupialization of a mesenteric cyst was performed in 1883.[5]

EPIDEMIOLOGY AND ETIOLOGY

- Very rare; incidence: 1 in 20 000 children[4]
- 25% of cases occur in children younger than 10 years[3]
- Etiology:
  - Lymphatic
  - Infectious
  - Neoplastic

- Traumatic
- Abnormal embryologic development
- Differ from duplication cysts because they lack a muscular layer. They are composed of a fibrous wall that is lined by a single layer of endothelial cells, with cuboidal or columnar cells[3]
- Histologic classification:[3]
  - Lymphangioma—lined by endothelium
  - Mesothelial cyst—lined by mesothelium
  - Enteric cyst—lined by enteric mucosa, but with no muscle layer
  - Pseudocyst—fibrous wall with epithelial lining

CLINICAL PRESENTATION

- Symptoms of partial bowel obstruction with palpable, free moving abdominal mass[3]
- May also present with volvulus, intestinal ischemia, or infarction[3]
- Most commonly occur in ileum or distal sigmoid

DIAGNOSIS

Imaging

- Abdominal ultrasound
  - localize cystic lesions; determine if cyst is simple or multiloculated
  - Water-dense homogenous mass displacing loops of bowel[3]

SURGICAL MANAGEMENT

- Mesenteric cysts require complete resection.[3]
- Partial resection with marsupialization of the remnant cyst is acceptable.[3]

POSTOPERATIVE CARE

- Recurrence risk after resection is 6% to 13%. Most recurrences occur in those with partial excision or retroperitoneal cysts.[3]
- For patients who undergo bowel resection and anastomosis, continue NGT decompression postop and await bowel function before initiating feeds.[4]

Complications

- Duplications or mesenteric or omental cysts found in adulthood are at risk for malignant degeneration.[4]

PEARLS AND PITFALLS

- Goal of surgery is complete resection when possible, otherwise mucosal stripping and marsupialization may suffice, ESPECIALLY if ectopic gastric or pancreatic mucosa present in the duplication.
- Duplications and mesenteric/omental cysts are very rare diseases, and lesions can be found incidentally during laparotomy, or remain asymptomatic.

REFERENCES

1. Holcomb GW, Murphy PJ. Alimentary tract duplications. In: *Ashcraft's Pediatric Surgery*. 5th ed. Saunders/Elsevier; 2010:517-525.
2. Grosfeld JL. Alimentary tract duplications. In: *Pediatric Surgery*. 6th ed. Vol 1. Mosby Elsevier; 2006:1389-1398.
3. Arensman RM. Gastrointestinal duplications and mesenteric cysts. In: *Pediatric Surgery*. 2nd ed. Landes Bioscience; 2009:281-288.
4. Mattei P. Abdominal cysts and duplications. In: *Fundamentals of Pediatric Surgery*. New York: Springer; 2011:365-371.
5. Grosfeld JL. Mesenteric and omental cysts. In: *Pediatric Surgery*. 6th ed. Vol 1. Mosby Elsevier; 2006:1399-1407.

Chapter 17

Gastroesophageal Reflux Disease

Kandace Kichler

- Many parents report that their infant will spit up or develop emesis of milk after feedings. This is usually inconsequential and considered normal, and infants often outgrow postprandial regurgitation by 2 years of age.
- Pathologic gastroesophageal reflux (GER), or gastroesophageal reflux disease (GERD), can be associated with failure to thrive, apnea, extreme irritability, and aspiration of gastric contents.

RELEVANT ANATOMY

- The esophagus has cervical, thoracic, and intra-abdominal segments that arise from the embryonic foregut.
- The esophagus travels through the esophageal hiatus in the diaphragm and is enveloped by the diaphragmatic crura on each side. Once inside the abdomen, the esophagus makes an acute angle (the angle of His) and enters the stomach.
- The lower esophageal sphincter (LES), not a true muscular sphincter, is located in the intra-abdominal esophagus adjacent to the body of the stomach. This is a physiologic high-pressure zone that, when diminished, can result in GER (Figure 17.1).
- Other anatomic contributors to GER include a shortened intra-abdominal esophagus, presence of hiatal or paraesophageal hernia, widened angle of His, and both functional and neurologic issues with esophageal and/or stomach motility.

EPIDEMIOLOGY AND ETIOLOGY

Incidence: Approximately 1 in 300 to 1000 children has excessive, passive reflux with an incompetent LES and requires medical or surgical therapy.[1]

Etiology: Many theories as to the exact etiology exist, but it is likely multifactorial.

- Children with neurologic impairments are more likely to be affected by GER as well as delayed gastric emptying.[1]
- Prolonged exposure of squamous esophageal mucosa to gastric acid and refluxed contents results in the symptoms.

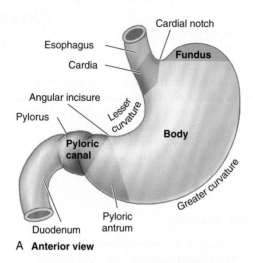

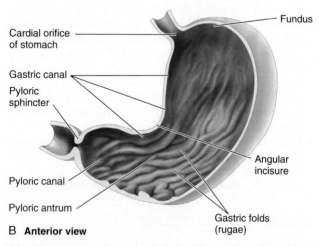

Figure 17.1 Esophagus (terminal part), stomach, and proximal duodenum. A, Parts of stomach. B, Internal surface of stomach. C, Radiograph of stomach and duodenum after barium ingestion (arrows, peristaltic wave). D, Coronal section of region of esophagogastric junction. D, diaphragm; E, esophagus; ST, stomach; Z, esophagogastric junction (Z-line). (Reprinted with permission from Moore KL, Agur AMR, Dalley AF. *Essential Clinical Anatomy*. 5th ed. Philadelphia, PA: Wolters Kluwer Health; 2015.)

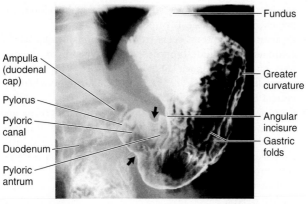

C AP view

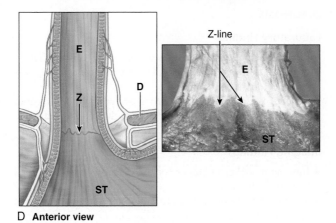

D Anterior view

Figure 17.1—cont'd

CLINICAL PRESENTATION

Classic presentation: A mother will complain that her infant has recurrent, severe postprandial regurgitation of milk and irritability.

- Patients with GERD also vomit with coughing, exertion, and crying.
- It is paramount to distinguish this from infants with bilious emesis, which can suggest a multitude of other pathologies that will be discussed in other chapters.
- Patients with GERD typically have either respiratory or esophageal symptoms. Infants usually present with

respiratory complications, whereas very young children will present with esophageal symptoms.

- Respiratory symptoms occur from aspiration of gastric acidic contents and include bronchospasm, laryngospasm, hoarseness, pneumonia, apnea, and choking spells.[1] This aspiration is usually right-sided and worsened at night or when the patient is in recumbent positions.
- Esophageal symptoms include irritability, heartburn, and esophagitis. Endoscopy can disclose columnar metaplasia in the distal esophagus secondary to prolonged GERD. Esophagitis can result in hematemesis, heme-positive stools, and chronic iron anemia.
- Malnutrition can be seen with prolonged GERD, as well as growth delays.

DIAGNOSIS

Laboratory Finding

- If a patient presents with signs or symptoms of dehydration or failure to thrive, it is essential to obtain intravenous access and check basic electrolytes.
- Patients with significant vomiting and regurgitation could potentially have a **hypokalemic, hypochloremic, metabolic alkalosis**.

Imaging Findings

- Imaging modality of choice for the diagnosis is an upper GI series with barium.
- The upper GI series is used to evaluate the reflux as well as visualize the infant's anatomy. This can identify reflux, hiatal hernias, esophageal strictures, and other disorders of the foregut contributing to the regurgitation. This study can be normal in up to 50% of patients, as barium is not a physiologic medium, reflux may not occur during the interval of the examination, and interpretation of the study can be radiologist-dependent.
- **The gold standard for diagnosing GER in children is a 24-hour pH probe study.**
- This study is more invasive than an upper GI series because a pH probe is endoscopically placed in the distal esophagus. This probe monitors the frequency of reflux episodes (marked by esophageal pH ≤ 4), the duration of the episodes, and the total percentage of time with a pH ≤ 4. It is useful to correlate the symptoms with the findings of the study.

However, a negative 24-hour pH probe study does not rule out symptomatic GER because there can be nonacidic reflux in pediatric patients.

- Esophageal manometry can be used to evaluate the pressure of the LES as well as the peristalsis of the esophagus with swallowing.
- Nuclear medicine scans and gastric scintiscans can be useful in diagnosis and operative planning. A quantity of radioisotope in ingested or placed into the stomach via nasogastric tube. The scans can then document reflux and gastric emptying.
- Finally, upper GI endoscopy can be used and can identify esophagitis, esophageal metaplasia or dysplasia, hiatal hernias, ulcers, strictures, or other anatomic issues, including occult neoplasms.

MEDICAL MANAGEMENT

- Rehydration and correction of any electrolytes is the first step in medical management of GERD. Electrolyte disturbances can be corrected with **normal saline boluses at 20 mL/kg**.
- In our practice, we then recheck the laboratory test results, and if the derangements are improved, patients are then placed on maintenance fluids.
- Diet modification is instituted, and this includes formula changes and thickened feeds, upright eating, and avoidance of positions in the postprandial period that can exacerbate symptoms or increase intra-abdominal pressure in the child.
- Patients with pathologic GER are placed on proton pump inhibitors and promotility agents. Proton pump inhibitors have better results and safety profile than H_2 receptor antagonists, and prokinetic agents assist in improving gastric emptying. The combination of prokinetic agents and acid-reducing medications results in control of GER in up to 90% to 95% of children.[1]
- Medical management of GERD should be attempted for at minimum 8 weeks, unless life-threatening symptoms or sequelae develop. Treatment is not usually lifelong, as most patients will have spontaneous resolution of their symptoms with time.[1]

SURGICAL MANAGEMENT

- Surgery for GERD is typically not an emergency, and it is **important to correct any electrolyte imbalances before operative intervention**.

Operative Intervention

- Antireflux surgery should be performed in patients with inadequate response to medical therapy, who are dependent on medical management despite attempts at weaning, and in those presenting with complication of GER including esophagitis, failure to thrive, aspiration pneumonia, and extreme metabolic derangements.

- The procedure of choice is a laparoscopic Nissen fundoplication with or without gastrostomy tube placement.

- This can be performed either laparoscopically or open depending on surgeon preference, and the gastrostomy can be completed laparoscopically, open, or endoscopically.

- Partial wraps can be used in patients with significant esophageal dysmotility, to potentially avoid postoperative dysphagia.

- The goals of surgical intervention include restoring normal anatomic relationship of the gastroesophageal junction in the abdomen, recreating the angle of His, increasing the length of intra-abdominal esophagus, repairing any hiatal hernia if present, and potentially improving gastric emptying.[1]

- In addition, gastrostomy tube can be used to secure positioning of the stomach within the abdomen and allow for supplemental feeding while the fundoplication heals and in the event that the patient suffers from postoperative dysphagia.

Laparoscopic Nissen Fundoplication

For the laparoscopic approach, the patient is placed supine. Typically, we enter the abdominal cavity through the umbilicus and initiate pneumoperitoneum, and this is our optical or camera port. In the right upper quadrant, 2 small stab incisions are made, and 1 to 2 left upper quadrant incisions are used as working ports. These are typically 2 to 5 mm trocars in size depending on the patient's age and body habitus. At least one of the left upper quadrant ports should be 5 mm in size for the surgeon to use a vessel sealing device in their right hand (Figure 17.2). Dissection along the greater curve using a vessel sealer for short gastrics is performed up to the angle of His, toward the left crus, and the spleen is separated from the stomach. A retroesophageal window is created bluntly until the right crus is identified. The gastrohepatic ligament is opened using blunt and sharp dissection with care to identify and avoid injury to a possible replaced left

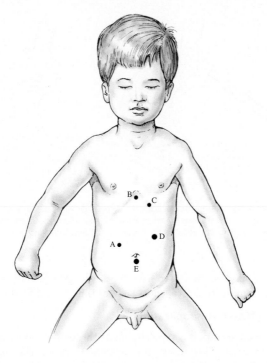

Figure 17.2 Trocar positioning in a pediatric Nissen fundoplication. (Reprinted with permission from Swanström LL, Soper NJ, Leonard M, eds. *Mastery of Endoscopic and Laparoscopic Surgery.* 4th ed. Philadelphia, PA: Wolters Kluwer; 2014.)

hepatic artery off the left gastric artery. If the surgeon prefers, a bougie can be placed at this time by anesthesia (with size dependent on age and body habitus of the patient). The crura are approximated posteriorly using 2-0 nonabsorbable interrupted sutures (usually 1-2 stitches total). The esophagus is anchored to the crura on each side using two to three 3-0 nonabsorbable sutures. Next, the Nissen fundoplication is performed by wrapping the proximal stomach through the retroesophageal window clockwise. The shoe-shine maneuver is used to ensure adequate mobilization of the stomach. Three interrupted 2-0 nonabsorbable sutures are then used to secure the wrap. The most superior stitch incorporates the anterior esophagus. Once this is completed, a gastrostomy tube can be placed, if desired. In general, laparoscopic

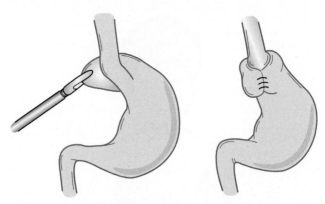

Figure 17.3 Nissen fundoplication. (Reprinted with permission from Shirkhoda A. *Variants and Pitfalls in Body Imaging: Thoracic, Abdominal and Women's Imaging.* Philadelphia, PA: Lippincott Williams & Wilkins; 2011.)

surgery has been found to have shorter lengths of stay, lower total complication rate, and a shorter time to full feeding.[2]

Open Nissen Fundoplication

The open approach is typically made through an upper midline incision. This allows for dissection around the hiatus while leaving adequate space laterally for possible gastrostomy tube placement. In a similar fashion to the laparoscopic approach, the stomach mobilization and near circumferential dissection of the hiatus are completed. A handheld liver retractor or sweetheart retractor may be helpful in the open approach. The fundoplication with or without gastrostomy tube placement is then performed as described (Figure 17.3).

POSTOPERATIVE CARE

- Postoperative care is similar after both open and laparoscopic approaches with some surgeons starting feeds sooner after laparoscopic repair.
- It is not uncommon for patients to have dysphagia or episodes of vomiting postoperatively, but this is usually self-limited.
- Pain is usually well controlled with acetaminophen, and patients are usually discharged within a few days of surgical intervention.

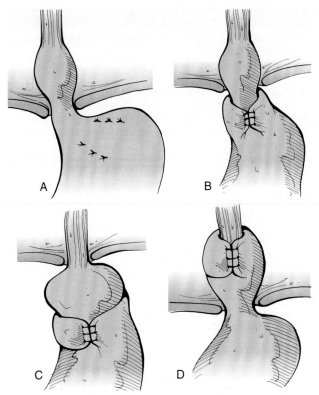

Figure 17.4 Types of fundoplication failures. A, Disrupted wrap. B, Sliding hiatal hernia with wrap in abdomen. C, "Slipped" fundoplication onto proximal stomach. D, Intrathoracic migration of the fundoplication. (Reprinted with permission from Desai KM, Soper NJ. Laparoscopic Nissen fundoplication. In: Soper NJ, Swanström LL, Eubanks WS, eds. *Mastery of Endoscopic and Laparoscopic Surgery*. 2nd ed. Philadelphia, PA: Lippincott Williams & Wilkins; 2005:193.)

Complications

- Nissen fundoplication is successful in relieving GERD in more than 90% of patients, but near 10% require revision (for slipped Nissen or loosening with recurrent reflux). Up to 30% of those with neurologic impairment require reoperation. Most reflux recurrence is able to be controlled with medical management (Figure 17.4).
- Other complications include postoperative dysphagia, gas bloat syndrome, esophageal or gastric perforation, and bleeding.

PEARLS AND PITFALLS

- Consider PGR in patients with recurrent, nonbilious regurgitation and irritability.
- Upper GI series and 24-hour pH probe studies are key to securing the diagnosis.
- Medical management is attempted unless life-threatening complications develop.
- Those refractory to medical management usually improve with Nissen fundoplication with or without gastrostomy tube placement.

REFERENCES

1. Cook M, Adolph V. Gastroesophageal reflux. In: Arensman RM, Bambini DA, Almond PS, Adolph V, Radhakrishnan J, eds. *Pediatric Surgery*. 2nd ed. Austin: Landes Bioscience; 2009:378-381.
2. St Peter SD, Holcomb GW. Nissen fundoplication. In: Saxena AK, Hollwarth ME, eds. *Essentials of Pediatric Endoscopic Surgery*. Germany: Springer; 2009:193-198.

SUGGESTED READING

Georgeson KE. Gastro-oesophageal reflux and hiatus hernia. In: Puri P, Hollwarth ME, eds. *Pediatric Surgery*. Germany: Springer; 2006:49-60.

Chapter 18

Bariatric Surgery in Children

Kandace Kichler

HISTORICAL BACKGROUND

- In 2013, the American Medical Association officially recognized obesity as a disease.
- Bariatric surgery is widely accepted as safe and effective in adults suffering from morbid obesity, and reduction in comorbidities has been established with operative intervention.[1]
- However, the transfer of this treatment option to the pediatric or adolescent population is limited and controversial.

DEFINITIONS

- The American Academy of Pediatrics (AAP) considers any child between the 85th and 95th percentile of BMI (body mass index) as "overweight." Above the 95th percentile of BMI is considered "obese"[2] (Figure 18.1).
- In 18-year olds, the 95th percentile of BMI for age corresponds to a BMI of 30 mg/kg^2.[1]
- The International Pediatric Endosurgery Group considers bariatric surgery for adolescents with BMI greater than or equal to 40, or greater than or equal to 35 with serious obesity-related comorbidities (similar to guidelines for adult patients with morbid obesity).

EPIDEMIOLOGY AND ETIOLOGY

Incidence: Over the past 30 years, the United States has seen an almost 3-fold increase in children who fall into the "overweight" category. Among children aged 2 to 19 years, more than 20% of the pediatric population is considered obese.[2]

- It is estimated that up to 80% of obese teenagers will go on to become obese adults as they continue to gain weight into adulthood.[1]

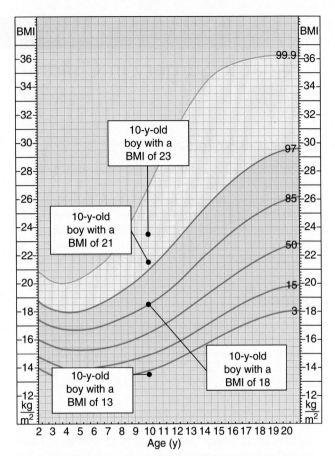

Figure 18.1 Body mass index–for-age percentiles for boys 2 to 20 years of age. Overweight in children and adolescents is defined by body mass index (weight in kilograms divided by the square of height in meters) at or above the 95th percentile for children of the same age and sex. (Source: Centers for Disease Control and Prevention. *About BMI in Children and Teens*. 2007. Available online at www.cdc.gov/nccdphp/dnpa/obesity/defining. htm. Calculator for determining BMI available at http://apps.nccd.cdc.gov/ dnpabmi/Calculator.aspx.)

- Obesity-related conditions and comorbidities increase with the prevalence of the disease in the pediatric population. These include, but are not limited to, diabetes, hypertension, obstructive sleep apnea, nonalcoholic fatty liver disease, and metabolic syndrome[2] (Figure 18.2).

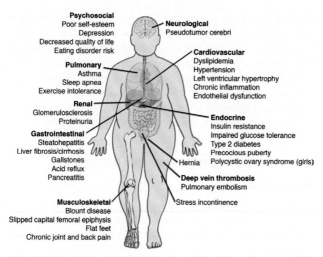

Figure 18.2 Health risks of obesity in adolescents and young adults. (Reprinted with permission from Neinstein LS, Katzman DK. *Neinstein's Adolescent and Young Adult Health Care: A Practical Guide*. Philadelphia, PA: Wolters Kluwer; 2016. Originally adapted from Xanthakos SA, Daniels SR, Inge TH. Bariatric surgery in adolescents: an update. *Adolesc Med Clin*. 2006;17(3):589-612.)

Etiology: Many theories are hypothesized for the etiology of obesity, but it is become more evident that this disease is multifactorial.

- Some environmental causes include decreased daily exercise and increased intake of fast food and processed foods.
- Familial predisposition is also evident, as many individuals suffering from obesity are not the sole member of their family with the disease.
- Few genetic syndromes such as Prader-Willi syndrome, melanocortin 4 receptor deficiency, and Albright's hereditary osteodystrophy are associated with childhood obesity.

PATIENT SELECTION

- Children suffering from obesity will have increased BMI, subcutaneous fat, and waist circumference.
- In many practices, bariatric surgery is not considered for the adolescent population until a BMI of 50 or greater, with obesity-related comorbid conditions, is identified.

- Guidelines from the National Institute of Health, American College of Surgeons, and American Society for Metabolic and Bariatric Surgery all recommend that at-risk patients be evaluated at a specialized center that incorporates a multi-disciplinary approach to obesity management. This includes bariatric surgeons, bariatric nurse specialists, nutritionists, behavioral therapists, exercise physiologists, and adolescent medicine physicians, among others.[1]

PREOPERATIVE WORKUP AND EVALUATION

Medical Evaluation

- Includes complete history and physical examination, usually performed by the surgeon, with extensive discussion into the risks, benefits, options, and alternatives to bariatric surgery.
- Nutritional evaluation and coaching are completed.
- Pediatric endocrinologists are consulted to assess for medically treatable causes of obesity. These physicians also screen for diabetes mellitus, polycystic ovarian disease, and insulin resistance.[1]
- Sexual and bone maturity are assessed using bone X-rays and endocrinologist consultation.
- Any other associated comorbidities are addressed and pertinent referrals to specialists, completed. This includes pulmonology evaluation for possible obstructive sleep apnea.
- A comprehensive psychologic assessment is imperative. The patient must display adequate emotional and cognitive development, reasonable expectations of surgery, understanding of risks and outcomes, and motivation to comply with postoperative recommendations.

Laboratory and Other Evaluations

- Preoperative laboratory tests include chemistry panel, complete blood count, hemoglobin A1c, hepatic function panel, lipid profile, fasting blood glucose and insulin levels; thyroid-stimulating hormone, thiamine, folate, and iron levels; and urinalysis, including pregnancy test for females
- Formal polysomnography—to confirm or rule out obstructive sleep apnea
- Upper gastrointestinal (GI) series—to confirm anatomy and rule out hiatal hernia or significant reflux disease
- Right upper quadrant ultrasound—to identify gallstones

MEDICAL MANAGEMENT

- Before any operative intervention and at the onset of diagnosis and recognition of obesity, all patients should undergo comprehensive medical therapy. This includes nutritional counseling, behavioral modification, and exercise programs, all under the guidance and direction of a physician.

SURGICAL MANAGEMENT

- Bariatric operations are typically either restrictive or restrictive plus malabsorptive. The most common purely restrictive operations performed today include laparoscopic adjustable gastric banding and laparoscopic sleeve gastrectomy. Laparoscopic Roux-en-Y gastric bypass is considered restrictive and malabsorptive. A very uncommon operation to be performed in adolescents that is both restrictive and malabsorptive is the duodenal switch. Historical operations for adults include biliopancreatic bypass, vertical banded gastroplasty, and minigastric bypass—all of which have fallen out of favor because of either weight regain or significant long-term complications.
- Data regarding the outcomes of each operation are limited because of the infrequency of the operations being performed in the adolescent population. The laparoscopic sleeve gastrectomy is currently the most often performed bariatric procedure in adult patients.
- **Contraindications to adolescent bariatric surgery include untreated glandular diseases, inflammatory GI tract diseases, severe cardiopulmonary disease, dependency on alcohol or drugs, mental retardation or emotional instability, or serious concerns about the compliance of the patient.**[3]

PERIOPERATIVE MANAGEMENT

- Clear liquid diet is recommended for 48 hours before operative intervention. Some centers use a 2-week very low-calorie liquid diet preoperatively in adult patients to shrink the liver volume and mesenteric fat density. This is carried out to make the operation technically easier by limiting visual and mechanical obstructive factors and potentially decrease intraoperative complications. However, this diet has not been studied in the pediatric population.

- Low-molecular-weight heparin (LMWH) is give preoperatively at a dose of 40 mg subcutaneously. This is continued twice daily while the patient is hospitalized. Sequential compression devices (SCDs) are also put in place before induction of anesthesia and continued throughout the hospital stay.
- Preoperative antibiotics are also give—usually 2nd generation cephalosporins—and continued until 24 hours postop.

SURGICAL INTERVENTIONS

- Nearly all primary bariatric operations are performed laparoscopically. Contraindications to laparoscopic technique include extensive previous abdominal surgery and/or inability to tolerate pneumoperitoneum.

Laparoscopic Adjustable Gastric Banding

The pars flaccida technique is used to create a window behind the stomach toward the angle of His. The band is put into positioning and gastrogastric sutures are used to secure its position and prevent band slippage. The port is fixated on the anterior rectus fascia or lowest part of the sternum. Postoperatively, band fills with saline are used to tighten the band and increase satiety (see Figure 18.3). This operation has fallen out of favor in adult patients because of limited long-term benefit and significant rate of revision or reoperation (up to 40%).

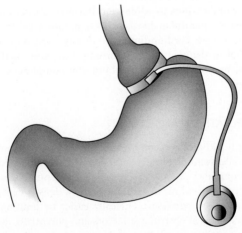

Figure 18.3 Laparoscopic adjustable gastric band. (Reprinted with permission from Singh A. *Gastrointestinal Imaging: The Essentials*. Philadelphia, PA: Wolters Kluwer; 2016.)

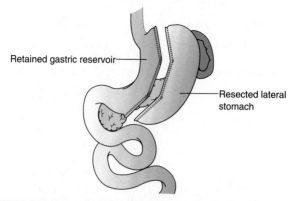

Figure 18.4 Sleeve gastrectomy. (Reprinted with permission from Mulholland MW, Lillemoe KD, Doherty GM, Upchurch GR, Alam HB, Pawlik TM. *Greenfield's Surgery: Scientific Principles and Practice.* 6th ed. Philadelphia, PA: Wolters Kluwer; 2017.)

Laparoscopic Sleeve Gastrectomy

Short gastric arteries and the omentum are dissected off the greater curve of the stomach all the way to the angle of His. The spleen is dissected off of the stomach. A linear stapler is used to create a "sleeve"-shaped stomach, usually under bougie guidance (size depending on patient size, age, and body habitus). The excess stomach is excised completely (Figure 18.4).

Laparoscopic Roux-en-Y Gastric Bypass

A Roux limb of 50 to 75 cm in length is created, depending on the patient's BMI and comorbid conditions. This can be placed retrocolic or antecolic, retrogastric or antegastric. Gastrojejunostomy (GJ) and jejunojejunostomy anastomoses are stapled or handsewn, depending on surgeon preference (Figure 18.5). Mesenteric defects can be closed to potentially prevent internal hernias. Intraoperative esophagogastroduodenoscopy or air-water leak tests with or without methylene blue can be performed to evaluate for patency and leak of the GJ anastomosis intraoperatively.

POSTOPERATIVE CARE

- Postoperative patients go to a monitored ward, get intravenous fluid, and patient-controlled anesthesia for pain control. SCDs and LMWH are used, and ambulation starts the evening of surgery.

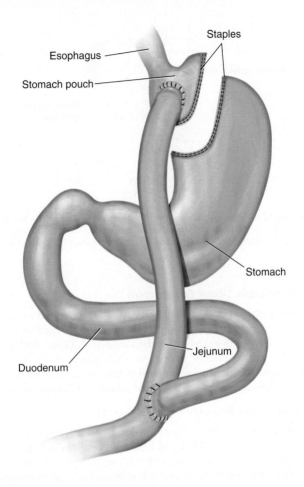

Figure 18.5 Roux-en-Y gastric bypass.

- Postoperative day 1 patients get an upper gastrointestinal series with water-soluble contrast to rule out anastomotic leak or obstruction. If negative, bariatric clear liquid diet is initiated.
- Most patients are discharged home on POD2 or POD3 on liquid diet with a follow-up appointment 1 week from surgery. Any drains, if present, are usually removed on the day of discharge or at the first postop visit.

- Follow-up visits are scheduled monthly for 6 months, every 3 months for 18 months, and yearly thereafter. Laboratory values including iron and vitamin levels are checked every 6 months. Diet and exercise assessment, as well as weight loss monitoring, is performed at each visit.[1]

Complications

- Mortality rate for bariatric surgery in adults is approximately 0.5%, and it is reportedly lower in adolescents.
- Operative complications vary slightly with each operation and can include bleeding, GI perforation, damage to band or tubing, twisting of Roux limb, devascularization of biliopancreatic limb or Roux limb, and anastomotic leak.
- Early postoperative complications include emesis, dehydration, food impaction, anastomotic leak, anastomotic bleeding, wound infection, esophageal obstruction, trocar site/band port site infection, deep venous thrombosis, pulmonary embolism, other pulmonary complications, and dumping syndrome.
- Late postoperative complications include emesis, dehydration, nutritional deficiencies, anemia, marginal ulceration, anastomotic stricture, bowel obstruction, dumping syndrome, internal hernia, gallstone formation, nephrolithiasis, food impaction, band herniation or slippage, band erosion, GERD, and port displacement or infection.[1]

▶ PEARLS AND PITFALLS

- A multidisciplinary team is crucial, and careful patient selection is essential. Extensive preoperative workup, evaluation, and counseling are required.
- A variety of surgical options exist for obesity in adolescents, but the most commonly performed are laparoscopic adjustable gastric banding and Roux-en-Y gastric bypass.
- Tachycardia is the first sign of a postoperative complication.
- Surgical weight loss can reduce comorbid conditions.
- Bariatric patients require lifelong follow-up.

REFERENCES

1. Collins JL. Bariatric surgery. In: Mattei P, ed. *Fundamentals of Pediatric Surgery*. New York: Springer; 2011:415-424.
2. Ibele AR, Mattar SG. Adolescent bariatric surgery. In: Martin RF, Kothari SN, eds. *Surgical Clinics of North America, Bariatric and Metabolic Surgery*. Vol 91(6). Philadelphia: W.B. Saunders Company; 2011:1339-1352.
3. Saxena AK. Gastric banding. In: Saxena AK, Hollwarth ME, eds. *Essentials of Pediatric Endoscopic Surgery*. Germany: Springer; 2009:215-220.

Chapter 19

Gallbladder Disease in Children

Allison Rice

- Gallbladder disease in children has evolved over the past 25 years.
- Historically, disease of the biliary tract was relatively uncommon in pediatrics and typically associated with hemolytic diseases.[1]
- The increase in incidence is due to multifactorial causes that parallel the rise in pediatric obesity, improved diagnostic modalities, and improved survival of critically ill patients.
- Cholelithiasis and biliary dyskinesia are increasing in frequency as well as a rise in cholecystectomy rates.[1,2]
- Definitions:
  - Cholecystitis: inflammation and distention of the gallbladder caused by obstruction of the cystic duct[6]
  - Acute cholangitis: ascending bacterial infection of the biliary tree caused by an obstruction[5]
  - Acute acalculous cholecystitis (AAC): inflammation of the gallbladder, without the presence of gallstones[6]
  - Biliary colic: postprandial abdominal pain, typically in the right upper quadrant (RUQ) or epigastric region, caused by failure of gallbladder to fully contract typically from the presence of a stone, without signs of inflammation[5]
  - Biliary dyskinesia: vague RUQ pain and a low ejection fraction on hepatobiliary iminodiacetic acid scan (<35%), in the absence of gallstones or gallbladder wall thickness[4]

RELEVANT ANATOMY

- The gallbladder is situated between the 9th and 10th costal cartilages along the anterior abdominal wall.
- Normal gallbladder wall thickness is <3 mm.[8]
- Normal common bile duct diameter in neonates to 1-year olds is <1.6 mm. In childhood to early adolescence, it is <3 mm.[8]

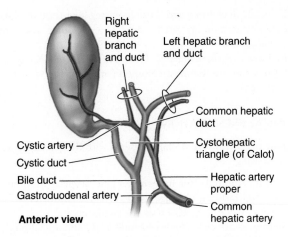

Figure 19.1 Blood supply of the gallbladder. (Reprinted with permission from Moore KL, Agur AMR, Dalley AF. *Essential Clinical Anatomy*. Philadelphia, PA: Wolters Kluwer Health; 2015.)

- Arterial supply to common bile duct is from the right hepatic and gastroduodenal artery branches at the 9- and 3-o'clock position, respectively (Figure 19.1).
- Bile excretion is increased by cholecystokinin (CCK), secretin, and vagal input. Excretion is decreased by somatostatin and sympathetic stimulation.[5]

EPIDEMIOLOGY AND ETIOLOGY

Incidence

- Gallstones are more common in Caucasian children compared with those of African American descent.

Etiology

- Congenital malformations of the biliary system.
- Pigmented gallstones are frequently seen in those with hemolytic disorders, which form when bilirubin is conjugated with calcium as a result of hemolysis. Specific conditions include sickle cell anemia, thalassemias, red blood cell enzymopathies, Wilson disease, and Gilbert syndrome.[4]
- Risk factors for cholesterol stones include obesity and oral contraceptive pills.

- Critically ill children and those requiring long-term total parenteral nutrition are predisposed to developing acalculous cholecystitis.[7]
- *Klebsiella, Escherichia coli, Enterobacter, Pseudomonas,* and *Citrobacter* are the most common pathogens found in acute cholangitis.[5]

CLINICAL PRESENTATION

Classic presentation: A child presents with RUQ pain, nausea, and vomiting.

- Younger children often have more vague, atypical symptoms.[7]
- Pain after fatty meals suggests cholelithiasis; however, >75% of patients with cholelithiasis are asymptomatic.[1]
- Signs of acute cholecystitis include RUQ abdominal tenderness, frequently with nausea and vomiting. Inspiratory arrest on palpation over the gallbladder, known as Murphy sign, is a classic physical examination finding.[1]
- Leukocytosis, fever, and a positive Murphy sign suggest infection.[7]
- Signs of obstruction to bile flow include jaundice and acholic stools.[7]
- Charcot triad (fever, RUQ pain, and jaundice) suggests cholangitis.[5]

DIAGNOSIS

Laboratory Findings

- WBC count, electrolytes, glucose, LFTs, lipase, and amylase are helpful for narrowing the differential.[7]
- A mild leukocytosis with normal LFTs is common in acute cholecystitis.
- A rise in LFTs may indicate more complicated forms of gallbladder disease, including choledocholithias and cholangitis.[6]
- An elevation of lipase and amylase is concerning for pancreatitis.

Imaging Findings

- Ultrasound is the best initial test with an accuracy of 95% in detecting many diseases of the gallbladder.[1]
  - Hyperechoic structures with acoustic shadowing are diagnostic of cholelithiasis.[1]

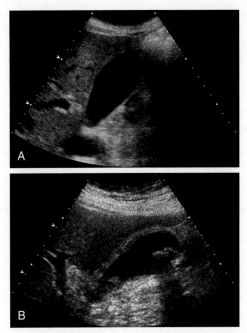

Figure 19.2 Gallbladder ultrasound. A, Demonstrates the normal ultrasound appearance of the gallbladder. B, The presence of gallstones, thickening of the gallbladder wall, and gallbladder wall edema are suggestive of acute cholecystitis. (Reprinted with permission from Hughes SJ, Mulholland MW. *Operative Techniques in Hepato-Pancreato-Biliary Surgery.* Philadelphia, PA: Wolters Kluwer Health; 2015.)

- The sonographic findings in acute cholecystitis include gallbladder wall thickening (>4 mm), distention, pericholecystic fluid, and presence of a gallstone within the neck (Figure 19.2).[6]
- These findings, without the presence of gallstones, are diagnostic of acalculous cholecystitis.[6]
- Increased gallbladder wall thickness (>4 mm), pericholecystic fluid, and mucosal membrane sludge, without the presence of gallstones, are diagnostic of AAC.[1]
- Ultrasound is usually normal in patients with biliary dyskinesia.[3]
- A nuclear medicine study is beneficial in patients with suspected acute cholecystitis.[3]
- Nuclear studies such as cholescintigraphy with CCK injection and are used less frequently, but helpful in assessing function of the gallbladder and diagnosing biliary dyskinesia.[7]

- If cholangitis is suspected, an endoscopic retrograde cholangiopancreatography (ERCP) or percutaneous transhepatic cholangiogram are both diagnostic and therapeutic.[5]
- CT is not a reliable imaging study because 60% of gallstones are radiolucent. It can show the location of the obstruction but unreliable for identifying the cause.[1,3]

SURGICAL MANAGEMENT

- A cholecystectomy should be performed within 72 hours in acute cholecystitis.[6]
- Medical management may be used for patients with moderate to severe comorbidities and mild acute cholecystitis.[6]
- Percutaneous drainage is used for patients who are poor surgical candidates with severe acute cholecystitis and failed medical therapy.[6]
- Early cholecystectomy (<7 d) is recommended for AAC, symptomatic choledocholithiasis, and mild gallstone pancreatitis.[1]
- Surgery is recommended for patients with symptomatic cholelithiasis.
- Prophylactic cholecystectomy should be strongly considered in the following:
  - Children with sickle cell disease and cholelithiasis or symptomatic biliary sludge
  - Children with hemolytic diseases undergoing a splenectomy[7]
- There are no reliable data on the efficacy of cholecystectomy for treatment of biliary dyskinesia.[1]

Operative Intervention

- This can be performed either laparoscopically or open; However, a laparoscopic cholecystectomy with attention to the "critical view" is the most common approach.
- Four-port technique versus single-site via umbilical trocar.

Open Approach

- Either an upper midline or right subcostal (Kocher) incision will provide good exposure.[6]
- A fundus-down technique is preferred, using electrocautery.
- The gallbladder serosa is incised at the fundus, and the gallbladder is removed from the fossa by dissecting the subserosal plane and applying downward traction.

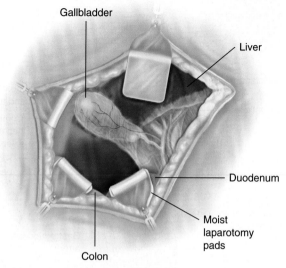

Figure 19.3 Placement of retractors. Correct application of a fixed retracting device (Bookwalter) is the key to a successful and safe open cholecystectomy. Inferiorly, moist laparotomy pads are carefully placed behind deep retractors to exclude the duodenum, colon, and small bowel from the operative field. Superiorly, additional retractors are placed to retain the liver. As the gallbladder is dissected free from its bed, the more lateral superior retractor can be progressively exchanged for deeper retractors placed over the dissected bed to improve visualization. (Reprinted with permission from Hawn MT, Mulholland MW. *Operative Techniques in Foregut Surgery*. Philadelphia, PA: Wolters Kluwer Health; 2015.)

- The medial and lateral peritoneal reflections are incised with cautery.
- Once at the infundibulum, exposure of the cystic artery and duct is attained by lateral retraction, which are then clipped and divided, and the gallbladder is removed from the field (Figure 19.3).

Laparoscopic Approach

- The conventional technique (Figure 19.4) involves 4 ports (Figure 19.5):
  - 12 mm periumbilical incision for the camera
  - 5 mm subxiphoid port located to the right of the falciform ligament
  - 5 mm subcostal port in the right midclavicular line
  - 5 mm subcostal port along the anterior axillary line for retraction

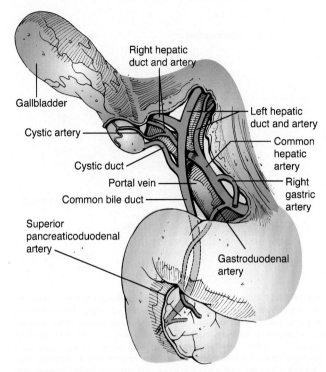

Figure 19.4 Surgical anatomy for laparoscopic cholecystectomy and common duct exploration. (Reprinted with permission from *Anesthesiologist's Manual of Surgical Procedures*. 5th ed. Philadelphia, PA: Lippincott Williams & Wilkins; 2014.)

1. The gallbladder fundus is grasped and retracted laterally and cephalad. The infundibulum is retracted laterally and slightly caudad.
2. The cystic artery and duct are identified using electrocautery and blunt dissection. This is the critical view. These structures are then clipped and divided.
3. The infundibulum is retracted cephalad, and the gallbladder is removed from the liver using electrocautery.[6]

POSTOPERATIVE CARE

Complications

- Bile leaks typically present within 1 week of surgery as abdominal pain, fever, or jaundice. Ultrasound or CT scan will show a biloma, or fluid collection, which should be

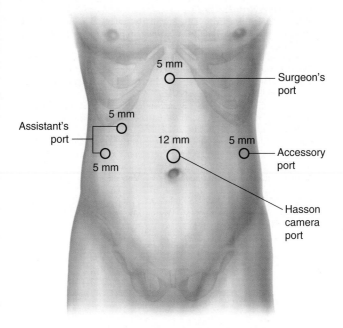

Figure 19.5 Trocar placement for a laparoscopic cholecystectomy. The surgeon stands on the patient's left. The subxyphoid port is the operating port; the 2 right upper quadrant ports are for gallbladder retraction. An accessory port can be placed in the left upper quadrant if needed. (Reprinted with permission from Lillemoe KD, Jarnagin W. *Hepatobiliary and Pancreatic Surgery*. Philadelphia, PA: Wolters Kluwer Health; 2013.)

followed by ERCP with stent placement, and percutaneous drainage of any collection.[5]

- A bile duct injury is the most devastating. Avoid this by careful dissection of the cystic structures with use of intraoperative cholangiography if necessary.[6]

PEARLS AND PITFALLS

- Always consider gallbladder disease in children who present with RUQ pain, nausea, and vomiting.
- Ultrasound is the best initial imaging modality for patients with suspected gallbladder disease.

REFERENCES

1. Rothstein DH, Harmon CM. Gallbladder disease in children. *Semin Pediatr Surg.* 2016:25:225-231.
2. Fishman DS, Gilger MA. Diseases of the gallbladder. In: Wyllie R, Hyams J, Kay M, eds. *Pediatric Gastrointestinal and Liver Disease.* 6th ed. Philadelphia: Elsevier; 2016:977-989.
3. Ashcraft KW, Holcomb GW, Murphy JP, Ostlie DJ, eds. *Ashcraft's Pediatric Surgery.* 5th ed. Philadelphia: Saunders Elsevier; 2010.
4. Suchy FJ. Diseases of the gallbladder. In: *Nelson's Textbook of Pediatrics.* 12th ed. Philadelphia: Elsevier; 2016.
5. Townsend CM, Evers BM, Beauchamp RD, Mattox KL, *Sabiston Textbook of Surgery: The Biological Basis of Modern Surgical Practice.* 20th ed. Philadelphia: Elsevier; 2017.
6. Fagenholz PJ, Velmahos G. The management of acute cholecystitis. In: *Current Surgical Therapy.* 12th ed. Philadelphia: Elsevier; 2017:430-441.
7. Arensman RM, Bambini DA, Almond PS, Adolph V, Radhakrishnan J, eds. *Pediatric Surgery.* 2nd ed. Austin, TX: Landes Bioscience; 2009.
8. William H. Paediatric liver and bile ducts, gallbladder, spleen and pancreas. In: Allan PL, Baxter GM, Weston MJ, eds. *Clinical Ultrasound.* 3rd ed. China: Elsevier; 2011.

Chapter 20

Choledochal Cyst

Ryan D. Reusche, Hibbut-ur-Rauf Naseem

HISTORICAL BACKGROUND

- Choledochal cysts were first described by Vater in 1723.[1]
- Anatomic variations of choledochal cyst were later classified by Alonso-Lej et al in 1959.[2] Subsequently, Todani et al classified choledochal cysts into 5 major types and multiple subtypes. This is the most commonly used classification system today.[3]
- Described in literature up through the 1970s a cholecystoenterostomy was considered a surgical management option for choledochal cysts.[4,5]
- Cyst excision with hepaticoenterostomy is now the favored procedure. This reduces the chance of pancreatitis,[6] malignancy in the remaining cyst,[6] and cholangitis.[7]

RELEVANT ANATOMY

- Type I (most common): consists of dilatation of the common bile duct, which may be cystic, focal, or fusiform (subtypes A, B, and C, respectively)
- Type II: a saccular diverticulum off the common bile duct
- Type III: a cystic dilatation of the intramural portion of the common bile duct (may represent a duodenal diverticulum rather than a choledochal cyst)
- Type IV-A (second most common): both intrahepatic and extrahepatic dilatation of the biliary tree
- Type IV-B: Multiple extrahepatic cysts
- Type V: "Caroli disease"; multiple intrahepatic biliary dilatations (Figure 20.1)

EPIDEMIOLOGY AND ETIOLOGY

Incidence: It varies depending on ethnic and geographic locations. There is higher incidence of choledochal cysts in Asian populations compared with other ethnicities.[8]
- 1 in 100 000 Western individuals[9]
- 1 in 13 000 people within the Japanese population[9]

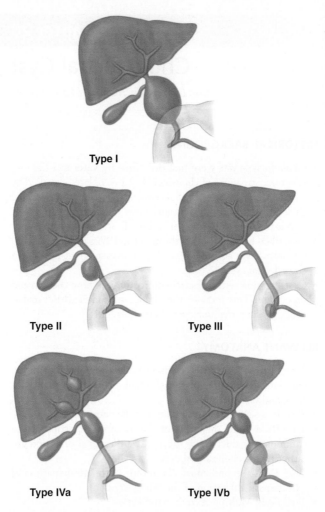

Figure 20.1 Artistic rendering of choledochal cyst types I-V and their prevalence. (Reprinted with permission from Lee EY. *Pediatric Radiology: Practical Imaging Evaluation of Infants and Children.* Philadelphia, PA: Wolters Kluwer; 2018.)

- Females are affected more frequently. Male-to-female ratio in both children and adults is approximately 1:4.[10,11]

Etiology: Many theories as to the exact etiology exist, but it is possibly multifactorial.

- The most universally accepted theory is that pancreatic juice refluxes into the biliary system, causing increased pressure within the common bile duct that leads to ductal dilatation.[12]
- They are associated with an anomalous pancreatobiliary junction with a long common channel (>15 mm).
- Additionally, abnormal function of the sphincter of Oddi has been reported to predispose to pancreatic reflux into the biliary tree, which may be associated with choledochal cysts.[13]

CLINICAL PRESENTATION

Classic presentation: classic triad (seen in 10%-20% of patients)—palpable right upper quadrant mass, jaundice, and abdominal pain

Infants

- Jaundice
- Acholic (gray/white) stools
- Palpable right upper duadrant mass

Children

- Recurrent pancreatitis
- Intermittent biliary obstruction
- Colicky abdominal pain
- Biliary peritonitis from cyst rupture[14]

DIAGNOSIS

Laboratory Findings

- They are generally nonspecific.
- In infants, laboratory findings tend to show biliary obstruction with conjugated hyperbilirubinemia and elevated alkaline phosphatase, transaminases, and gamma-glutamyl transferase.
- The coagulation profile may be deranged in chronic biliary obstruction because of vitamin K malabsorption.[15]
- Adults may present with elevated amylase levels because of pancreatitis.[16]

Imaging Findings

- Ultrasound is the initial screening to define the intrahepatic and extrahepatic biliary systems, gallbladder, and pancreaticobiliary system.
- Relevant findings include common bile duct size, intrahepatic biliary dilation, and intraluminal stones.[17]

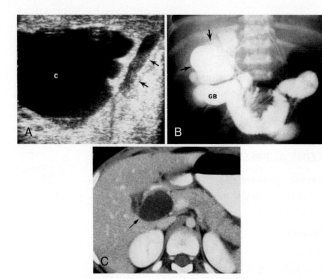

Figure 20.2 Choledochal cyst. A, Ultrasound shows a large, multilobulated anechoic cyst (C) that is adjacent to, but separate from, the gallbladder (arrows). B, Cholangiography confirms the presence of a large intrahepatic choledochal cyst (arrows) involving the right hepatic duct. GB, gallbladder. C, CT scan of a different child shows a well-defined cyst in the porta hepatis (arrow) associated with dilated central hepatic ducts. (Reprinted with permission from Brant WE, Helms CA. *Fundamentals of Diagnostic Radiology*. Philadelphia, PA: Lippincott, Williams & Wilkins; 2007.)

- Presence of intrahepatic biliary dilation is indication for further imaging.
- Percutaneous transhepatic cholangiography and endoscopic retrograde cholangiopancreatography are not used frequently because of invasiveness and associated risks, although there is still a role in the setting of obstructive jaundice.[18]
- Magnetic resonance cholangiopancreatography is the preoperative imaging of choice and excellent for anatomic imaging with high sensitivity and specificity in the diagnosis of choledochal cyst disease (Figure 20.2).[18]

SURGICAL MANAGEMENT

- Mortality is 97% with medical therapy alone.[16]
- Cyst excision is the definitive treatment for choledochal cyst disease.

- Surgical procedure of choice is total cyst excision with restoration of biliary enteric drainage.
- Surgical intervention should be elective. Prior treatment of cholangitis or pancreatitis should take place with intravenous antibiotics and biliary decompression.[18]

Open Approach

- The most common approach is right upper quadrant incision or transverse abdominal incision.
- The cyst, depending on its location, may be readily evident.
- Further exposure can be gained with medial and inferior reflection of the hepatic flexure of the colon and a Kocher maneuver with lateral division of the gastrohepatic ligament, as the cyst frequently extends behind the proximal duodenum.
- The gallbladder is mobilized from the liver bed, and the cystic artery is ligated.
- The degree of pericystic inflammation dictates circumferential dissection of the porta hepatis structures versus partial excision with posterior mucosectomy.
- For circumferential dissection, medial reflection of the gallbladder exposes the posterior plane between the cyst and portal vein.
- The dissection is carried inferiorly to the head of the pancreas.
- The distal duct is transected and oversewn.
- Using cephalad retraction of the cyst, the portal vein and hepatic artery are dissected from the back wall of the cyst.
- The dissection is carried proximally to the hepatic duct bifurcation, at which point the duct is usually normal caliber.
- The common hepatic duct is transected, and the specimen (gallbladder and choledochal cyst), passed off the field.

Internal Approach

- If the degree of pericystic inflammation precludes safe dissection of the porta hepatis structures, intramural dissection may be performed.
- After exposure of the cyst, an anterior transverse incision is made in the cyst and the contents, evacuated.
- The dissection is carried out in the submucosal plane from a lateral to posterior approach.
- A bridging incision is made in the posterior wall of the cyst from which the dissection is completed.

- Biliary continuity is restored with a Roux-en-Y hepaticojejunostomy.
- The jejunal conduit is brought through a retrocolic window.
- A tension-free hepaticojejunostomy is then perfomed in an end-to-end fashion.
- Fixation of the jejunal serosa to the transverse mesocolon avoids tension on the hepaticojejunostomy and internal herniation.
- A suction drain is usually left in proximity to the anastomosis and externalized.
- The abdominal wound is closed in layers.[16]

Laparoscopic Approach

- The technique is similar to that of the open approach.
- The operation can be carried out with 4 or 5 ports.
- Again, if there is substantial inflammation, the anterior wall of the cyst can be opened to provide a safe internal window for dissection.
- The hepaticojejunostomy technique is the same as the open technique.
- Laparoscopic operation is safe and effective for pediatric choledochal cyst excision.
- It carries the advantage of less blood loss, shorter postoperative recovery time, and improved cosmetic features.[19]
- Intraoperative endoscopy can also be used for safe excision of the pancreatic portion of a fusiform choledochal cyst and in evaluating the dilated intrahepatic bile duct for presence of debris.[17]

POSTOPERATIVE CARE

- Postoperative care is similar after both open and laparoscopic approaches with some surgeons starting feeds sooner after laparoscopic repair.
- The drain is removed several days after resumption of an oral diet without concomitant bilious drainage.

Complications

- Intrahepatic ducts: residual stones/strictures—may lead to cholangitis
- Common channel: residual tones/debris—may lead to pancreatitis
- Residual biliary mucosa: possible long-term risk of malignancy

PEARLS AND PITFALLS

- Vague abdominal pain leads to delayed diagnosis.
- Other abnormalities seen on imaging (eg, hepatic cyst) may cause choledochal cyst to be overlooked.
- Extent of cystic disease may be underrecognized, leading to incomplete/wrong operative procedure.

REFERENCES

1. Vater A. *Dissertation in auguralis medica, poes diss. Qua Scirris viscerum dissert*, C.S. *Ezlerus*. Edinburg, TX: University Library; 1723.
2. Alonso-Lej F, Rever W, Pessagno D. Congenital choledochal cysts, with report of 2, and an analysis of 94 cases. *Int Abstr Surg.* 1959;108:1-30.
3. Todani T, Watanabe Y, Narusue M, Tabuchi K, Okajima K. Congenital bile duct cysts: classification, operative procedures, and review of thirty-seven cases including cancer arising from choledochal cyst. *Am J Surg.* 1977;134:263-269.
4. Spitz L. Choledochal cyst. *Surg Gynecol Obstet.* 1978:147444-147452.
5. Muakkasah K, Obeid S, Slim M. Congenital choledochal cysts. *Arch Surg.* 1976:1112-1114.
6. Nagorney DM, McIlrath DC, Adson MA. Choledochal cysts in adults: clinical management. *Surgery.* 1984:96656-96663.
7. Kouraklis G, Misiakos E, Glinavou A, Karatzas G, Gogas J, Skalkeas G. Cystic dilatations of the common bile duct in adults. *HPB Surg.* 1996:1091-1099.
8. Yamaguchi M. Congenital choledochal cyst: analysis of 1,433 patients in the Japanese literature. *Am J Surg.* 1980;140(5):653-657.
9. Huang CS, Huang CC, Chen DF. Choledochal cysts: differences between pediatric and adult patients. *J Gastrointest Surg.* 2010;14(7):1105-1110.
10. Shah OJ, Shera AH, Zargar SA, et al. Choledochal cysts in children and adults with contrasting profiles: 11-year experience at a tertiary care center in Kashmir. *World J Surg.* 2009;33(11):2403-2411.
11. Edil BH, Cameron JL, Reddy S, et al. Choledochal cyst disease in children and adults: a 30-year single-institution experience. *J Am Coll Surg.* 2008;206(5):1000-1005.
12. Zhao L, Li Z, Ma H, et al. Congenital choledochal cyst with pancreatitis. *Chin Med J (Engl).* 1999:112637-112640.
13. Schweizer P, Schweizer M. Pancreaticobiliary long common channel syndrome and congenital anomalous dilatation of the choledochal duct: study of 46 patients. *Eur J Pediatr Surg.* 1993:315-321.
14. Samuel M, Spitz L. Choledochal cyst: varied clinical presentations and long-term results of surgery. *Eur J Pediatr Surg.* 1996:678-681.
15. Cameron J, Cameron A. *Cameron's Current Surgical Therapy.* 11th ed. Saunders; 2014:407-409.
16. Ziegler, Azizkhan, Allmen, Weber. *Operative Pediatric Surgery.* 2nd ed. McGraw Hill; 2014:716-723.
17. Holcomb G, Murphy J. *Ashcraft's Pediatric Surgery.* 5th ed. Saunders; 2009:566-573.
18. Soares KC, Goldstein SD, Ghaseb MA, et al. Pediatric choledochal cysts: diagnosis and current management. *Pediatr Surg Int.* 2017;33:637-650.
19. Song G, Jiang X, Wang J, et al. Comparative clinical study of laparoscopic and open surgery in children with choledochal cysts. *Saudi Med J.* 2017;38(5):476-481.

Chapter 21

Appendicitis

Rennier A. Martinez

- Accounts for about one-third of childhood admissions for abdominal pain[1]
- Peak incidence during adolescence[2]
- Diagnosis is difficult especially in younger children
- Definite diagnosis only in 50% to 70% of cases[3]
- Variable diagnostic algorithms depend on physician and institutional factors
- Appendectomy is still the treatment of choice; however, in select patients nonoperative management can be attempted

RELEVANT ANATOMY

- Location:
  - Intraperitoneal (95%)
    - Pelvis (30%) and Retrocecal (65%)
  - Retroperitoneal (5%)
- Size: average 8 cm and 5 to 10 mm wide
- Blood supply: appendiceal branch of ileocolic artery (lies behind ileum)
- Base of the appendix arises from confluence of the 3 taeniae coli (useful landmark to find appendix)[4]
- McBurney point: most common location of the appendix; one-third of the distance from the anterior superior iliac spine to the umbilicus (Figure 21.1)

ETIOLOGY AND EPIDEMIOLOGY

- Appendicitis is due to obstruction of the appendiceal lumen leading to vascular congestion, ischemic necrosis, and subsequent infection[2,4]
  - Commonly due to fecalith (20%)[4,5]
  - Other causes include lymphoid hyperplasia, carcinoid or other tumors, foreign bodies, and parasites[5]

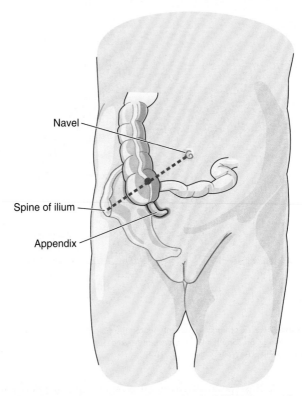

Navel

Spine of ilium

Appendix

Figure 21.1   Location of appendicitis on a female child. McBurney point is indicated as a dot on the center of a dashed line drawn between the anterior spine of ilium and the navel. (Reprinted with permission from Nath JL. *Using Medical Terminology*. 2nd ed. Philadelphia, PA: Lippincott Williams & Wilkins/ Wolters Kluwer Health; 2012.)

- Pathophysiology:[4]
  - Obstruction of appendiceal lumen → distention due to accumulating mucus
  - Distention activates T-10 visceral nerve fibers referring to periumbilical region
  - As pressure increases, lymphatic, venous, and, later, arterial flow are compromised; thus, ischemia ensues
  - Localized inflammation activates somatic parietal peritoneum pain fibers causing pain in right lower quadrant (RLQ)
    - Localized abscess or peritonitis occurs late in the process (>24-36 h)

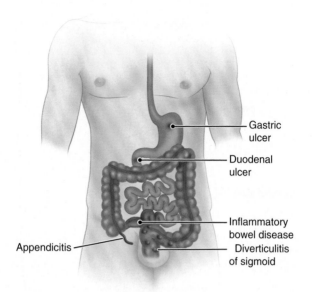

Figure 21.2 Common causes of peritonitis. (Reprinted with permission from Timby BK, Smith NE. *Introductory Medical-Surgical Nursing.* 12th ed. Philadelphia, PA: Wolters Kluwer; 2018.)

- Diffuse peritonitis is more common in young children and infants owing to proportionally smaller omentum that is less able to contain advancing inflammatory process (Figure 21.2)
- Rare in children <2 years of age
- Children <5 years of age more likely to present with perforation[2]

CLINICAL PRESENTATION

- Appendicitis can affect any age group; however, it is extremely rare in neonates and infants.
- This rarity as well as inability of young children to voice complaints leads often to delay in diagnosis.[4,5]

Classic presentation: a child with periumbilical pain that over past 12 hours has migrated to RLQ with associated nausea, anorexia, low-grade fever, and leukocytosis.

- This presentation however is not very common especially in younger children.

- Pain in the RLQ is the most common symptom.
- Midabdominal pain migrating to RLQ, and fever increases probability of appendicitis.[6]
- Fever, if not present, decreases probability of appendicitis by two-thirds.[6]
- Anatomic variability of appendix (ie, retrocecal, pelvic) is common and can alter presentation.
- Children often lie in bed with minimal movement.
  - A squirming, screaming child rarely has appendicitis.[4]
    - Exception is the retrocecal appendicitis inflaming the ureter and causing renal colic-type symptoms.
- Older children will often limp or flex trunk.
- Referred testicular pain or urinary frequency is often seen in the cases of pelvic appendicitis because of inflammation of the ureter.[4]
- Anorexia is another classic presenting symptom. Emesis is mild, and diarrhea may be due to ileocecal inflammation.
  - Severe GI symptoms before onset of pain usually indicate another diagnosis other than appendicitis.[5]
- Low-grade fever with temperature <38.6°C is the norm in nonperforated appendicitis.
- Higher temperature suggests severe inflammation or perforation.

Differential Diagnosis

- Acute appendicitis can mimic any intra-abdominal process.
- Have to keep in mind other inflammatory, infectious, vascular, congenital, and genitourinary conditions including the following:
  - Gastroenteritis, Crohn disease, mesenteric adenitis (ie, *Campylobacter*, viruses), pancreatitis, peptic ulcer, cholelithaisis, cholecystitis, Meckel diverticulitis, constipation, intussusception, ovarian torsion, ovarian cysts, pelvic inflammatory disease, renal stones, pyelonephritis, cystitis, etc.[5]
    - Systemic disorders that may present with acute abdominal pain include porphyria, sickle cell disease, diabetic ketoacidosis, measles, and parasitic infections.

DIAGNOSIS

Physical Examination

- Principal means of diagnosis is history and physical examination.
  - Serial examination by the same examiner is perhaps the most accurate diagnostic tool.[4,5]
    - It decreases number of unnecessary laparotomies without increased risk to the patient.

- Signs during physical examination depend on the time course of the disease as well as anatomic location of the appendix.[5]
  - Initially tenderness is mild and vague over RLQ.
  - As the parietal peritoneum becomes irritated, tenderness becomes localized over McBurney point.
    - Retrocecal appendicitis may cause pain midway between 12th rib and posterior superior iliac spine.
    - Pelvic appendicitis produces rectal tenderness, testicular pain, or urinary frequency by causing inflammation to surrounding tissues.[4]
  - Once appendicitis has progressed beyond 24 hours, there may be a period of pain relief, which may be due to rupture of the appendix where the intraluminal pressure is relieved.[5]
  - Peritonitis manifests as muscle rigidity, guarding, and rebound tenderness.
    - *Rovsing sign*: palpation of LLQ produces RLQ pain.
    - *Psoas sign*: right hip extension or raising straight leg against resistance.
    - *Obturator sign*: passive internal rotation of the right thigh.
    - Above signs are all nonspecific findings.
    - Only rebound tenderness has been found to have increased likelihood of appendicitis.[7]
    - Lack of RLQ tenderness reduces probability by half.[7]
  - Rectal examination may reveal a palpable, tender extrinsic mass or abscess; however, it is not routinely performed.

Laboratory Findings

- Leukocytosis >10k (90%); the addition of a left shift adds sensitivity.
- Only 3.7% of pediatric patients without a left shift have appendicitis.
- C-reactive protein and ESR useful when positive but do not rule out disease if negative.
- Normal WBC count in children younger than 4 years has an negative predictive value (NPV) of 95.6%; this decreases as children get older.[7]
- Urinalysis excludes urologic causes (mild hematuria/pyuria can be seen with appendicitis near ureter).
- B-HCG in appropriate pediatric patients.

Scoring

- Two scoring systems are commonly used to predict likelihood of appendicitis in pediatric patients.

- They use a combination of aforementioned symptoms; physical examination findings and laboratory values arrive at a score—total of 8 components in each system (total of 10 points).[7,8]
- Alvarado score and Pediatric Appendicitis Score (PAS): Both have divided their scores into low, medium, and high range to guide management.[9]
  - Intermediate scores typically precipitate further imaging.
  - Low score warrant no CT imaging, as appendicitis is unlikely.
  - High score mandates surgical consultation.
  - Both systems have sensitivity, specificity, and negative and positive predictive values in high 90s.[7]
  - Large validation studies however have found these numbers to be closer to the 70s and 80s.[7]

Imaging Findings

- Plain film radiograms are of limited value.
  - Radiopaque fecalith is seen only 5% to 20% of time.[4]
  - Sentinel loop in RLQ, mass effect from a pelvic abscess, lumbar scoliosis concave to RLQ, and loss of psoas shadow may be seen.
- Ultrasonography (US) has about 85% sensitivity and 90% specificity in the diagnosis of acute appendicitis.
  - Noncompressible appendix larger than 7 mm diameter, fecalith, or periappendiceal fluid is also helpful in diagnosis.[2,5]
  - It may be used to exclude other diagnoses particularly in the female population.[2]
  - Efficiency depends on the ability of US technician, patients' body habitus, and ability to tolerate test.
- CT imaging is excellent; however, to reduce radiation in the pediatric population, it is reserved when the diagnosis is unclear.
  - Sensitivity and specificity are 96% and 98%, respectively.[5]
  - IV contrast improves sensitivity and specificity, and oral contrast/rectal contrast improves sensitivity over IV alone.
  - Nonvisualization of the appendix has an NPV of 98.7%.[7]
  - Pediatric-specific protocol CT (often carried out in pediatric centers) reduces radiation.
  - In obese patients, or those suspected of having abscesses, CT is the diagnostic test of choice.
- MRI has high diagnostic accuracy for appendicitis and does not expose child to ionizing radiation; HOWEVER, it is expensive, time consuming, not universally available, and in young children may require sedation or anesthesia (Figures 21.3 and 21.4).
- For these reasons, it is not commonly used.[7]

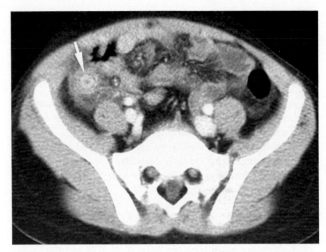

Figure 21.3 Acute appendicitis. CT scan of a 12-year-old boy with right lower quadrant pain shows a thick, dilated appendix (arrow) with enhancing walls. There is surrounding inflammation. (Reprinted with permission from Siegel MJ, Coley BR. *The Core Curriculum: Pediatric Imaging.* Philadelphia, PA: Lippincott Williams and Wilkins; 2005.)

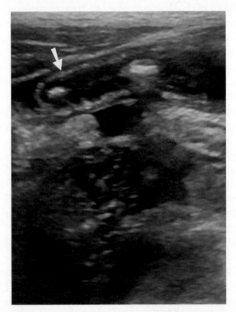

Figure 21.4 Acute appendicitis on ultrasonography (US). US demonstrates a dilated, noncompressible, blind-ending tubular structure (arrow) containing 2 appendicoliths in the right lower quadrant. (Reprinted with permission from Singh A. *Gastrointestinal Imaging: The Essentials.* Philadelphia, PA: Wolters Kluwer; 2016.)

MEDICAL AND SURGICAL MANAGEMENT

Acute Appendicitis

- For most patients, immediate surgical intervention is not mandatory. Adequate resuscitation is paramount, as well as antibiotics and bowel rest.[2]
  - If peritonitis is present, then emergent intervention is required.
  - Piperacillin/tazobactam and cefoxitin are started once the diagnosis is made. Flagyl may be started as well to cover for anaerobes.[7]
- Appendectomy is the treatment of choice. Outcomes are same whether the performed appendectomy is emergent (within 5 h of diagnosis) or urgent (6-16 h).[2,5,7]

Perforated Appendicitis

- Perforation is defined as hole in the appendix or a fecalith in the abdomen.[7]
- In children incidence of perforation is 25% to 75% with younger population at greatest risk.[2]
  - Children younger than 3 years have an 80% perforation rate versus 20% of those aged 10 to 17 years.[6]
- Perforated appendicitis is at higher risk for complications than nonperforated.
  - 50% of children with perforated appendicitis have complications as opposed to 2% to 4% of those without perforation.[2]
  - Factors associated with rupture include male sex, extremes of ages, and retroperitoneal position.[4]
- For late (days-weeks) appendicitis with well-localized abscess or phlegmon, prolonged IV antibiotics (2-3 wk) and CT-guided drainage are another option.[2]
  - Recent studies have shown that in patients with well-localized abscess early appendectomy, although more difficult, is a better option.[7,10]
    - During the interval from percutaneous drainage until eventual appendectomy, percutaneous drainage was associated with multiple drainage procedures, higher cost, and worse quality of life.
    - Some authors recommend early appendectomy in this group.[7]
  - Failure of nonoperative management should prompt surgical intervention.

- Early appendectomy, interval appendectomy, and "watchful waiting":
  - Early appendectomy has improved outcomes compared with delayed appendectomy.[11]
  - Interval appendectomy is typically performed 4 to 6 weeks versus "watchful waiting."[2]
  - Risk of recurrent appendicitis averages 10% versus risk of complications from interval appendectomy being 12%.
  - Some surgeons and parents decide to forgo interval appendectomy.[7]
- Nonoperative management is relevant because 30-day complication rate is as high as 10% in children and negative appendectomy rate is as high as 4.3%, making appendectomies unnecessary in these patients.[7]
  - Currently in adult studies nonoperative approaches have been found to have fewer complications, sick leaves, and better pain control, but when compared with combined failure rates and recurrence, it has been shown to be a less effective approach than appendectomy.[7]
  - However, there is increasing evidence of feasibility of nonoperative management of appendicitis in pediatric patients. Current international randomized trials are underway.
- Open versus laparoscopic approach has no difference in cost, cosmesis, or length of stay.
  - Laparoscopic approach may allow for better intra-abdominal visualization and makes it easier to find the appendix if it is at an unusual location.[2]
  - Currently more than 90% of appendectomies are performed laparoscopically.
  - Meta-analysis and multi-institutional reviews have found no differences in intra-abdominal abscess rates and continued low rates of wound infection at port sites in laparoscopic versus open approach.

Open Approach

- Abdomen is explored via transverse or oblique RLQ incision. Appendix is delivered into wound if possible and assessed. Appendectomy is all that is needed whether perforation is present or not. Occasionally small portion of cecum may be gangrenous, in which cases a limited ileocecectomy is indicated with primary anastomosis. For gross contamination, the abdomen is irrigated with warm saline and wound, closed.
  - In children wound can be closed regardless of findings.

- If normal appendix is found (5%-15%),[5] systematically inspect abdomen for evidence of inflammatory bowel disease, Meckel diverticulum, mesenteric adenitis, peptic ulcer disease, ovarian cysts, torsion, etc.

Laparoscopy-Assisted Approach

- Many different methods exist, but most commonly 3 approaches are used:
  - Complete laparoscopic approach: 3 ports; variation in trocar placement and practice[2,3,5]
  - Transumbilical laparoscopic approach: 1 or 2 ports
    - Cosmetically the initial advantages fade with longer interval follow-up[7]
- Irrigation has not shown to neither decrease or increase intra-abdominal abscess rates.[7]
- Incidental appendectomies are not routinely advocated except in the setting of RLQ incisions (ie, Meckel diverticulum, intussusception reduction).[7]

POSTOPERATIVE CARE

- Recent evidence shows that postop care is best protocolized.[7]
- Children with acute appendicitis can be discharged a few hours after operative intervention.
- For perforated or gangrenous appendicitis, patients are kept on broad-spectrum antibiotics until they are afebrile, asymptomatic, and tolerating diet.
- Normalization of WBC count is not required before discharge; however, a WBC evaluation is performed, and if still elevated, the patient is sent home on antibiotics.
  - No evidence arguing for or against a 3 or 5 days' course exists.[7]
  - Some surgeons are more aggressive with antibiotic use and use 7 to 14 days' course.[2]
- For nonperforated appendicitis, postop antibiotics are usually continued for 24 hours.[2]

Outcomes

- Mortality from appendicitis in children is less than 0.2% because of early diagnosis and appropriate fluid resuscitation before operation.
- Complication rates vary with severity of appendicitis.
  - Wound infections (5%-10%), abscess, and bowel obstruction[5]

PEARLS AND PITFALLS

- Appendicitis is frequent in adolescence, but a surgeon needs a high incidence of suspicion in younger patients.
- Classic symptoms are not common. Use diagnostic score for guidance but acknowledge their drawbacks.
- US imaging is the study of choice; however, in equivocal patients, CT imaging is an excellent modality.
- Laparoscopic approaches are the indicated procedures in most cases.
- Nonoperative management in select children is possible.
- Complex appendicitis with perforation and absence of a well-defined abscess is best managed with minimally invasive operative technique.

REFERENCES

1. Glass CC, Rangel SJ. Overview and diagnosis of acute appendicitis in children. *Semin Pediatr Surg*. 2016;25(4):198-203.
2. Mattei P, ed. *Fundamentals of Pediatric Surgery*. New York: Springer; 2011.
3. Puri P, Hollwarth M, eds. *Pediatric Surgery*. New York: Springer-Verlag Berlin Heidelberg; 2006. Lumley JSP, Siewert JR, eds. *Springer Surgery Atlas Series*.
4. Grosfeld JL, O'Neil JAJ, Fonkalsrud EW, Coran AG, eds. *Pediatric Surgery*. 6th ed. Philadelphia: Mosby; 2006 [No. 1].
5. Arensman RM, Bambini DA, Almond PS, Adolph V, Radhakrishnan J, eds. *Pediatric Surgery*. 2nd ed. Austin, Texas: Landes Bioscience; 2009.
6. Pearl RH, Hale DA, Molloy M, Schutt DC, Jaques DP. Pediatric appendectomy. *J Pediatr Surg*. 1995;30(2):173-178 [discussion 178-181].
7. Rentea RM, St Peter SD. Pediatric appendicitis. *Surg Clin North Am*. 2017;97(1):93-112.
8. Alvarado A. A practical score for the early diagnosis of acute appendicitis. *Ann Emerg Med*. 1986;15(5):557-564.
9. Di Saverio S, Birindelli A, Piccinini A, Catena F, Biscardi A, Tugnoli G. How reliable is Alvarado score and its subgroups in ruling out acute appendicitis and suggesting the opportunity of nonoperative management or surgery? *Ann Surg*. 2017;265(6):E84-E85.
10. Holcomb G III, Murphy JP, eds. *Ashcraft's Pediatric Surgery*. 5th ed. Philadelphia: Saunders; 2010.
11. Blakely ML, Williams R, Dassinger MS, et al. Early vs interval appendectomy for children with perforated appendicitis. *Arch Surg*. 2011;146(6):660-665.

Chapter 22

Intussusception

Paige E. Finkelstein

- Intussusception was first described in 1674 by Paul Barbette of Amsterdam, but it was defined by Treves in 1899.[1]
- Cornelius Velse successfully operated on an adult with intussusception in 1742, but John Hutchinson was the first person to operate successfully on an infant in 1873.[1,2]
- Samuel Mitchell reported the first case of successful air enema reduction in childhood in 1836.[2]

RELEVANT ANATOMY

- Certain anatomic features in the GI tract may dispose a patient to intussusception, including the anterior insertion of the ileum with respect to the cecum, decreased rigidity of the cecum secondary to abnormal taeniae coli, and abnormal muscle fibers at the ileocecal valve.[3]
- Hypertrophy of Peyer patches and/or mesenteric lymphadenopathy may act as a lead point for intussusception after infection.[1,3]
- Many other anatomic anomalies have been identified as lead points, including Meckel diverticulum, appendix, duplication cyst, heterotrophic tissues, lipoma lymphoma, ganglioneuroma, Kaposi sarcoma, hamartomas secondary to Peutz-Jeghers syndrome, cystic fibrosis, hemorrhagic edema, pseudomembranous colitis, bacterial infections, and hematomas due to trauma.[4]
- Anatomic location breakdown of intussusception[5]:
  - 77% Ileocolic
  - 12% Ileoileocolic
  - 5% Ileoileal
  - 2% Colocolic
  - 4% other

EPIDEMIOLOGY AND ETIOLOGY

Incidence: It is 56 per 100 000 children, with increased incidence during the winter months.[4]

- The mean age of intussusception in children is 6 to 18 months, with a male predominance of 2:1.[3,4]
- Intussusception is uncommon below 3 months or above 3 years of age.[1]
- In the pediatric population, ileocolic intussusception is the most common type.[3]

Etiology: An alteration of normal peristalsis by a lesion in the bowel that creates a telescoping effect (Figure 22.1). It can occur anywhere in the small bowel or colon. Most etiologies are unknown; only 10% have identifiable cause.[1,3]

- Intussusception is the most common abdominal emergency in early childhood and second most common cause of obstruction after pyloric stenosis.[1,3]

CLINICAL PRESENTATION

Classic presentation: A child with acute, colicky abdominal pain, knees drawn up to chest, with excessive irritability. Child may either return to normal state after episodes or appear lethargic as the pain begins to intensify again (episodes occur about every 15-25 min).[1,3]

- Shortly after onset of pain, vomiting or "currant jelly" stool may appear, a sign of impending bowel ischemia.[1,3]
- Physical examination may reveal sausage-shaped mass in right upper quadrant.[3]
- Intussusception may spontaneously reduce, but the natural progression is to bowel ischemia and necrosis, leading to sepsis and shock. Thus, the condition should be recognized and treated as soon as possible.[1,6]

DIAGNOSIS

Laboratory Findings

- Laboratory derangements are a LATE finding.[1]
- May be useful to order a CBC and metabolic panel, although no consistent findings have been defined. Increased white count and bandemia should be a red flag for necrotic bowel.[4]
- Signs of dehydration or metabolic alkalosis may be present because of dehydration and prolonged vomiting.
- Serum lactate may be indicative of bowel injury.

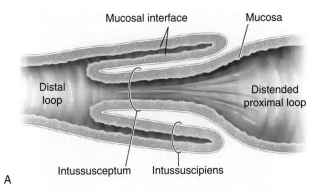

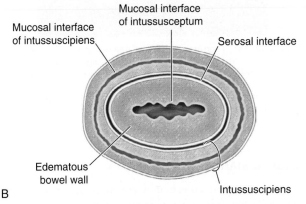

Figure 22.1 Telescoping of the bowel. A, Illustration of intussusception caused by the proximal bowel loop telescoping into the lumen of the adjacent distal portion. B, Cross-sectional illustration of intussusception. (Reprinted with permission from Kawamura D, Lunsford B. *Abdomen and Superficial Structures*. 4th ed. Philadelphia, PA: Wolters Kluwer; 2018.)

Imaging Findings

- Ultrasound diagnostics for intussusception approaches 100% sensitivity and specificity.[3]
- Classic "donut sign" or "target sign" can be seen on ultrasound (Figure 22.2).[1,3]
- In about half the cases, diagnosis can be made on plain flat and upright radiographs. Abnormalities will include an abdominal mass, abnormal bowel gas/fecal content distribution, and air fluid levels due to obstruction.[1]
- CT scan may demonstrate compromised vascular perfusion, edema, or air due to necrosis. However, CT with contrast may delay proper diagnosis, limiting its use.[3]
- MRI is not routinely used.[3]

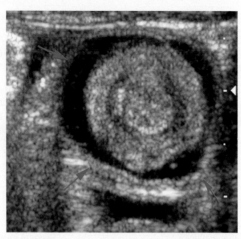

Figure 22.2 Target sign of intussusception. Ultrasound of a child with eosino-philic gastroenteritis, which demonstrated the classic target sign seen with intus-susception. The bowel within the intussusception (arrows) was thin-walled and echogenic, and the intussusception resolved during the examination. (Reprinted with permission from Brant WE, Helms CA. *Fundamentals of Diagnostic Radiology.* 4th ed. Philadelphia, PA: Lippincott Williams & Wilkins; 2012.)

SURGICAL MANAGEMENT

- Nonoperative reduction of intussusception via air or contrast enema should be considered before surgery.[3]
- Persistent small bowel intussusception likely requires surgical intervention.[3]
- Signs of bowel necrosis and peritonitis are indications for surgery as well.[3,4]

Operative Intervention

- Preoperative preparation includes broad-spectrum antibiotics, IV fluids, urinary catheter, and nasogastric tube placement.[1]
- Typically, the terminal ileum and cecum are involved and must be reduced. This can be performed either laparoscopically or open.

Open Approach

- An incision in the lower right abdomen in made.
- The leading edge of the intussusceptum is identified and manipulated back toward its normal anatomic position.

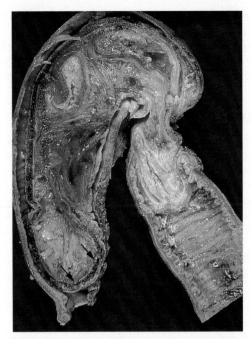

Figure 22.3 Resected bowel status post intussusception. Bowel of an adenovirus-induced intussusception in an 8-year-old child. The lead point of the intussusception (black arrows) is an area of lymphoid hyperplasia secondary to an infection. One loop of bowel completely telescopes into another. (Reprinted with permission from Noffsinger A. *Fenoglio-Preiser's Gastrointestinal Pathology*. 4th ed. Philadelphia, PA: Wolters Kluwer; 2017.)

- Ischemic bowel or lead points should be resected (Figure 22.3) followed by bowel anastomosis or diversion, depending on the patient.
- Incidental appendectomy is often performed as well.[1]

Laparoscopic Approach

- Most minimally invasive approaches describe the use of 3 abdominal ports: 1 in the infraumbilical region with 2 other ports along the left side of the abdomen.
- Laparoscopic reduction is accomplished by applying gentle pressure distal to the intussusceptum using atraumatic graspers.
- Although counterintuitive to the conventional open method, traction is usually required proximal to the intussuscipiens to complete the reduction.

- Appendectomy is not routinely performed with laparoscopic reduction but is up to the surgeon's discretion.
- Careful inspection of the bowel is performed to evaluate for any signs of ischemia, necrosis, or perforation.
- If necessary, the procedure may be converted to open.[1]

POSTOPERATIVE CARE

- Postoperative care is similar after both open and laparoscopic approaches, although feeds may be able to be resumed sooner and there may be a shorter hospital stay associated with laparoscopic approach.[4]
- Patients who undergo nonoperative enema reductions can be started on liquid diet immediately and be advanced as tolerated; some may be immediately discharged home.[4]

Complications

- Intestinal necrosis is associated with a longer duration of symptoms. Missed necrotic bowel has high rates of morbidity and mortality[7]
- Chronic or recurrent intussusception[6]
- Bowel perforation, although rates are low in developed countries, with estimates ranging from 0% to 3%[6]
- Adhesion and volvulus are late surgical complications, seen in 3% to 6% of cases[6]
- Consider lymphoma workup for a child older than 6 years presenting with intussusception[8]

PEARLS AND PITFALLS

- Ultrasound sensitivity and specificity approach 100% when it comes to diagnosing intussusception. Consider as first-line imaging study when intussusception is suspected.
- Surgery is not the initial treatment modality. Consider air or contrast enemas first.
- Surgery should be performed when nonsurgical treatment modalities fail, if there are recurrent intussusceptions, or if signs of necrotic bowel are present.
- Patients tend to do very well postop.
- Missed or late diagnosis of intussusception can lead to necrotic bowel, which can be fatal. Timely diagnosis is key.

REFERENCES

1. Holcomb GW III, Murphy JD, Ostlie DJ. *Ashcraft's Pediatric Surgery*. Elsevier Health Sciences; 2014.
2. Davis CF, McCabe AJ, Raine PAM. The ins and outs of intussusception: history and management over the past fifty years. *J Pediatr Surg*. 2003;38:60-64.
3. Marsicovetere P, Ivatury S, White B, Holubar S. Intestinal intussusception: etiology, diagnosis, and treatment. *Clin Colon Rectal Surg*. 2016;30:030-039.
4. Pepper VK, Stanfill AB, Pearl RH. Diagnosis and management of pediatric appendicitis, intussusception, and Meckel diverticulum. *Surg Clin North Am*. 2012;92:505-526 [vii].
5. Kumar R, Nayak P. *Elsevier Comprehensive Guide to Combined Medical Services: UPSC Simplied*. Elsevier; 2014.
6. del-Pozo G, Albillos JC, Tejedor D, et al. Intussusception in children: current concepts in diagnosis and enema reduction. *Radiographics*. 1999;19:299-319.
7. Huang H-Y, Huang XZ, Han YJ, et al. Risk factors associated with intestinal necrosis in children with failed non-surgical reduction for intussusception. *Pediatr Surg Int*. 2017;33:575-580.
8. Young G, Toretsky JA, Campbell AB, Eskenazi AE. Recognition of common childhood malignancies. *Am Fam Physician*. 2000;61:2144-2154.

Chapter 23

Meckel Diverticulum

Jessica L. Buicko

- The first description of a small bowel diverticulum was in 1598 by a German surgeon Wilhelm Hildanus.
- Alexis Littre also noted a small bowel diverticulum, this time in an inguinal hernia in 1745.
- Nevertheless, this entity was ultimately named after anatomist Johann Meckel in 1809 after he further described the anatomy and embryology of this unique structure.[1]

RELEVANT ANATOMY

- The Meckel diverticulum is a true diverticulum containing all layers of the intestinal wall (Figure 23.1).
  - It is located on the antimesenteric border of the ileum.
- The "rule of 2's" is a helpful way to remember the general anatomic features of a Meckel diverticulum.
- Meckel diverticulum is usually located within 2 feet of the ileocecal valve, approximately 2 inches in length, and contains 2 distinct types of heterotopic mucosa, gastric (the more common) and pancreatic (Figure 23.2).

EPIDEMIOLOGY AND ETIOLOGY

- Meckel diverticulum is the most common congenital abnormality of the small intestine.
- Approximately 2% of the population has a Meckel diverticulum, but only approximately 4% of patients with a Meckel diverticulum become symptomatic.[1]
- The risk of developing symptoms decreases with increasing age.
- There does not appear to be a familial link.
- Males are twice as likely as females to have a Meckel diverticulum.
- It is noted that the prevalence is increased in children with malformations of the umbilicus, alimentary tract, nervous system, and cardiovascular system.[2]

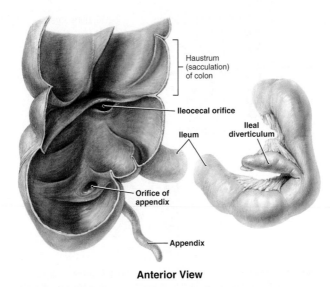

Haustrum (sacculation) of colon

Ileocecal orifice

Ileum

Ileal diverticulum

Orifice of appendix

Appendix

Anterior View

Figure 23.1 Meckel diverticulum seen on the antimesenteric border of the ileum. (Reprinted with permission from Agur AMR, Dalley AF. *Grant's Atlas of Anatomy.* 14th ed. Philadelphia, PA: Wolters Kluwer; 2017.)

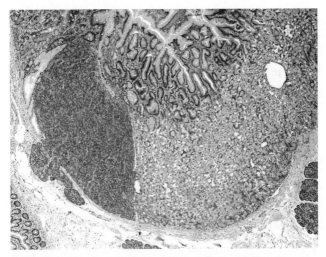

Figure 23.2 Ectopic gastric fundic and pancreatic tissue in the mucosa line the diverticulum, 100×. (Reprinted with permission from Husain AN, Stocker JT, Dehner LP. *Stocker & Dehner's Pediatric Pathology.* 4th ed. Philadelphia, PA: Wolters Kluwer; 2016.)

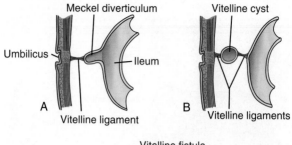

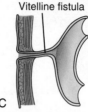

Figure 23.3 Remnants of the vitelline duct. A, Meckel, or ileal, diverticulum combined with the fibrous cord (vitelline ligament). B, Vitelline cyst attached to the umbilicus and wall of the ileum by vitelline ligaments. C, Vitelline fistula connecting the lumen of the ileum with the umbilicus. (Reprinted with permission from Sadler TW. *Langman's Medical Embryology*. 13th ed. Philadelphia, PA: Wolters Kluwer; 2014.)

- A Meckel diverticulum is a remnant of the omphalomesenteric (vitelline) duct, which in the fetus connects the midgut to the yolk sac.
- The omphalomesenteric duct usually involutes between the fifth to seventh weeks of gestation.
- Failure of this involution can lead to a wide variety of pathologies, most commonly a Meckel diverticulum (Figure 23.3A).
- Other anatomic varieties seen secondary to a persistent omphalomesenteric duct include omphalomesenteric cysts (Figure 23.3B), fistulae (Figure 23.3C), umbilical polyps, and persistent fibrous cords.
- The blood supply to the Meckel diverticulum is from the vitelline artery off the superior mesenteric artery.[1]

CLINICAL PRESENTATION

- The majority of patients with Meckel diverticulum are clinically asymptomatic.
- The most common presentations in children include intestinal bleeding, obstruction, or diverticular inflammation.[1]

- Meckel diverticula that have gastric mucosa are more likely to present with bleeding.
- Adults are more likely to present with obstructive symptoms when symptomatic from a Meckel diverticulum.
- The classic presentation of a Meckel diverticulum in a child is painless rectal bleeding.
- Meckel diverticulum is the cause of more than 50% of all lower intestinal bleeding in children.[1]
- The bleeding is usually due to ulceration of the normal ileal mucosa adjacent to the Meckel diverticulum.
- Usually in these patients, the physical examination is not helpful in making a diagnosis.
- A Meckel diverticulum can also present with obstructive symptoms, especially when it acts as a lead point in an intussusception or volvulus.
- For further information on intussusception in children, please see chapter 22.
- In addition to cramping abdominal pain, these patients may pass "currant jelly" stool and may have a palpable mass on examination.

DIAGNOSIS

- In patients presenting with obstruction or inflammation secondary to a Meckel diverticulum, the diagnosis is often not known before operative exploration.
- If the Meckel diverticulum is causing an intussusception, this can often be diagnosed on ultrasound.
- If this is the case, air enemas are rarely successful in reducing intussusception due to this etiology.

Imaging Studies

- The diagnosis of a bleeding Meckel diverticulum can be made with the technetium-99m pertechnetate radionuclide study or "Meckel scan."
- This isotope has a high affinity for gastric mucosa.
- Meckel diverticulum without ectopic gastric mucosa will not be visualized on this study.
- The positive predictive value of a Meckel scan is almost 100%, yet the sensitivity can be as low as 60%.[1,3]
- If a Meckel scan is negative, yet there is a high suspicion for bleeding, one can consider diagnostic laparoscopy (Figure 23.4).

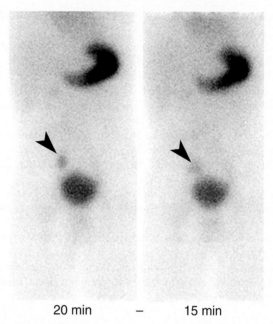

20 min — 15 min

Figure 23.4 Tc-99m pertechnetate Meckel scan performed in a 3-year-old male child with painless rectal bleeding demonstrates a focus of radiotracer activity (arrowheads) in the right lower quadrant compatible with ectopic gastric mucosa. (Reprinted with permission from Singh A. *Gastrointestinal Imaging: The Essentials*. Philadelphia, PA: Wolters Kluwer; 2016.)

MEDICAL AND SURGICAL MANAGEMENT

- The treatment for a symptomatic Meckel diverticulum is resection via either an open or laparoscopic approach (Figure 23.5).
- Preoperatively, patients should be started on intravenous fluids.
- If the patient presents with obstructive symptoms, consideration should be given to placing a nasogastric tube.
- If the patient presents severely anemic with active bleeding, consideration should be given to blood transfusion.
- The extent of necessary resection depends on the presenting pathology.
- If the diverticulum is causing obstruction, a simple diverticulectomy can be performed.[1]
- If ectopic tissue is encountered, it should also be removed.

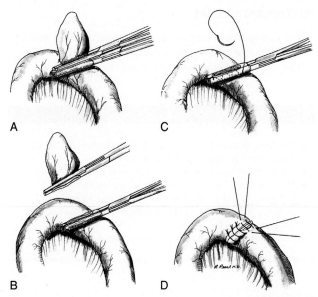

Figure 23.5 A, Base of Meckel diverticulum clamped. B, Specimen excised between clamps with cautery. C, Full-thickness sutures placed beneath the clamp. D, Inverting interrupted Lembert sutures placed in the seromuscular layer. (Reprinted with permission from Fischer JE, Jones DB, Pomposelli FB, Upchurch GR, eds. *Fischer's Mastery of Surgery.* 6th ed. Philadelphia, PA: Wolters Kluwer Health/Lippincott Williams & Wilkins; 2012.)

- If surgery is being performed for bleeding, a segmental resection is recommended as an ulcer is often present on the mesenteric side of the diverticulum.
- The management of an incidentally noted asymptomatic Meckel diverticulum is a topic of debate.
- Generally, if identified incidentally on imaging studies, no intervention is warranted.
- If the diverticulum is recognized intraoperatively, there are some data to support resection due to the small risk of malignancy and future complications.[4,5]
- On the other hand, some authors argue that the risks of future complications is less than the actual complications of resection in general and recommend leaving any incidentally noted Meckel diverticulum.
- Park et al, from the Mayo Clinic, recommend a selective approach for resection depending on 4 main characteristics: patient age less than 50 years, male sex, diverticulum length more than 2 cm, and the presence of histologically abnormal tissue.[6]

POSTOPERATIVE CARE

- The postoperative care is relatively straightforward and similar to that for an appendectomy or small bowel resection.
- The overall rate of postoperative complications is low.

PEARLS AND PITFALLS

- The Meckel diverticulum is a TRUE diverticulum located on antimesenteric border of the small bowel.
- Classic presentation in children is painless rectal bleeding.
- Remember the rule of 2's: usually located within 2 feet of the ileocecal valve, approximately 2 inches in length, and contains 2 distinct types of heterotopic mucosa, gastric and pancreatic.
- The treatment for patients who are symptomatic is resection.

REFERENCES

1. Leys CM. Chapter 40: Meckel diverticulum. In: *Ashcraft's Pediatric Surgery*. N.p.: Elsevier Health Sciences; 2014:548-552 [Print].
2. Simms MH, Corkery JJ. Meckel's diverticulum: its association with congenital malformation and the significance of atypical morphology. *Br J Surg*. 1980;67(3):216-219.
3. Swaniker F, Soldes O, Hirschl RB. The utility of technetium 99m pertechnate scintigraphy in the evaluation of Meckel diverticulum. *J Pediatr Surg*. 1999;34:760-765.
4. Thirunavukarasu P, Sathaiah M, Sukumar S, et al. Meckel diverticulim—A high-risk region for malignancy in the ileum. *Ann Surg*. 2011;253:223-230.
5. Onen A, Cigdem MK, Ozturk H, et al. When to resect and when not to resect an asymptomatic Meckel diverticulum: an ongoing challenge. *Pediatr Surg Int*. 2003;19:57-61.
6. Park JJ, Wolff BG, Tollefson MK, et al. Meckel diverticulum: the Mayo Clinic experience with 1476 patients (1950-2002). *Ann Surg*. 2005;241(3):529-533.

SUGGESTED READING

Yahchouchy EK, Marano AF, Etienne JC, Fingerhut AL. Meckel's diverticulum. *J Am Coll Surg*. 2001;192(5):658.

Chapter 24

Intestinal Atresia

Kara Baker

- Intestinal stenosis and atresia are usually grouped together as a spectrum of congenital disorders that cause narrowing or complete obstruction anywhere along the intestine.
- These disorders are generally classified by anatomic location: duodenal, jejunoileal, or colonic.
- The first case report describing duodenal atresia was published by Calder in 1733.
- Clinical findings were further described by Cordes in 1901, but it was not until 1905 and 1914 that the first surgical repairs were reported by surgeons in France and the Netherlands, respectively.[1]
- The first enterostomy to correct jejunoileal atresia was performed by Voisin in 1804.
- The first attempted resection and anastomosis was performed by Wanitschek in 1894, but Fockens is credited with the first successful anastomosis in 1911.[1]
- Colonic atresia was the earliest to be described in 1673 by Binninger.
- In 1922, Gaub treated a patient with sigmoid atresia with a proximal diverting colostomy, documenting the first record of a survivor of the condition.
- In 1947, a surgeon by the name of Potts performed the first known primary anastomosis of the transverse colon in a newborn.[1]

RELEVANT ANATOMY

- The small intestine is composed of 3 parts: the duodenum, jejunum, and ileum.
- The duodenum is mostly retroperitoneal, outside of the proximal 2.5 cm.
- It extends from the end of the pyloric canal to the duodenojejunal junction.

- There is no clear boundary between the jejunum and ileum, but instead a gradual transition is noted by decreases in both wall thickness and presence of plicae circularis.[2]
- The jejunum and ileum lie within the boundary of the colon and are attached to the posterior abdominal wall by mesentery, which also carries the blood and lymphatic supply.

EPIDEMIOLOGY AND ETIOLOGY

- The duodenum is the most common site of neonatal intestinal obstruction, accounting for nearly half of all cases (Table 24.1).
- The incidence of small bowel stenosis and atresia is believed to be 1:5000 to 1:10 000 live births, and they affect males more commonly than females.
- Colonic stenosis and atresia are less common, occurring in 1:20 000 live births.
- The etiology is believed to be due to failure of recanalization in the fetal gastrointestinal (GI) tract, which typically occurs during the 11th week of gestation.
- They may also be due to intrauterine vascular disruption during fetal development, causing ischemia, necrosis, and reabsorption of affected segments of small or large bowel.
- Intestinal stenosis and atresia are commonly associated with other congenital and chromosomal abnormalities, including trisomy 21 (30% of patients), Hirschsprung disease, cystic fibrosis, malrotation, neural tube defects, congenital heart diseases, and other GI atresias.
- Fetal risk is increased by conditions that decrease fetal blood supply, such as vasoconstrictive medications and maternal smoking in the first trimester. Use of methylene blue has also been associated with intestinal atresia.[3]
- Small bowel atresias are further classified into types I to IV (Figure 24.1).

CLINICAL PRESENTATION

- Most cases will present with signs of obstruction: polyhydramnios in utero, abdominal distention, feeding intolerance, and vomiting after birth.
- Emesis may be bilious or nonbilious based on the location of the obstruction relative to the ampulla of Vater.

TABLE 24.1		
Classification of Duodenal and Jejunoileal Atresias		
Classification	Occurrence (% of Cases)	Description
Stenosis	12	Narrowing of intestinal lumen.
Type I	23	Mucosal and submucosal defect with no damage to the muscularis layer.
Type II	10	Two blind ends of intestine connected by fibrous band. Mesentery is usually intact.
Type IIIa	16	Complete separation of 2 blind ends of intestine, usually with a V-shaped mesenteric defect.
Type IIIb	19	Coiling of diseased intestine around mesentery, causing "apple-peel" or "Christmas tree" appearance.
Type IV	20	Multiple areas of atresia. Can be any combination of types I-III.

Adapted from Puri P, Hollwarth M, eds. *Pediatric Surgery.* 1st ed. Berlin: Springer; 2006.

- Patients will also have failure to pass meconium with complete obstruction. Incomplete obstruction may allow passage of mucous plugs or blood per rectum.

DIAGNOSIS

- Diagnosis is usually made with an abdominal ultrasound, which can be performed prenatally in suspected cases.
  - With duodenal stenosis and atresia, it will typically show the classic "double bubble."
  - Jejunoileal atresia has less specific findings and usually only shows dilated loops of bowel.
  - Polyhydramnios may or may not be present, based on the gestational age and level of obstruction. Prenatal diagnosis of jejunoileal stenosis or atresia is rare.
- Upright plain abdominal films may also be obtained.

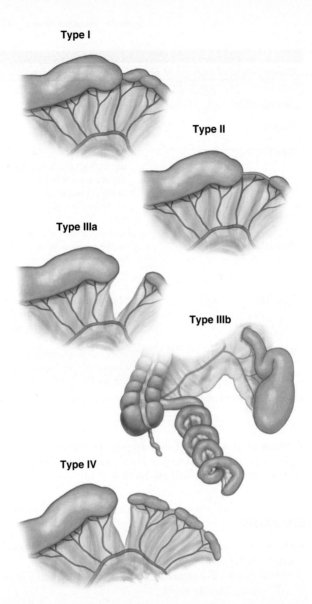

Figure 24.1 Small bowel atresias. Type I: atresia of the mucosa with sparing of the other layers of the bowel wall. Type II: 2 atretic segments attached by fibrous cord with intact mesentery. Type IIIa: atretic segments with mesenteric defect, typically V-shaped. Type IIIb: coiling of intestines around mesentery, often called "apple-peel atresia." Type IV: multiple atretic segments of any type. (Reprinted from Frischer JS, Azizkhan RG. Jejunoileal Atresia and Stenosis. In: Coran AG, ed. *Pediatric Surgery*. 7th ed. Philadelphia, PA: Saunders; 2012:1059-1071. Copyright © 2012 Elsevier. With permission.)

- These may also show the double bubble and absence of gas in the distal bowel.
- In some cases, thickened meconium has a "ground glass" appearance.
- A contrast enema may also be ordered to identify a small or large bowel obstruction.
- Typically, there will be dilated segments that abruptly transition to a small diameter at the level of the obstruction.
- Bowel distal to the obstruction often appears gasless and unused (Figure 24-2).

EPIDEMIOLOGY AND ETIOLOGY

- Preoperatively, patients are managed with gastric decompression via nasogastric (NG) or orogastric (OG) tube, as well as fluid and electrolyte replacement.
- Urgent correction of small or large bowel obstruction is usually mandated in cases where malrotation and volvulus cannot be ruled out.
- All surgical approaches to correction of intestinal stenosis and atresia begin with an inspection of the abdomen to classify the type of atresia and rule out other congenital abnormalities, such as annular pancreas or malrotation, which may be present in up to 30% of cases.[4]
- It is also paramount to identify and avoid injury to the ampulla of Vater and common bile duct throughout the procedure.

Surgical Intervention

- The procedure of choice for duodenal stenosis or atresia is laparoscopic or open duodenoduodenostomy, with a proximal transverse to distal longitudinal, or diamond-shaped anastomosis preferred over the traditional side-to-side anastomosis.

Open Approach

- Right upper quadrant supraumbilical transverse incision is made.
- Duodenum is exposed and mobilized to allow a tension-free anastomosis.
  - Gastric tube is advanced to localize the obstruction and identify a wind sock deformity if present.

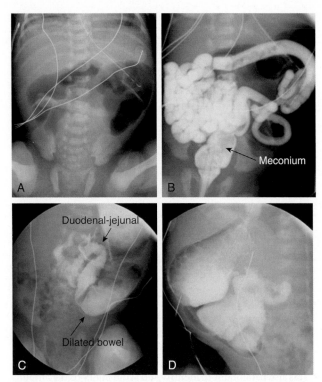

Figure 24.2 High intestinal obstruction. A, Jejunal atresia. X-ray abdomen: Few dilated bowel loops in the upper abdomen with paucity of gas distally concerning for upper GI (UGI) obstruction. B, Ileal atresia. Lower GI study: Contrast enema image demonstrates a normal caliber rectum containing some meconium. Contrast refluxed freely into the terminal and distal ileum. Contrast was not refluxed into the more proximal distended loops of the small bowel. The patient was found to have proximal ileal atresia at surgery. C, Jejunal stenosis. Contrast UGI study: The duodenum is normal in caliber, with a normally positioned duodenal-jejunal junction. There is gradual dilatation of jejunum distal to the ligament of Treitz, with a markedly dilated loop at least 7 cm from the ligament of Treitz. D, Lateral view demonstrating the same dilated proximal jejunal loop. There was delay in contrast emptying distal to this dilated loop. However, the contrast eventually filled multiple normal caliber small bowel loops. (Reprinted with permission from Nichols DG, Shaffner DH, eds. *Rogers' Textbook of Pediatric Intensive Care.* 5th ed. Philadelphia, PA: Wolters Kluwer; 2016.)

- A transverse incision is made in the proximal segment, and a longitudinal incision is made in the distal segment bordering the obstruction.
- If a windsock presentation is suspected, a 2.5- to 3-cm longitudinal excision may be made to enter the duodenal lumen.

- A small catheter may be passed into the distal segment to rule out distal atresias.
- A single-layer anastomosis is made using 5-0 or 6-0 Vicryl sutures.

Laparoscopic Approach

- Insufflation of the abdomen through the umbilicus.
- Ports can be placed at infant's right lower quadrant and right midepigastric region with a liver retractor in the right or left upper quadrant if necessary.
- Alternatively, the liver can be elevated using a transabdominal wall suture around the falciform ligament and tied or clamped into place.
- The duodenum is identified and mobilized, and the obstruction is localized.
- The surgery proceeds in the same fashion as the open procedure.
- Surgical clips may also be used to make the anastomosis with the laparoscopic approach.
- The surgical management of jejunoileal stenosis or atresia is largely based on the location of the lesion, but the most commonly performed procedure is resection of the abnormal bowel with primary end-to-end anastomosis.
- Once the small bowel is accessible, repair of any perforations should be performed, and the peritoneal cavity should be irrigated as necessary with warm saline.
- The bowel should be inspected in its entirety to identify the site of obstruction as well as any other abnormalities.
- The distal bowel segment should be cannulated with a catheter and used to rule out any distal obstruction.
- If malrotation is present, it should be corrected with a Ladd procedure.
- Care should be taken to limit the length of bowel resection as much as possible to avoid short bowel syndrome.
- Ideally, the resection should include all of the proximal dilated bowel, leaving only normal-caliber bowel for the anastomosis.
- An adequate length is at least 80 cm and includes the ileocecal valve.
- Multiple options exist for the anastomosis, but the most commonly accepted is a single-layer, end-to-back technique using 5-0 or 6-0 absorbable monofilament sutures.

- The resection line should be slightly shorter on the antimesenteric border to ensure that proximal and distal openings are approximately equal in size.
- Colonic stenosis or atresia is typically managed with a staged surgical approach of colostomy with mucous fistula.

POSTOPERATIVE CARE

- Duodenal repairs usually require a transanastomotic jejunal feeding tube and NG or OG tube for post-op gastric drainage.
- Most patients will require immediate parenteral nutrition, which should be continued until the infant is tolerating enteral feeds.
- These can be restarted once the patient has minimal clear gastric aspirate and bowel function has returned.
- Early postoperative mortality has been reported at 3% to 5%, with the majority due to complications of associated congenital abnormalities, usually involving the heart, lungs, and brain.[3]
- Complications include transient GI dysfunction, prolonged feeding intolerance, blind loop syndrome, delayed gastric emptying, bleeding peptic ulcers, and intestinal obstruction due to adhesions or incorrect identification of obstruction site.
- If the infant does not return to normal function after 2 to 3 weeks, a GI series should be obtained to look for a new or missed obstruction and stenosis of the anastomosis.
- Persistently poor peristalsis may also be a cause of continued poor function.
- Colonic atresia has an excellent prognosis if diagnosed within the first 72 hours.
- Late diagnosis can cause massive dilation and perforation.

PEARLS AND PITFALLS

- Techniques no longer recommended for correction of intestinal atresia include simple transverse enteroplasty, excision of membranes, bypassing techniques, and side-to-side anastomosis.
- These techniques fail to remove the abnormal dysfunctional segments and thus increase the risk of blind loop syndrome.
- The side-to-side anastomosis has a higher incidence of breakdown and prolonged obstruction, compared with the "diamond-shaped" anastomosis, which has been shown to allow for early feeding, early discharge, and good long-term results.

REFERENCES

1. Grosfeld JL, O'Neill JA, Coran AG, Fonkalsrud EW, eds. *Pediatric Surgery*. 6th ed. Philadelphia: Mosby Elsevier; 2006.
2. Standring S, ed. *Gray's Anatomy*. 41st ed. London: Elsevier; 2016.
3. Holcomb GW, Murphy JP. *Ashcraft's Pediatric Surgery*. 5th ed. Philadelphia: Saunders Elsevier; 2010.
4. Puri P, Hollwarth M, eds. *Pediatric Surgery*. 1st ed. Berlin: Springer; 2006.

Chapter 25

Malrotation

Erica Davanian

- First described around 1898, William Edwards Ladd standardized the evaluation and surgical management of malrotation in 1932.
- The principles from Ladd's landmark article and textbooks still hold true today.[1,2]
- Although an open surgical technique is still used in most cases of malrotation, the first laparoscopic procedure was attempted in 1995 and has become more commonly used since that time.[3,4]
- However, laparoscopic management is controversial for reasons discussed in the surgery section later in this chapter.

RELEVANT ANATOMY

- Between the 4th and 10th weeks of gestation, normal development of the midgut proceeds via herniation through the umbilicus.
- This involves a 90° counterclockwise rotation, retraction with 180° counterclockwise rotation, and fixation to the retroperitoneum.[2,5]
- The superior mesenteric artery (SMA) and superior mesenteric vein (SMV) course through the root of the mesentery, acting as a fulcrum around which the embryologic intestine makes its total 270° counterclockwise rotation.
- Ultimately, the SMA lies to the left of the SMV.
- The duodenojejunal junction is fixated in the left upper quadrant (LUQ) by the ligament of Treitz.
- The cecum is fixed to the retroperitoneum in the right lower quadrant (RLQ), within the right iliac fossa.[2,5]
- The term "malrotation" encompasses a spectrum of disorders that occur when less than 270° of rotation is achieved during embryologic development resulting in abnormal location of the cecum and the duodenojejunal junction.
- In the classic malrotation patient, the duodenojejunal junction lies to the right of the midline and the cecum lies to the left of the midline.

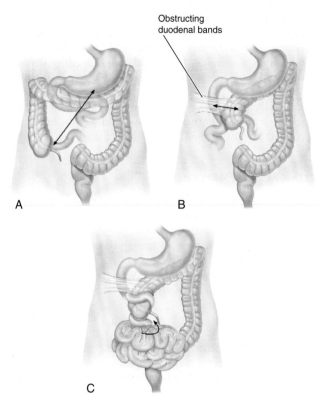

Figure 25.1 Malrotation with volvulus. A, Normal small bowel mesenteric attachment (as demonstrated by the arrow). This prevents twisting of small bowel because of the broad fixation of the mesentery. B, Malrotation of colon with obstructing duodenal bands (arrow, shortened mesenteric attachment). C, Midgut volvulus around the superior mesenteric artery caused by the narrow base of the mesentery (arrow shows twisting of bowel). (Reprinted with permission from Stephenson SR. *Diagnostic Medical Sonography*. 3rd ed. Philadelphia, PA: Wolters Kluwer/Lippincott Williams & Wilkins; 2012.)

- Additionally, a relatively long and narrow mesenteric root results as well as a peritoneal band that crosses from the right to left, from the cecum to duodenojejunal junction (Figure 25.1).[2,5]

EPIDEMIOLOGY AND ETIOLOGY

- The actual incidence of malrotation is estimated to be between 0.2% and 1% of the population but becomes symptomatic in approximately 1 of 2500 live births.[3,5]

- There is no gender preponderance.
- Etiology is thought to be multifactorial, as it is often associated with additional developmental abnormalities (eg, heterotaxy syndrome, congenital diaphragmatic hernias, anorectal malformations, duodenal webs, and intestinal atresias).[2,5,6]
- Generally, presentation is early, with 75% of patients presenting within 1 month of age. The majority of the remaining patients present within their first year of age.[2,5,6]

CLINICAL PRESENTATION

- Malrotation can present at any age and with a wide variety of symptoms of both acute and chronic nature.
- Age often correlates to symptomology.
- Bilious emesis is the most common presenting symptom in neonates with malrotation.
- However, older children and adults have a broader spectrum of symptoms, most commonly abdominal pain, but also emesis, diarrhea, and nausea.[6]
- Patients of any age can present with volvulus and acute abdomen.
- In these patients, the abdomen is distended and peritonitic and the overlying skin may have erythema.
- Patients will most likely have laboratory test results representative of metabolic acidosis.[2]
- There is also a subset of patients who are diagnosed with malrotation incidentally or who only have mild symptoms that are not life altering.
- These patients are generally not considered surgical candidates but must be educated on their disorder and instructed to seek emergency medical care if they begin to develop severe abdominal pain or if other symptoms worsen.[6,7]
- Malrotation exists as a spectrum of rotational disorders and abnormal anatomic orientations from reversed rotation to paraduodenal hernias (Table 25.1).
- The presentation is also dependent on the physical degree of malrotation.[2,6]
- This variation of presentation may lead to delayed diagnosis, most often in older children and adults, **so high clinical suspicion should always be maintained to avoid the devastating results of an undiagnosed volvulus**.[6]

TABLE 25.1

Spectrum of Anatomic Variations Associated With the Term "Malrotation"

	Rotational Abnormality	Anatomic Orientation	Associated Complications
Reversed rotation	90° clockwise rotation	Transverse colon to the right and dorsal to the SMA within a retroduodenal tunnel and within the small bowel mesentery	Volvulus with transverse colon obstruction
Nonrotation	Failure to rotate (0°)	Cecocolic limb at the left hemidiaphragm and duodenojejunal limb at the right hemidiaphragm	Midgut volvulus
Incomplete rotation	Arrested counterclockwise rotation at about 180°	Cecum at RUQ	Obstructing peritoneal bands
Mesocolic/paraduodenal hernias	Normal rotation (270°)	Failure of the right and left mesocolon to fuse with the posterior body wall creating a potential space	Small bowel sequestration and obstruction within aberrant potential space

RUQ, right upper quadrant; SMA, superior mesenteric artery.

DIAGNOSIS

- Historically, barium enema was used to evaluate the cecal position.[6]
- However, upper gastrointestinal (UGI) series is now accepted as the gold standard of diagnosis.[2,6,8]
- Ultrasound is becoming a more commonly used modality of diagnosis, especially in neonates and younger children.[9]
- In older children and adults, CT scan can be used to diagnose malrotation, as radiation concern is not as significant in older patients.
- CT will show the duodenojejunal junction to the right of the midline and the cecum to the left.
- Axial cuts also highlight the relatively anterior position of the duodenum.[6]
- As with most abdominal complaints, radiographic diagnosis usually begins with plain films, which will show a paucity of air within the distal small bowel.
- A "double-bubble" sign may also be seen, although this is nonspecific.[9]
- In an UGI contrast study, the duodenojejunal junction should be seen to the left of the vertebral column and take a posterior course within the abdomen on lateral films.
- In malrotation, the duodenojejunal junction is to the right of the midline and the distal duodenum takes an anterior course on lateral views.
- Redundant duodenum and severely distended bowels can mimic malrotation and result in a false-positive study.[8]
- Jejunal obstruction can also have a "coiled spring" or "corkscrew" appearance on an UGI series (Figure 25.2).[2]
- Color Doppler ultrasound can show dilated loops of duodenum and inversion of the SMA relative to the SMV, with the SMV lying to the left of the SMA.[9]
- This abnormal orientation of vessels can also be seen during prenatal ultrasounds, allowing for diagnosis of malrotation in utero.[9]
- Additionally, twisting of the mesentery and the vessels contained therein results in a swirling pattern of fat and vessels known as a "whirlpool" sign, which is indicative of acute volvulus (Figure 25.3).[2,9]

SURGICAL MANAGEMENT

- Symptomatic intestinal malrotation is most commonly managed today via an open surgical technique.[4]
- Since being described by Ladd in 1941, the procedure has remained relatively unchanged.[4,5]

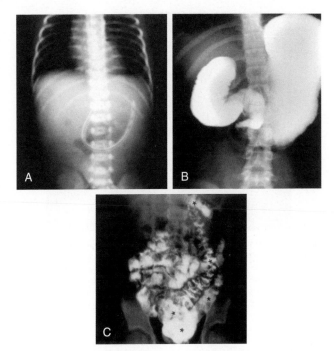

Figure 25.2 A, Plain radiograph of an infant with malrotation. There is a paucity of small bowel gas. B, Upper gastrointestinal contrast study demonstrating malrotation with midgut volvulus and duodenal obstruction. The position of the duodenojejunal junction is abnormal. C, Plain film showing a contrast-filled colon and cecum on the patient's left (asterisks). The entire small bowel is to the right of the midline. These are typical radiographic findings of malrotation. (Reprinted with permission from Mulholland MW, Lillemoe KD, Doherty GM, Upchurch GR, Alam HB, Pawlik TM. *Greenfield's Surgery: Scientific Principles and Practice.* 6th ed. Philadelphia, PA: Wolters Kluwer; 2017.)

- It is controversial whether laparoscopic technique should be used in the management of malrotation.
- There are significantly higher rates of postoperative volvulus associated with laparoscopic surgery.
- This is thought to be due to incomplete detorsion during laparoscopic procedure.
- Furthermore, decreased formation of adhesions during laparoscopic surgery result in insufficient fixation of bowels after detorsion.[4]
- However, advantages to laparoscopic surgery include earlier return to oral feeding, decreased length of hospital stay, and fewer postoperative complications overall.[3,4]

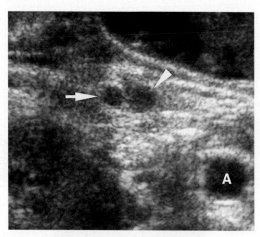

Figure 25.3 Transverse sonogram of a 6-week-old boy with vomiting shows inverted positioning of the mesenteric vessels. The superior mesenteric artery (arrow) lies to the right of the superior mesenteric vein (arrowhead). Subsequent upper gastrointestinal series confirmed malrotation (A, aorta). (Reprinted with permission from Siegel MJ, Coley BD. *Pediatric Imaging.* Philadelphia, PA: Lippincott Williams & Wilkins; 2006.)

- Additionally, laparoscopy can be used as an initial intervention when the diagnosis of malrotation is uncertain to avoid a negative exploratory laparotomy.[4]

Open Approach

- The patient is positioned supine, and the bowels and bladder are decompressed.[5]
- The abdomen is entered through an upper midline incision that extends below the umbilicus.
- The small bowel and its mesentery are eviscerated and any visible adhesive bands are lysed.
- If a volvulus is present, the bowel is then detorsed via counterclockwise rotations until it is decompressed and the mesentery appears to be completely untwisted.
- The right colon is mobilized by dividing the Ladd bands binding the cecum and duodenum to the right upper quadrant.
- The colon is also freed from the greater omentum and greater curvature of the stomach.
- Any adhesions between the mesentery and the jejunum or ileum are lysed, allowing the small bowels to fan out within the abdominal cavity.[5]

- The anterior mesenteric leaflet at the base of the SMA/SMV is incised, which allows for broadening of the mesentery and prevents recurrence of volvulus.[2]
- At this point, any bowel that appears dusky and devitalized after detorsion in cases of volvulus is resected, but care is taken to resect only as much bowel as necessary.
- Bowel may be left in discontinuity or primarily anastomosed depending on certainty of viability, which may be reassessed with a second-look laparotomy.[2]
- Then, the duodenojejunal junction is mobilized by freeing the third portion of the duodenum from the uncinate process of the pancreas, allowing the proximal jejunal loops to lie in the infrahepatic fossa.
- The rest of the bowel is placed inferiorly in an axial trajectory to ensure no twisting or angulation occurs.[5]
- Appendectomy is also performed to avoid misdiagnosis in the future given abnormal positioning.[2,4,5]
- Finally, the ileocecal junction is positioned in the left lower quadrant to further maximize mesenteric broadening.[5]
- No sutures are used to secure the bowel.[2]
- The abdomen is then closed if no bowel resection is necessary or left open to allow for second look 24 hours later, to be closed after definitive management has been achieved (Figure 25.4).[2]

Laparoscopic Approach

- The patient is again positioned supine with decompression of the stomach and bladder.[5]
- The patient is placed in reverse Trendelenburg with a 30° tilt.
- The physician can stand at the patient's feet or right side with the first assistant at the patient's left.[2,5]
- The abdomen is entered by inserting a 10-mm trocar via Hassan technique at the umbilicus and a camera is placed into the port.[2,5]
- Two additional 5-mm ports are placed via stab incisions at the RLQ and left subcostal locations to be used as working ports.
- A third 5-mm trocar can also be placed at the subxiphoid position for liver retraction if necessary.[2,5]
- With 2 graspers, the bowel is run and inspection of the abdomen is performed beginning with the second portion of the duodenum.[2]
- Peritoneal bands are lysed as they are encountered and volvulus is reduced if present.
- Any portions of bowel that appear ischemic are resected; conversion to open may be necessary.[2]

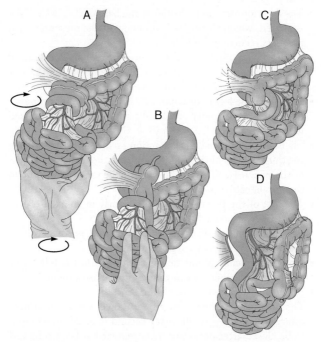

Figure 25.4 Correction of malrotation. A and B, Detorsion of midgut. C and D, Division of peritoneal attachments (Ladd bands) of the cecum to the abdominal cavity. (Reprinted with permission from Mulholland MW, Lillemoe KD, Doherty GM, Upchurch GR, Alam HB, Pawlik TM. *Greenfield's Surgery: Scientific Principles and Practice.* 6th ed. Philadelphia, PA: Wolters Kluwer; 2017.)

- Duodenum and jejunum are mobilized, and the anterior mesenteric leaflet is incised to broaden the mesenteric base.
- Laparoscopic appendectomy is then performed.
- If no bowel of questionable viability is encountered, exit of the abdomen would proceed as in a typical laparoscopic case.[2]

POSTOPERATIVE CARE

- Postoperative care is similar after both open and laparoscopic cases, although return to normal feeding is shorter with the laparoscopic approach.[4]
- For patients who had bowel resections or who were severely distended, NGT is left in place.
- Fluid resuscitation should continue and should be guided by urine output.[2]

- For patients with acute obstruction, return of bowel function can usually be expected within 5 days[4]
- For patients with chronic obstruction, postoperative ileus may be expected and should be managed accordingly.[4]

PEARLS AND PITFALLS

- Malrotation consists of a spectrum of disorders and presentation can vary widely depending on age and anatomic abnormality.
- Consider malrotation in any infant with acute onset bilious emesis and abdominal distention.
- An UGI series is the study of choice to diagnose malrotation in neonates and children.
- A CT is often used for diagnosis in adults.
- Ladd open procedure is still considered the standard of care by most pediatric surgeons, but the laparoscopic approach is gaining popularity and often results in earlier return to normal activities.

REFERENCES

1. Tan V, Kotobi H, Parc Y. Ladd procedure for malrotation with total intestinal volvulus. *J Visc Surg*. 2017(17):30043-30047 [pii:S1878-S7886].
2. Little DC, Smith S. In: Holcomb GW, Murphy JP, eds. *Ashcroft's Pediatric Surgery*. 5th ed. Philidelphia: Saunders Elsevier; 2010:416-424.
3. Kinlin K, Shawyer AC. The surgical management of malrotation: a Canadian association of pediatric surgeons survey. *J Pediatr Surg*. 2017;52(5):853-858.
4. Catania VD, Lauriti G, Pierro A, et al. Open vs laparoscopic approach for intestinal malrotation in infants and children: a systematic review and meta-analysis. *Pediatr Surg Int*. 2016;32(12):1157-1164.
5. Adams SD, Stanton MP. Malrotation and intestinal atresias. *Early Hum Dev*. 2014;90(12):921-925.
6. Nehra D, Goldstein AM. Intestinal malrotation: varied clinical presentation from infancy through adulthood. *Surgery*. 2011;149(3):386-393.
7. Graziano K, Islam S, Dasgupta R, et al. Asymptomatic malrotation: diagnosis and surgical management: an American pediatric surgical association outcomes and evidence-based practice committee systematic review. *J Pediatr Surg*. 2015;50(10):1783-1790.
8. Birajdar S, Rao SC, Bettenay F. Role of upper GI contrast studies for suspected malrotation in neonatal population. *J Paediatr Child Health*. 2017;53(7):644-649.
9. Orzech N, Navarro OM, Langer JC. Is US a good screening test for intestinal malrotation? *J Pediatr Surg*. 2006;41(5):1005-1009.

Chapter 26

Necrotizing Enterocolitis

Olga Zhadan

- Necrotizing enterocolitis (NEC) is an acquired inflammatory disease affecting the gut of newborns, predominantly premature infants.
- Incidence in infants weighing less than 1500 g is 10%.
- It is the most common newborn surgical emergency and leading cause of infant morbidity and mortality in neonatal intensive care units (NICUs).[1]

HISTORICAL BACKGROUND

- Pathologic findings of intestinal perforation in neonates as the cause of death were first described in 1888.
- Agerty in 1943 did the first report of successfully treated infant with localized ileal perforation.
- In 1953 Schmid and Quaiser first used the term *necrotizing enterocolitis*.
- In 1964 Berdon reported clinical and radiographic findings of 21 patients with NEC.

PATHOPHYSIOLOGY

- NEC is rare in full-term infants and those who have never been fed.
- Premature infants lack mature barrier defense owing to poorly developed mucosal cells; goblet cells produce scant amount of mucus; gastric, pancreatic, and intestinal secretions are reduced. Secretory IgA levels are low or absent.
- Three components are essential in the development of NEC: presence of bacteria, injury to intestinal mucosa, and availability of metabolic substrate (enteral feedings).
- Bacteria gain access to macrophages and dendritic cells of the innate immune system, which recognizes pathogenic bacteria toll-like receptors (TLRs). Based on the results of experiments in cell culture and in mice, it appears that NEC is a TLR4-driven process.

CLINICAL PRESENTATION

- Several days after feeds are started, abdomen becomes distended and large amount of bilious gastric residual is produced.
- Physical examination: distended abdomen, palpable bowel loops, and lethargy.
- **Erythema** of the abdominal wall is ominous sign developing when underlying gangrene or perforation of the bowel is present. It occurs because thin abdominal wall and lack of subcutaneous fat allow the inflammatory reaction to produce cellulitis.

DIAGNOSIS

Laboratory Findings

- Anemia, thrombocytopenia, neutropenia, and acidosis (resulting from hypovolemia and sepsis).
- Levels of IL-6, IL-10, and C-reactive protein are increased. The highest levels of IL-10 were documented in the patients who did not survive.
- Blood cultures are positive in 30% to 35% of patients and commonly grow *Escherichia coli*, *Klebsiella pneumoniae*, *Proteus mirabilis*, *Staphylococcus aureus*, *Staphylococcus epidermidis*, enterococci, *Clostridium perfringens*, and *Pseudomonas aeruginosa*. Peritoneal cultures are most commonly positive for *Klebsiella* species, *E. coli*, coagulase-negative staphylococci, *Enterobacter* species, and yeast.

Imaging Findings

- **Abdominal X-ray** (anteroposterior and left lateral decubitus views) is the current standard for diagnosing. **Pneumatosis intestinalis** (intramural gas) is the hallmark of NEC (Figure 26.1). **Portal venous air** is present in case of extensive intestinal injury, but it is **not** necessarily an indication for operation (Figure 26.2).
- **Abdominal ultrasound**: evaluation of bowel wall thickness and echogenicity, free and focal fluid collections, peristalsis, and the presence or absence of bowel wall perfusion by using Doppler imaging.

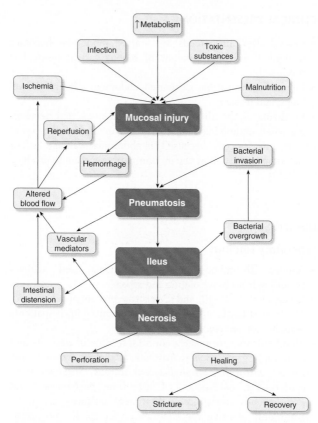

Figure 26.1 Necrotizing enterocolitis. This schematic is a composite of the theories about factors thought to be involved in the pathogenesis of NEC. Large boxes denote the progression of this disease, whereas small boxes denote the factors thought to initiate or propagate the disease process. (Reprinted with permission from Alldredge BK, et al. *Applied Therapeutics: The Clinical Use of Drugs.* 10th ed. Philadelphia, PA: Lippincott Williams & Wilkins; 2013. Originally adapted from Crouse DT. Necrotizing enterocolitis. In: Pomerance JJ, Richardson CJ, eds. *Neonatology for the Clinician.* Norwalk, CT: Appleton & Lange; 1993:364.)

INITIAL MANAGEMENT

- Over the past several decades, the management of infants with NEC evolved from early operation to supportive care, with the increasing realization that most infants can be managed nonoperatively.
- Initial treatment includes bowel rest, antibiotics, and supportive care.

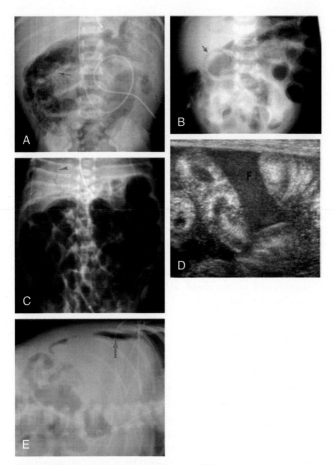

Figure 26.2 Necrotizing enterocolitis. A, Multiple loops of distended bowel have bubbly and linear radiolucencies in the bowel wall, representing pneumatosis intestinalis (arrows). B, Another patient with linear pneumatosis of the wall of the intestines (arrows). C, Another infant showing pneumatosis intestinalis and branching radiolucencies (arrowheads) within the liver representing air within the portal venous system. D, Ultrasound of another infant with perforation following necrotizing enterocolitis shows free intraperitoneal fluid (F) containing echogenic debris and punctated areas of high echogenicity within the intestinal wall (arrows), consistent with pneumatosis intestinalis. E, Left lateral decubitus radiograph shows free intraperitoneal air (arrow) indicating perforation in an infant with necrotizing enterocolitis. (Reprinted with permission from Brant WE, Helms C. *Fundamentals of Diagnostic Radiology*. 4th ed. Philadelphia, PA: Wolters Kluwer Health/Lippincott Williams & Wilkins; 2012.)

- **Bowel rest**: All feeds are held, Salem sump-type oro- or nasogastric tube should be placed to intermittent suction.
- Broad-spectrum **antibiotics** (7-14 d) should be given to cover both gram-negative and gram-positive microorganisms.
- Combinations of vancomycin and gentamicin or vancomycin and a third-generation cephalosporin are recommended owing to the reports of patients with stool and blood cultures positive for coagulase-negative staphylococci.
- Consider antifungal therapy if the patient's clinical course is prolonged.
- **Supportive care** includes intravenous fluid resuscitation, transfusions of red blood cells and platelets, endotracheal intubation, and blood pressure support with dopamine if necessary.
- Infants are monitored for abdominal distention, vomiting, or nonspecific signs and symptoms of NEC.
- Feedings are initiated with clinical improvement and return of bowel function.
- When feedings resume, stools are tested for reducing substances and occult blood. If the result is positive, feedings are discontinued.[2]

OPERATIVE TREATMENT

- The timing of operative treatment is based on experience and good clinical judgment.
- **Absolute indications** for operation in NEC: free intraperitoneal air, abdominal wall erythema, discolored abdomen due to meconium peritonitis, and meconium in processus vaginalis.
- **Relative indications** for operation in NEC: persistent or worsening acidosis or thrombocytopenia despite adequate resuscitation and fixed bowel loop (due to severe ischemia) on abdominal radiograph.
- Surgical intervention **does not halt** the pathologic process but rather treats the end result of NEC.
- In a single randomized prospective study, infants treated by peritoneal drain or laparotomy had the same outcomes.

GOALS OF OPERATIVE TREATMENT

- Effective preoperative volume resuscitation
- Correction of coagulopathy (with platelet transfusions)
- Removal of septic foci (stool, necrotic tissue)
- Diversion of the fecal stream
- Preservation of viable bowel

SURGICAL TECHNIQUE

Peritoneal Drainage

- If the infant remains septic and cannot be stabilized, bedside procedure should be considered.
- Peritoneal drainage is not a definitive treatment but can facilitate resuscitation efforts.
- It can be performed at the bedside with local anesthesia or with intravenous sedation.
- The abdominal skin is prepared and small skin incision is made in the right lower quadrant.
- The peritoneum is entered bluntly with a curved hemostat, and the meconium and air are evacuated.
- Irrigation with 10 to 15 mL/kg of warm saline is used to remove intraperitoneal meconium and wash out the peritoneal cavity with red rubber catheter.
- A 0.25-inch penrose drain is then placed into the peritoneal cavity aiming for the left upper quadrant.
- The drain is sutured in place including the muscle of the abdominal wall with a nylon suture.

Laparotomy

- In the stable infant or if the infant shows no improvement over the next 8 to 24 hours after the peritoneal drainage, laparotomy should be performed.
- Transverse supraumbilical incision provides access to the entire abdomen in small infants.
- As the liver capsule is poorly developed, incidental injury can easily lead to life-threatening exsanguination.
- If there are no umbilical lines in place, the falciform ligament should be transected and ligated to avoid inadvertent liver injury.
- Care should be taken entering the peritoneal cavity, as the bowel is usually distended, is friable, and requires careful handling.
- Bloody ascites is the sign of bowel gangrene.
- The bowel is delivered from the abdomen and examined.
- The goal of operative treatment of NEC is to preserve intestinal length.
- Resection is performed only when the bowel is gangrenous.
- Several approaches exist to preserve the intestinal length and avoid more than one ostomy.
- If only a **single segment of bowel** is involved, the best option is to resect the clearly dead bowel and create an ostomy of the proximal end.

- The ostomy is brought out through one end of the primary incision and does not need to be formally matured.
- The ostomy is sutured to the fascia of the abdominal wall, and the edges will roll back on their own over time.
- If the part of the proximal jejunum is resected, it can be closed with a large hemoclip.
- Primary anastomosis can be created in several days when the infant is taken back to the operating room (OR) hemodynamically stable and no further affected bowel is encountered.
- Any infant instability or additional bowel compromise should warrant an ostomy, regardless of how proximal it will be.
- In case of multiple bowel segments involved, a **"clip and drop back"** technique (introduced by Jay Grosfeld) is used.
- The gangrenous bowel segments are resected, and the ends of each segment are closed with a large hemoclip.
- The abdomen is closed, and the infant is brought back to the NICU for further resuscitation.
- The abdomen is reexplored 24 to 72 hours later.
- The patients who remain persistently hypotensive, acidotic, or thrombocytopenic should be taken back to the OR earlier, as they likely have additional gangrenous segments.

POSTOPERATIVE CARE

- Supportive care with IV fluids and parenteral nutrition; treatment of sepsis with antibiotics (7-14 d) and vasopressors.
- Intestinal decompression with a nasogastric tube until return of bowel function; antibiotics continued.
- Frequent early complication is **necrosis of the ostomy**. It can be caused by ongoing intestinal ischemia at the level of the ostomy, small size of the fascial defect, postoperative edema, or use of epinephrine for blood pressure support. Necrosis of the ostomy below the level of the skin warrants early revision if the infant is stable.
- Recurrent NEC occurs 5 to 6 weeks postoperatively in 5% of cases. Intestinal stricture must be ruled out.
- Symptoms of **intestinal strictures** include feeding intolerance, abdominal distention, and intestinal obstruction. Strictures can occur in the defunctionalized colon, most commonly in the sigmoid. Remember to perform routine radiographic examination of the colon before reversal of any ostomy. The strictures should be resected with creation of primary anastomosis.

- The most severe complication in NEC survivors is **short bowel syndrome**. The likelihood of achieving full enteral feeds is good if there is 15-cm bowel remaining with the ileocecal valve or 30-cm bowel remaining without the ileocecal valve.
- **Malabsorption, liver failure, line infections, ostomy complications, total parenteral nutrition (TPN) dependence,** and **neurodevelopmental delays** are common complications developing in the infants with NEC.
- Overall survival for infants with NEC treated medically is 65% to 90%; for those requiring surgery, it is 50% to 75%. It remains largely unchanged from 30 years ago.[3]

PEARLS AND PITFALLS

- NEC is the most common intra-abdominal emergency in infants.
- The incidence is lower in babies who are breastfed.
- First-line therapy is conservative management: bowel rest and decompression, IV fluids resuscitation, and antibiotics.
- Infants who require surgery have worse prognosis.
- The goals of surgery are to remove the septic foci and preserve intestinal length.
- Numerous surgical options exist, such as bowel resection, ileostomy, clip and drop back, and placement of drains.
- Infants treated by peritoneal drain or laparotomy have the same outcomes.
- Malabsorption, liver failure, line infections, stricture, ostomy complications, TPN dependence, short bowel syndrome, and neurodevelopmental delays are common in patients with NEC.
- There is need in development of preventive strategies for NEC (probiotics, toll-like receptor blockade).

REFERENCES

1. Henry MCW, Moss RL, Necrotizing enterocolitis. In: *Ashcraft's Pediatric Surgery*. 5th ed. Philadelphia: Elsevier Saunders; 2010:1006-1007.
2. Gingalewski CA. Necrotizing enterocolitis. In: Mattei P, ed. *Fundamentals of Pediatric Surgery*. New York: Springer; 2011:381-386.
3. Sylvester KG, Liu GY, Albanese CT. Necrotizing enterocolitis. In: *Pediatric Surgery*. 7th ed. Elsevier; 2012:1187-1207.

Chapter 27

Inflammatory Bowel Disease

Sana Ahmad Qureshi

- Inflammatory bowel disease (IBD) is a spectrum involving Crohn disease (CD) and ulcerative colitis (UC).
- CD was first written about by Dr Crohn in 1932 describing terminal ileitis.
- UC was described first in 1859 by Wilks and Moxon.
- Initially fecal diversion and end ileostomy were recommended earlier in the 1900s, but in 1944 Strauss and Strauss introduced proctocolectomy and ileostomy for severe UC.[1]

EPIDEMIOLOGY AND ETIOLOGY

- The annual incidence of UC varies between 0 and 19.2 per 100 000 in North America.
- CD has a similar incidence of 0 to 20.2 per 100 000 in North America.[3]
- There has been a general increase in incidence globally since World War II.[2]
- Approximately 25% of IBD cases present in childhood.
- Pediatric CD is slightly more dominant in males (1.5:1 ratio), but UC is equal.
- There is also a significantly higher ratio of CD to UC in children compared with adult populations.[4]
- Etiology of CD is unknown, but it is likely induced by multiple environmental and genetic factors.
- Mutations of *NOD2* and *CARD15* on chromosome 16 have been noted in 30% to 43% of CD patients.
- Also gene *IBD5* on chromosome 5q31 has been associated with perianal disease.
- A gene variant of *ATG16L1* has been recently noted to be related to increased abnormal inflammatory response.[2]
- UC is also not fully understood but is a chronic immune-mediated inflammatory condition.
- Recent genetic research has noted increased risk with presence of HLA-B27 and some association with *NOD2* and *IL23R* genes.

TABLE 27.1

Comparison of Crohn Disease and Ulcerative Colitis

	Crohn Disease	Ulcerative Colitis
Epidemiology	More common in whites vs blacks	More common in whites vs blacks
	More common in Jews vs non-Jews	No sex predilection
	More common in women	Affects young adults
	Affects young adults	
Extent	Transmural	Mucosal and submucosal
Location	Terminal ileum alone (30%)	Mainly the rectum
	Ileum and colon (50%)	May extend into descending colon
	Colon alone (20%)	May involve entire colon
	Involves other areas of GI tract (mouth to anus)	Does not involve other areas of GI tract
Gross features	Thick bowel wall and narrow lumen (leads to obstruction)	Inflammatory pseudopolyps
	Aphthous ulcers (early sign)	Areas of friable, bloody residual mucosa
	Skip lesions, strictures, and fistulas	Ulceration and hemorrhage
	Deep linear ulcers with cobblestone pattern	
	Fat creeping around the serosa	
Microscopic findings	Noncaseating granulomas	Ulcers and intestinal gland abscesses with neutrophils
	Lymphoid aggregates	Dysplasia of cancer may be present
	Dysplasia or cancer less likely	
Clinical findings	Recurrent right lower quadrant colicky pain with diarrhea	Recurrent left-sided abdominal cramping with bloody diarrhea and mucus
	Bleeding occurs with colon or anal involvement	

(continued)

TABLE 27.1 (CONTINUED)		
Comparison of Crohn Disease and Ulcerative Colitis		
	Crohn Disease	**Ulcerative Colitis**
Radiography	"String" sign in terminal ileum due to luminal narrowing	"Lead pipe" appearance chronic state
Complications	Fistulas, obstruction	Toxic megacolon
	Calcium oxalate renal calculi	Primary sclerosing cholangitis
	Malabsorption due to bile deficiency	Adenocarcinoma
	Macrocytic anemia due to vitamin B12 deficiency	

Reprinted with permission from Dudek RW, Louis TM. *High-Yield Gross Anatomy*. 5th ed. Philadelphia, PA: Lippincott Williams & Wilkins; 2015.

CLINICAL PRESENTATION

- Pediatric CD presents with colonic or ileocolonic involvement in 80% to 90% cases.
- They generally present with inflammatory disease and then progress into structuring and penetrating disease.[4]
- CD patients usually present with crampy abdominal pain usually in right lower abdomen, diarrhea, loss of appetite, weight loss, and failure to thrive (50%).
- 10% will have perianal fistulas or other perianal diseases such as fissures and abscesses.
- UC also presents mainly as pancolitis in children (80%-90%).[4]
- Initial symptoms usually are persistent diarrhea with blood, mucus, and pus, along with abdominal cramping, tenesmus, and anemia.
- Anorexia, weight loss, and growth retardation occur in up to 38% of UC patients.
- About 3% of patients develop colorectal cancer in the first 10 years of disease, which increased to 10% to 15% afterward.
- Extracolonic manifestations of IBD are arthralgias, skin lesions (erythema nodosum, pyoderma gangrenosum), osteoporosis, primary sclerosing cholangitis, nephrolithiasis, uveitis, and stomatitis.[1,2]

DIAGNOSIS

- During a thorough history and physical examination, rectal examination is important especially if there is any concern for perianal disease.

- An exam under anesthesia would be thorough and helpful in anxious patients.
- A tool to assess UC clinically was recently developed called the Pediatric Ulcerative Colitis Activity Index (PUCAI), which scores abdominal pain, rectal bleeding, stool consistency, number of stools, nocturnal stools, and activity level with a maximum score of 85.
- It has been helpful with guiding treatment progress and has been validated as a research tool.[1]

Laboratory Findings

- Complete blood count can show anemia, elevated WBC count, and thrombocytosis. Erythrocyte sedimentation rate and C-reactive protein are elevated in acute disease.
- Children may develop hypokalemia and hyponatremia from prolonged diarrhea.
- While stool cultures are sent and usually negative, *Clostridium difficile* infection may coincide and delay diagnosis.[1]
- IgA and IgG anti–*Saccharomyces cerevisiae* antibody (ASCA) is specific in CD.[2]

Imaging Findings

- Upper GI and small bowel follow through can assess location and extent of disease (Figure 27.1).
- CT and ultrasound can also help evaluate ileitis and intra-abdominal abscesses.
- MRI has been shown to be highly specific and sensitive for proximal small bowel disease (Figure 27.1).
- Barium enema can show diagnostic images of shortened, narrow, and rigid colons for UC but can also stimulate acute colitis, so the test is now less used (Figure 27.2).
- Colonoscopy and esophagogastroduodenoscopy are necessary for visualization and biopsy of diseased bowel.
- Capsule endoscopy (after ruling out stricture disease with upper GI) can evaluate small bowel disease.[2]

MEDICAL AND SURGICAL MANAGEMENT

Medical

- Systemic corticosteroids are the standard for moderate to severe CD and exacerbated UC.
- It is effective in inducing remission in 54% to 77% of UC and up to 90% in CD. Prednisone of 1 to 2 mg/kg per day with maximum of 40 to 60 mg/d can be administered.

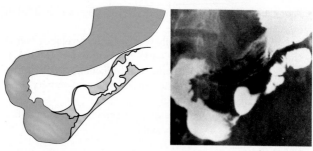

Figure 27.1 Crohn stricturing disease of the third and fourth parts of duodenum. (Reprinted from Block GE, Michelassi F, Tanaka M, et al. Crohn's disease. *Curr Probl Surg.* 1993;30(2):183-265. Copyright © 1993 Elsevier. With permission.)

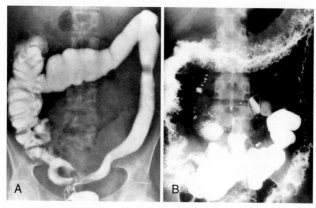

Figure 27.2 A, Chronic ulcerative colitis (UC) with shortening and loss of haustra. B, Severe UC with nodular, edematous mucosa. (Reprinted with permission from (A) Eisenberg RL. *Clinical Imaging: An Atlas of Differential Diagnosis.* 5th ed. Philadelphia, PA: Lippincott Williams & Wilkins; 2010; (B) Swischuk LE. *Emergency Imaging of the Acutely Ill or Injured Child.* 4th ed. Philadelphia, PA: Lippincott Williams & Wilkins; 2000:215.)

- It decreases production of proinflammatory cytokines (IL-1, IL-6, TNF-α).
- Owing to long-term side effects, it is not for maintenance therapy, although 50% of patients develop steroid dependency.
- It should be supplemented with calcium and vitamin D.
- **Mesalamine** is the first-line treatment for mild to moderate CD, unknown mechanism of action. Adverse effects (AE): rash, elevated LFTs, renal injury.

- **Azathioprine** (AZA) and **6-mercaptopurine** (6-MP), **thiopurine antimetabolite immunomodulators**, are the most effective treatments for long-term maintenance of CD and induction and maintenance of UC.
- AE include leukopenia, pancreatitis, and hepatotoxicity.
- **Methotrexate, dihydrofolate reductase inhibitor**, is the second-line immunomodulator therapy for CD.
- AE include bone marrow, pulmonary, and liver toxicity.
- **Infliximab and adalimumab** are monoclonal antibodies against TNF-α.
- They can be used for induction and maintenance therapy in CD and UC.
- Total liquid formula diet is used for nutritional support and can treat pediatric CD.[2]
- Antidiarrheal medications can help with decreased bowel movements but can occasionally lead to toxic megacolon.

Surgical

- Operative intervention for CD is recommended when there are failure of medical therapy, complications, severe dysphagia, cancer, and growth retardation.
- Obstruction is the most common indication in CD usually from strictures and is treated with an aim of minimal bowel loss.[2]
- Strictures <7 cm can be treated with Heineke-Mikulicz strictureplasty, which is performed by making a longitudinal incision on the antimesenteric side of the bowel about 2 cm distal and proximal to the stricture (Figure 27.3A).
- Intermediate segments between 7 and 15 cm can be managed with resection or Finney strictureplasty (Figure 27.3B).
- This is performed by folding the strictured loop, making a longitudinal incision halfway between the mesentery and antimesenteric border and sowing the bowel side to side as an anisoperistaltic anastomosis.
- For longer segments >15 cm, a side to side isoperistaltic strictureplasty can be performed.[5]
- Recently, endoscopic balloon dilation has been attempted with reasonable success for ileal and colonic strictures.[2]
- For perianal disease with CD, generally abscesses can be incised and drained and can either be packed with gauze or have a small drain placed.
- For fistula, a noncutting seton or a self-retaining catheter can be placed.[2]

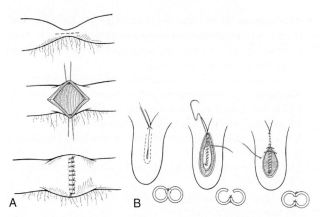

Figure 27.3 Heineke-Mikulicz (A) and Finney (B) strictureplasties. (From Scott-Conner CEH. Current surgical management of inflammatory bowel disease. *South Med J.* 1994;87(12):1232-1241. Reproduced with permission of Southern Medical Association in the format Book via Copyright Clearance Center.)

- For UC, total proctocolectomy is a curative procedure.
- It is usually performed for patients with refractory UC or emergent cases with fulminant colitis, extensive rectal bleeding, or toxic megacolon.
- Colectomy rates for UC in children used to be 50% after 5 years and are more recently down to 25% after 5 years.
- Total proctectomy and end ileostomy used to be the standard surgical treatment for UC, but because of ileostomy issues and complications, ileoanal pull through is the current recommended approach.[1]
- The patient is placed in lithotomy position, and initial subtotal colectomy from terminal ileum to rectosigmoid junction is performed through a midline incision.
- Then a mucosectomy from the proximal rectum is performed down to about 1 cm above the dentate line to prevent injury to the nervi erigentes and for sphincter preservation.
- The ileum is brought down for either a straight ileal-anal anastomosis or ileal pouch anastomosis hand sown or with a circular stapler.
- A diverting temporary ileostomy is created.
- There are 4 ileal pouch configurations with S- and W-shaped pouches, which are hand sewn, and J and lateral are created with stapling (Figure 27.4).

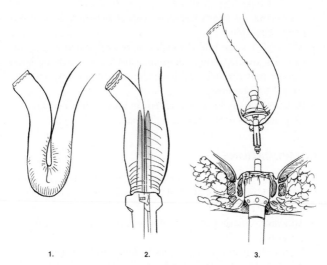

Figure 27.4 J pouch creation. 1, Loop of terminal ileum, 2, The antimesenteric border is stapled together, 3, An ileoanal anastomosis with a circular stapler. (From Fazio VW, Tjandra JJ, Lavery IC. Techniques of pouch construction. In: Nicholls J, Bartolo D, Mortensen N, eds. *Restorative Proctocolectomy.* 1st ed. Oxford, UK: Blackwell; 1993. Copyright © 1993 Blackwell Science Ltd. Adapted by permission of John Wiley & Sons, Inc.)

- The J pouch is most common because it is the simplest to create and has the fewest long-term complications.
- One key recommendation is to keep the total length of the pouch around 8 cm to allow adequate emptying of stool and lower chance of pouchitis.
- The procedure can be performed laparoscopically with a lower abdominal transverse incision to remove the colon.

POSTOPERATIVE CARE

- With an end ileostomy, patients generally have a hard time accepting it for long term and struggle with appliance-related issues.
- Although an ileoanal straight pull through is technically easier, patients have high urgency initially, but this normalizes after 2 years and is similar to a pouch.
- Also there is less chance of pouchitis as a complication.
- With an ileoanal pouch, patients have less bowel movements than a straight pull through and have normal sphincter function within 3 months.

- A diverting ileostomy decreases risk of anastomotic leak and pelvic infection.
- Although 1-stage pull through can be performed in polyposis cases, owing to inflammation, most UC patients undergo 2-stage pull through and have the loop ileostomy reversed after 2 to 3 months.
- Patients initially have 6 to 15 bowel movements per day, but they decrease in the next 2 to 3 years.[2]

COMPLICATIONS

- Pouchitis is most common after a pull through in about 10% to 50% of patients and is treated with 2 to 4 weeks of metronidazole.
- Adhesive obstruction can also occur in 10% to 30% of patients.
- Nocturnal incontinence occurs in about 40% initially.
- Pouch failure (stricture, leak, intractable pouchitis) can be caused by CD in 5% to 10%.[2]

PEARLS AND PITFALLS

- Differentiating CD and UC is vital when it comes to management because CD is not curable like UC with total proctocolectomy.
- Perioperative steroids and nutrition play major roles in patient health and complications.
- Continual follow-up with gastroenterologist and surgeon after surgery is highly important because of increased risk of colon cancer from chronic inflammation.
- A colonoscopy after 10 years from CD diagnosis is recommended, then every 3 years for the second decade, and then every 2 years.
- Postproctocolectomy and ileal-anal anastomosis for UC require sigmoidoscopy every 3 years.[1]

REFERENCES

1. Adler J, Coran AG, Tietelbaum DH. Ulcerative colitis. In: Coran A, Arnold G, Anthony C, Scott N, eds. *Pediatric Surgery*. 7th ed. N.p; 2012 [Print].
2. Adibe OO, Georgeson KE. Crohn's disease. In: Coran A, Arnold G, Anthony C, Scott N, eds. *Pediatric Surgery*. 7th ed. N.p; 2012 [Print].
3. Ananthakrishnan AN. Epidemiology and risk factors for IBD. *Nat Rev Gastroenterol Hepatol*. 2015;12(4):205-217 [Web].

4. Sauer CG, Kugathasan S. Pediatric inflammatory bowel disease: highlight-ing pediatric differences in IBD. *Med Clin North Am*. 2010;94(1):35-52 [Web].
5. Maggiori L, Michelassi F, Cameron J. Strictureplasty in Crohn's disease. In: *Current Surgical Therapy*. 11th ed. N.p; 2014 [Print].

Chapter 28

Pediatric Abdominal Wall Hernias

Sarah Simko

INGUINAL HERNIAS

- Inguinal hernias were first described in the Ebers Papyrus in 1550 BC.
- In AD 150, Galen defined hernias as a rupture of the peritoneum, and in the 16th century, Ambrose Paré documented the need for repair of hernias in childhood.[1]
- In the 1800s, the involved anatomic structures were discovered and surgical techniques for repair were developed.
- Gross performed a large series of hernia repairs in 1953, reporting a recurrence rate of 0.45%.[1]

EMBRYOLOGY

- The processus vaginalis forms during the third month of gestation from an outpouching of the peritoneum, creating a diverticulum at the internal ring.
- In males, the processus vaginalis obliterates spontaneously after the descent of the testes, usually by 2 years of age.
- In females, the processus vaginalis correlates to the diverticulum of Nuck and normally obliterates at 7 months' gestation.

RELEVANT ANATOMY

- The inguinal canal is a channel through the abdominal wall through which
  - The spermatic cord extends from the abdomen into the scrotum in males (Figure 28.1).
  - The round ligament extends from the abdomen into the labia majora in females.
- The canal is bordered by the aponeurosis of the external oblique muscle anteriorly and the transversus abdominus muscle and the transversalis fascia posteriorly.

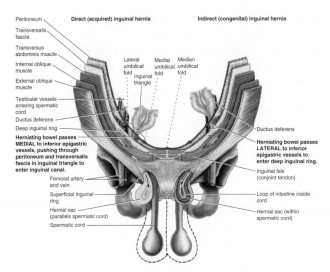

Figure 28.1 Inguinal hernia anatomy. (Reprinted with permission from Moore KL, Dalley AF, Agur AMR. *Clinically Oriented Anatomy.* 6th ed. Philadelphia, PA: Lippincott Williams & Wilkins; 2010:213.)

- Hesselbach triangle is an area of risk for direct herniation and is bounded by the inferior epigastric vessels, the inguinal ligament, and the rectus abdominus.
- The external inguinal ring, formed by the external oblique muscle, is located superior and lateral to the pubic tubercle.
- The internal inguinal ring is located in the transversalis fascia.
- In infants the external ring lies almost directly over the internal ring, which leads to increased risk of herniation.
- A congenital indirect inguinal herniation is the protrusion of fat or bowel through the processus vaginalis through the internal and external rings.
- A direct inguinal herniation is the protrusion of fat or bowel through the Hesselbach triangle and through the external ring.
- An incarcerated hernia is one that can no longer be reduced, while a strangulated hernia is one that has a compromised vascular supply.

EPIDEMIOLOGY AND ETIOLOGY

Incidence: The overall incidence of inguinal hernias in children is 4/100 live births.
- Males are affected approximately 10 times more frequently than females.

- Of inguinal hernias, 60% to 75% occur on the right side, and 15% to 20% of cases are bilateral.
- Preterm infants also have an increased risk with 30% of infants weighing less than 1 kg developing inguinal hernias.[2]
- The rate of incarceration is between 5% to 15% in the pediatric hernia population, with preterm infants having higher rates of up to 31%.[2]
- Peak incidence is during the first 3 months of life.[4]
- Most inguinal hernias are indirect; direct hernias are rare at this age.

Etiology:

- The predominance of congenital inguinal hernias is due to failure of the proximal processus vaginalis to close (Figure 28.2).
- This closure is thought to be hindered by the persistence of smooth muscle.[3]

CLINICAL PRESENTATION

Classic presentation: An infant presents with an intermittent bulge in the groin, scrotum, or labia.

- The bulge is often exacerbated by increased intra-abdominal pressures, for example, when an infant cries or has a bowel movement.
- Examiners should palpate the external ring with 1 finger to feel for the spermatic cord and associated structures.
- If a hernia is present, often the "silk glove sign" or thickening of the spermatic cord/associated structures will be evident.
- This clinical sign has a diagnostic sensitivity of 91% and a specificity of 97.3%.[2]
- Diagnosis of an inguinal hernia is often a clinical diagnosis.

DIAGNOSIS

Laboratory Findings

- Routine laboratory work is not helpful in the evaluation of patients with inguinal hernias.
- One study of 69 infants with incarcerated hernias found no correlation between white blood cell count and degree of vascular compromise.[3]

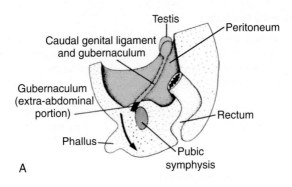

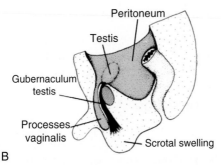

Figure 28.2 Patent processus vaginalis. A, When the uterus forms, the caudal ligament is interrupted in its course by growth of the uterus and becomes attached to the uterine wall. The part of the ligament from the ovary to this wall forms the proper ligament of the ovary, while the part extending from the wall to the labia majora forms the round ligament of the uterus. In addition, a cranial ovarian ligament, the suspensory ligament, forms from urogenital ridge mesoderm to hold the ovary in place at this pole. In males, the caudal genital ligament becomes surrounded by a band of mesenchyme tissue called the gubernaculum testis. B, Initially, this tissue band terminates in the inguinal region, but later it grows down to the floor of the scrotum. The gubernaculum is largely responsible for pulling the testes into the scrotum. Thus, outgrowth of the gubernaculum from the inguinal region to the scrotum pulls the testes to the inguinal area; then, as organ growth occurs and intra-abdominal pressure increases, the testes are pushed into and through the inguinal canal. The testes reach the inguinal region by 12 weeks, pass through the inguinal canal by 28 weeks, and reach the scrotum by 33 weeks. To pass from their intra-abdominal position of origin to the scrotum, the testes must migrate through the abdominal wall via the inguinal canal. They are preceded in this maneuver by an outpocketing of peritoneum called the processes vaginalis (B). (Reprinted with permission from Sadler TW, Langman J, Sadler TW. *Langman's Essential Medical Embryology*. Philadelphia, PA: Lippincott Williams & Wilkins; 2005.)

Imaging Findings

- Although not typically used, ultrasound may be useful in the diagnosis of inguinal hernias when the etiology of groin swelling cannot be determined on clinical examination.
- The diagnostic accuracy of ultrasound for groin conditions is 93%.[3]
- One study reported that a full hernia was found on surgical exploration when a groin width of 7.2 ± 2 mm was detected via ultrasound.[5]

SURGICAL MANAGEMENT

- Surgical management varies based on the age and presentation of the infant.
- Preterm infants have a higher rate of incarceration; therefore, these hernias are often repaired before discharge.
- Most inguinal hernias can be repaired electively.

OPERATIVE INTERVENTION

- The classic surgical procedure for pediatric inguinal hernia repair is high ligation and excision of the processus vaginalis.
- This can be performed either laparoscopically or open depending on surgeon preference.
- Open surgery is considered to be the gold standard; however, laparoscopic surgery is beneficial in that the surgeon is able to look for defects bilaterally and may be less traumatic to the spermatic cord.

Open Approach

- To begin, the external ring is identified inferior and lateral to the pubic tubercle.
- An incision is made along the inguinal crease superior and lateral to the pubic tubercle, cutting through the skin, dermis, Camper fascia, and Scarpa fascia, being careful to avoid the inferior epigastric vein.
- The external oblique muscle is identified and incised after clearing the inguinal ligament, and blunt dissection is used to visualize the inguinal canal.
- The inguinal canal contains the spermatic cord, the hernia sac, the iliofemoral and ilioinguinal nerves, and the cremasteric muscle.
- The cremasteric muscle fibers are spread to visualize the hernia sac, and the sac is dissected away from the spermatic cord.

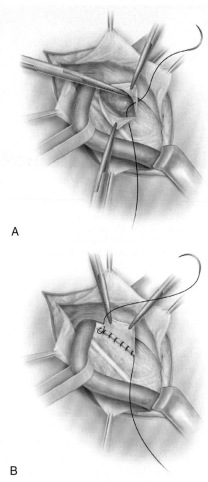

A

B

Figure 28.3 Open inguinal hernia repair. A, Only the defect in the posterior inguinal floor is opened. B, The defect is repaired primarily by 2 overlapping rows of suture. (Reprinted with permission from Jones DB. *Master Techniques in Surgery: Hernia*. Philadelphia, PA: Wolters Kluwer/Lippincott Williams & Wilkins; 2013.)

- The sac is opened, and the proximal portion is dissected free up to the internal ring.
- Next, the sac is twisted to prevent future herniation and ligated with a stick tie.
- The incision is then closed in layers (Figure 28.3).

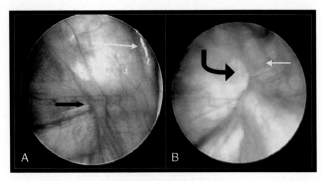

Figure 28.4 Laparoscopic images of normal anatomy versus inguinal hernia. A, Normal anatomy of the inguinal region. Black arrow indicates the closed deep inguinal ring; white arrow indicates the inferior epigastric vessels. B, An indirect inguinal hernia. Black arrow indicates the mouth of the hernial sac; white arrow indicates the inferior epigastric vessels. (Courtesy of NS Adzick. Reprinted with permission from Snell RS. *Clinical Anatomy by Regions.* 9th ed. Philadelphia, PA: Wolters Kluwer/Lippincott Williams & Wilkins; 2012.)

Laparoscopic Approach

- There are 2 laparoscopic approaches that are performed—intracorporeal repair and percutaneous ligation; however, many variations of these procedures exist.
- Figure 28.4 shows the visualization of normal anatomy versus an inguinal hernia via laparoscopic approach.
- For intracorporeal repair, 3 ports and nonabsorbable sutures are used.
- The peritoneum is closed primarily with interrupted sutures in a Z, W, or purse-string fashion, lateral to the cord structures.[6]
- The extracorporeal or percutaneous repair has grown more popular, as it is simpler and has lower recurrence rates.[5]
- In this repair, a suture held on the tip of a sharp instrument is introduced percutaneously and placed around the processus vaginalis extraperitoneally at the level of the internal inguinal ring.
- The sutures are advanced carefully between the peritoneum and the cord structures to avoid ligation of these structures, and the sutures are tied extracorporeally.
- This allows for ligation of the patent processus vaginalis.

POSTOPERATIVE CARE

- Most infants in the postoperative period can go home as soon as they are awake and able to drink fluids.

- If the infant is premature, they may be kept in the hospital to monitor their breathing as the anesthesia wears off.
- Pain can be managed with Motrin or Tylenol at home.

Complications

- The major complications after surgery for inguinal hernia repair are rare but include hematoma, infection, gonadal complications, and intestinal resection.
- Testicular atrophy occurs in 2% to 9% of patients after emergent operative reduction of incarceration because of vascular compromise.[3]
- Intestinal resection is necessary in 3% to 7% of patients in whom the hernia becomes strangulated.[4]
- The largest study of open repairs reports a recurrence rate of 1.2%.[2]
- The recurrence rates for laparoscopic hernia repairs ranged between 1% to 4%.[2]

PEARLS AND PITFALLS

- The majority of inguinal hernias are due to failure of the processus vaginalis to close.
- Diagnosis of hernias is a clinical diagnosis, but ultrasound can be used if the diagnosis is unclear.
- Extracorporeal laparoscopic surgery is gaining popularity for inguinal hernia repair.

UMBILICAL HERNIAS

- Like inguinal hernias, umbilical hernias have been studied for thousands of years.
- The diagnosis and various treatments for hernias were described by the Egyptians, Phoenicians, and ancient Greeks.
- The word "hernia" is derived from the Greek word for a bud or shoot.

EMBRYOLOGY

- At 5 weeks' gestation, the umbilical vessels are formed from mesenchymal tissue and enter the body through the umbilical ring.
- The umbilical cord consists of 2 arteries, 1 vein, the omphalomesenteric duct, urachal remnants, and connective tissue.

- After birth the umbilical ring generally closes as the rectus abdominis fuses into the linea alba and the umbilical arteries are obliterated.

RELEVANT ANATOMY

- An umbilical ring can persist and allow for direct or indirect herniation.
- The hernia sac is peritoneum and is often attached to the dermis of the umbilical skin.
- Layers of the abdominal wall from the inside out are the peritoneum, muscular layer, fat, and skin (Figure 28.5).

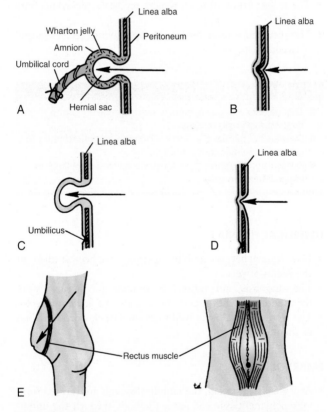

Figure 28.5 Umbilical hernia anatomy. A, Congenital umbilical hernia. B, Infantile umbilical hernia. C, Paraumbilical hernia. D, Epigastric hernia. E, Separation of recti abdominis. (Reprinted with permission from Snell RS. *Clinical Anatomy by Regions*. 9th ed. Philadelphia, PA: Wolters Kluwer/Lippincott Williams & Wilkins; 2012.)

EPIDEMIOLOGY AND ETIOLOGY

Incidence: The incidence of umbilical hernia is between 10% and 30% in children.

- African Americans are affected approximately 6 to 10 times more frequently than Caucasian infants.
- Newborns who weigh less than 1200 g are about 4 times more likely to have an umbilical hernia than those who weigh greater than 2500 g.[2]
- Infants with Down or Beckwith-Wiedemann syndrome have a higher risk as well.

Etiology:

- All neonates are born will a small umbilical defect; however, the umbilical ring generally closes within days to weeks of birth.
- Umbilical hernia occurs due to incomplete closure of the umbilical ring or weakness of the fascia at the ring through which peritoneal contents can herniate.

CLINICAL PRESENTATION

Classic presentation: An infant presents with a bulge at his/her umbilicus.

- The hernia is usually asymptomatic and rarely becomes incarcerated or strangulated.
- The bulge may only be present when the baby is crying, straining, or coughing.

DIAGNOSIS

Laboratory Findings

- Routine laboratory work is generally not helpful in the evaluation of patients with umbilical hernias, and diagnosis is generally made by history and physical examination.

Imaging Findings

- Imaging studies are usually not used for umbilical hernias.

SURGICAL MANAGEMENT

- Umbilical hernias can be observed or surgically repaired.
- Most resolve spontaneously by the age of 5 years and can be managed with observation and consistent follow-up.
- Surgical indications include persistence of defects beyond ages 3 to 4 years and incarceration or enlargement of fascial defects.[7]

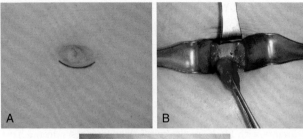

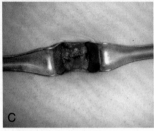

Figure 28.6 Repair of a small umbilical hernia. A, Curvilinear incision (may be either infra- or supraumbilical). B, Hernia sac circumferentially dissected and fascial defect defined. C, Hernia sac reduced and fascial defect closed with interrupted sutures in transverse fashion. (Reprinted with permission from Scott-Conner CEH, Dawson DL, eds. *Scott-Conner & Dawson Essential Operative Techniques and Anatomy*. 4th ed. Philadelphia, PA: Wolters Kluwer/Lippincott Williams & Wilkins; 2014.)

OPERATIVE INTERVENTION

- Umbilical hernias are surgically reduced and repaired via an open approach under general anesthesia.

Open Approach

A semicircular infraumbilical incision is made, and the subcutaneous layers are dissected to expose the hernia sac. Next, the hernia sac is divided and the hernia reduced, and the fascial defect is closed with interrupted transverse sutures. The skin is then closed with interrupted sutures (Figure 28.6).

POSTOPERATIVE CARE

- After the operation, most infants can go home as soon as they are awake and able to drink fluids.
- If infants are premature, they made be kept in the hospital to monitor their breathing as the anesthesia wears off.
- Pain can be managed with Motrin or Tylenol at home.

Complications

- Complications from umbilical hernia repair include local wound infection, effects of anesthesia, and strangulated bowel.
- Postoperative pain is generally mild and improves over a few days.
- Strangulation occurs in 8 in 1000 infants, and wound infection occurs in 7 in 1000.[8]

PEARLS AND PITFALLS

- Umbilical hernias are very common in the pediatric population and typically close spontaneously by the age of 3 to 4 years.
- Diagnosis of umbilical hernias is a clinical diagnosis and can normally be made by a physical examination alone.
- Hernia repair can usually be performed electively, unless the bowel becomes incarcerated.

REFERENCES

1. Holcomb GW, Murphy JP. *Ashcraft's Pediatric Surgery*. Saunders Elselvier; 2010:646-680.
2. Kelly KB, Ponsky TA. Pediatric abdominal wall defects. *Surg Clin*. 2013;93:1255-1267.
3. Ramsook C. Inguinal hernia in children. *Uptodate*. 2017.
4. Tovar JA. Hernias – inguinal, umbilical, epigastric, femoral and hydrocele. In: Puri P, ed. *Pediatric Surgery*. 1st ed. New York: Springer-Verlag; 2006:139-152.
5. Erez I, Rathause V, Vacian I, et al. Preoperative ultrasound and intraoperative findings of inguinal hernias in children: a prospective study of 642 children. *J Pediatr Surg*. 2002;37(6):865-868.
6. Lukong CS. Surgical techniques of laparoscopic inguinal hernia repair in childhood: a critical appraisal. *J Surg Tech Case Rep*. 2012;4(1):1.
7. Marinković S, Bukarica S. Umbilical hernia in children. *Med Pregl*. 2003;56(5-6):291-294.
8. *Pediatric Umbilical Hernia Repair*. American College of Surgeons; 2013.

SUGGESTED READING

Chirdan LB, Uba AF, Kidmas AT. Incarcerated umbilical hernia in children. *European J Pediatr Surg*. 2006;16(1):45-48.

Chapter 29

Meconium Ileus

Ann Alyssa Kurian

- Karl Landsteiner first described meconium ileus in 1905. He noted the association of meconium obstructing the small bowel with pathologic pancreatic enzyme deficiency.[1]
- Guido Fanconi coined the term *cystic fibrosis of the pancreas* in 1936, in patients with chronic pulmonary disease of infancy and pancreatic insufficiency.[1]
- In 1938, Dorothy H Andersen discovered similar histologic features of the pancreas in infants with cystic fibrosis (CF) and meconium ileus and described meconium ileus as an early and severe presentation of CF.[1]

EPIDEMIOLOGY AND ETIOLOGY

Incidence

- Present in up to 20% of infants with CF
- Incidence of CF is 1 in every 1000 to 2000 live births[2]
- Heterozygous carrier rate of CF mutation in Caucasian population is 5% to 6%[2]

Etiology

- CF is inherited in an autosomal recessive pattern
- Mutation in the CF gene on the long arm of chromosome 7q[2]
- Most common mutation is ΔF508, which results in the loss of a single phenylalanine amino acid on the cAMP-activated chloride channel protein encoded by the CF transmembrane conductance regulator gene *(CFTR)*[2]
- Meconium ileus can also be associated with RARE conditions, pancreatic aplasia or total colonic aganglionosis, rather than CF[3]
- Pathophysiology: An increase in protein concentration of meconium from 7% (normal infants) to 80% to 90% (CF) results in abnormally viscous meconium. Abnormal small intestinal glands and concentrating mechanisms also contribute to the adherence of this thickened meconium to ileal mucosa, and this leads to inspissated pellets within the lumen of distal ileum/proximal colon[2]

CLINICAL PRESENTATION

- Presentation is classified as simple or complicated. About half the cases present as simple bowel obstruction, and half present with complications such as volvulus, gangrene, atresia, perforation, meconium peritonitis, or giant cystic meconium peritonitis.[3]
- Maternal polyhydramnios is present in 20% of cases.[2]

Simple Meconium Ileus

- Newborn may appear healthy at first, then in the first 1 to 2 days of life presents with abdominal distention, bilious vomiting, and failure to pass meconium.[3]
- Terminal ileum is small in caliber and molds around inspissated meconium, with proximal bowel being dilated and filled with thick meconium, gas, and fluid.[3]

Complicated Meconium Ileus

- Neonate presents with more severe symptoms, such as peritonitis and sepsis, within 24 hours of birth.[3] Patients can have abdominal distention, with palpable "doughy" meconium impacted bowel. They can also present with respiratory distress, hypovolemia, and hemodynamic instability.[2]
- Segmental volvulus of distended segment of ileum → occlusion of mesenteric blood flow → ischemic bowel necrosis → intestinal atresia with mesenteric defects or perforation.[3]
- Prenatal perforation: Most sterile meconium reabsorbed with residual meconium forms calcifications.[3]
- Meconium peritonitis: It results from perforation, especially when perforation fails to seal before birth. Meconium is sterile before birth but becomes colonized after birth, and meconium peritonitis can become superinfected with bacteria.[3]
- Types of meconium peritonitis include adhesive, giant cystic (pseudocyst), meconium ascites, and infected meconium peritonitis.[3]

DIAGNOSIS

Diagnostic Testing

- Confirmatory testing for CF is required for any infant presenting with meconium ileus.[3]
- Tests include chloride sweat test, in which sweat production is stimulated using pilocarpine and an electrical current.[2] 100 mg of sweat must be collected, and a chloride

concentration of 60 mEq/L is diagnostic of CF.[1] This test is performed several weeks after birth.[1-3]

- Genetic testing of the *CFTR* gene also commonly performed; however, most panels will test for only the most common mutations. Amniocentesis may be offered for prenatal genetic testing if parents are known carriers.[1]

- Meconium can be tested for increased albumin concentration, with meconium of neonate with CF containing 80 mg albumin per gram of stool versus 5.0 mg/g of stool in normal neonates.[1]

- Stool trypsin and chymotrypsin levels can also be tested, with concentration of less than 80 mg trypsin/g of stool along with operative findings of meconium ileus being diagnostic of CF.[1,3]

Imaging Findings

- Third trimester prenatal ultrasound can show dilated, hyperechoic bowel.[1,3] Intra-abdominal mass and nonvisualization of the gallbladder can also be present.[3]

- Plain film radiography of the neonate will show unevenly dilated loops of bowel with relative absence of air-fluid levels. The bowel wall can have a "ground glass" appearance because of bubbles of swallowed air suspended in viscous meconium, also known as Neuhauser sign.[1-3]

- Abdominal X-ray in complicated meconium ileus can show calcifications, indicating extravasation of meconium, massive bowel dilation, mass effect due to pseudocyst, and ascites.[2]

- Contrast enema is used to further assess findings of intestinal obstruction in the newborn with suspected simple meconium ileus. Water soluble contrast is used, and it usually reveals a small caliber colon (microcolon of disuse), which can contain small, inspissated pellets of meconium.[3]

MANAGEMENT

Nonoperative Management

- First, stabilize the patient, and treat the bowel obstruction with volume resuscitation, nasogastric tube (NG) tube decompression, replete electrolytes, and respiratory support if needed. Also, correct coagulopathy and administer broad-spectrum antibiotics.[3]

- Many cases of **simple meconium ileus** can be treated with hyperosmolar contrast enema washout, which draws fluid into the lumen of the bowel and allows for osmotic diarrhea and diuresis.[2,3]

- A rectal catheter is placed under fluoroscopic guidance; balloon inflation of the catheter is avoided to minimize perforation risk.
- 25% to 50% Gastrografin solution is gently instilled through the catheter. Enema is administered under fluoroscopy to visualize reflux of contrast into the proximal dilated small bowel. Pellets of meconium followed by thick meconium will begin to pass and continue for the next 24 to 48 hours.
- Abdominal X-ray should be taken after enema and then every 8 to 12 hours post enema to evaluate for resolution of obstruction and monitor for signs of perforation.
- After hyperosmolar enema, patient should be transferred to NICU for monitoring, and serial enema can be performed with 1% N-acetylcysteine solution in warm saline.
- In cases of incomplete evacuation of meconium or absence of reflux of contrast into the proximal dilated bowel, a second Gastrografin enema can be performed. After 2 failed attempts, operative exploration is likely required.
- Patients require aggressive volume resuscitation during hyperosmolar enema, 1 to 3 times maintenance rate or 150 mL/kg per day.[1,3]

Operative Intervention

- Operative interventions include enterotomy or appendicostomy for simple meconium ileus, which failed to resolve with nonoperative management.
- A catheter is placed through either the enterotomy or the appendiceal stump; the distal ileum containing inspissated meconium is irrigated with saline, N-acetylcysteine, or Gastrografin.
- The enterotomy can either be closed primarily or a T-tube can be left in place for continued irrigation postoperatively.
- If the aforementioned method is inadequate, or patient has complicated meconium ileus, enterostomy with or without a bowel resection may be required.
- Enterostomy allows for continued irrigation of the distal ileum and infusion of pancreatic enzymes into the distal ileum.
- The following enterostomy methods have been described:
  - Mikulicz double-barreled side-to-side enterostomy: A loop of bowel is exteriorized, then enterotomy is made; a spur-crushing Mikulicz clamp is applied to create side-to-side anastomosis.
  - Benefits include avoidance of enterotomy until abdominal incision is closed, being a quick procedure that does not

require irrigation of meconium at time of operation, and potential for spontaneous closure of the anastomosis and enterocutaneous fistula.

- Bishop-Koop procedure: It includes resection of distal ileum containing inspissated meconium, creation of a proximal end to distal side anastomosis, and creation of stoma with open end of distal ileum.
- This allows for decompression of distal obstruction and infusion of pancreatic enzymes or irrigation.
- This can potentially be closed at bedside.[1]
- Santulli procedure: It is the reverse of the Bishop-Koop procedure.
- After resection, proximal side to distal end anastomosis is created, and the end of the proximal limb is brought to the anterior abdominal wall as an ostomy.
- This allows for enhanced proximal decompression and irrigation, although it results in a high-output stoma.
- Complicated meconium ileus must be treated urgently with adhesiolysis, resection of necrotic bowel, debridement and resection of pseudocyst if present, and distal irrigation.
- If there is no bacterially infected ascites, there is potential for primary anastomosis, with or without a enterostomy as described earlier.
- In the setting of bacterially infected ascites, avoid primary anastomosis.[1,2]
- Attempt should be made to reverse enterostomy in 4 to 6 weeks, to avoid complications of high-output stoma and electrolyte imbalance.[3]

POSTOPERATIVE CARE

- Once the obstruction is resolved, conservatively or operatively, administer 5 mL of 10% N-acetylcysteine solution via NG tube every 6 hours and initiate feeding when obstruction is resolved with pancreatic enzyme supplementation.[3]
- If enteral feeding not feasible, total parenteral nutrition should be initiated.[1,3]
- Prophylactic chest physiotherapy is initiated immediately postoperatively in the setting of CF.[1,3]

Complications

- Complication of hyperosmolar enema include perforation, early perforation from rectal catheter, or late perforation from repeated enema or bowel distention, and also hypovolemic shock due to osmotic diarrhea and diuresis.[3]

- One-year survival rates for simple meconium ileus are 92% to 100% and of complicated meconium ileus are 75% to 89%. Late complications are due to complications of CF including respiratory failure, distal intestinal obstructive syndrome, appendicitis, intussusception, rectal prolapse, colonic stricture due to pancreatic insufficiency, and gallbladder disease.[2]

PEARLS AND PITFALLS

- Consider meconium ileus in neonate with bowel obstruction and failure to pass meconium.
- Simple meconium ileus can often be treated nonoperatively, whereas complicated meconium ileus requires operative intervention.
- Meconium ileus is often a severe and early onset presentation of CF.
- Long-term treatment of CF is key to overall survival.

REFERENCES

1. Grosfeld JL. Meconium ileus. In: *Pediatric Surgery*. 6th ed. Vol 1. Mosby Elsevier; 2006:1289-1303.
2. Arensman RM. Meconium ileus. In: *Pediatric Surgery*. 2nd ed. Landes Bioscience; 2009:270-273.
3. Holcomb GW, Murphy JP. Meconium disease. In: *Ashcraft's Pediatric Surgery*. 5th ed. Saunders/Elsevier; 2010:425-434.

Chapter 30

Hirschsprung Disease

Sana Ahmad Qureshi

- Although there were sporadic case reports of pediatric colonic obstruction since 1691, Dr Harald Hirschsprung, a pediatrician from Copenhagen, first published observation of the pathologic megacolon in 1886.
- In 1920 Dalla Valle described the local absence of ganglion cells in the sigmoid colon in 2 brothers.
- Dr Swenson, Neuhauser, and Picket in Boston in 1948 noted the area of rectal spasm using barium enema, and Dr Swenson went on to perform the first colonic resection and coloanal anastomosis for Hirschsprung disease.
- Dr Soave in 1963 from Italy described the endorectal pull-through procedure to approximate normal innervated bowel with the perineum.[1]

RELEVANT ANATOMY

- The ascending and proximal two-thirds of the transverse colon receive blood supply from the superior mesenteric artery (SMA) and vein, which is derived from the midgut.
- The distal third of the transverse colon and descending colon and rectum receive blood supply by the inferior mesenteric artery (IMA) and vein derived from the hindgut.
- The rectum forms as the sigmoid colon's taeniae converge and is supplied by the superior rectal arteries (from the IMA) and middle and inferior rectal arteries (from the internal iliac arteries).
- Preganglionic sympathetic nerves from T6-T12 → preaortic ganglia → postsympathetic nerves → right vagus nerve → right and transverse colon.
- Preganglionic sympathetic from L1-L3 → preaortic plexus → postganglionic nerves → left colon, sigmoid, and rectum.
- Vagus nerve → parasympathetic nerves → right and transverse colon.

- Nervi erigentes (pelvic parasympathetic nerves S2-S4) → left colon, sigmoid, and rectum.[2]

EPIDEMIOLOGY AND ETIOLOGY

- Vagus nerve → parasympathetic nerves → right and transverse colon.
- Nervi erigentes (pelvic parasympathetic nerves S2-S4) → left colon, sigmoid, and rectum.[2]
- **Incidence:** occurs in 1 in 5000 lives births in both hemispheres and is still undefined in other races, although studied in Caucasians.
- Males are 4 times more affected than females.[3]
- The genetic component has relation not only to the RET proto-oncogene mutation, but also to the endothelin, SOX-10, S1P1, and Phox2B.[5]
- It is also associated with Down syndrome (100 times greater risk).
- **Etiology:** developmental disorder of enteric nervous system with failure of neural crest cell (NCC) migration caudally toward rectum.[3]
- Another theory is that the NCCs fail to survive or proliferate after migration.[5]
- Aganglionosis starts from anorectal line and affects rectosigmoid in 80% of patients, splenic and transverse colon in 17%, and the entire colon in 8%.[2]

CLINICAL PRESENTATION

- More than 90% present with worsening abdominal distention and bilious vomiting, as well as failure to pass meconium in the first 24 hours of life.
- They may present at an older age with poor feeding, chronic distention, and constipation.
- Enterocolitis is the most common cause of death in untreated patients.[2]

DIAGNOSIS

- Contrast imaging such as a barium enema is helpful with diagnosing Hirschsprung disease (Figure 30.1).
- Anorectal manometry can also identify absence of rectoanal inhibitory reflex to balloon distention.[4]

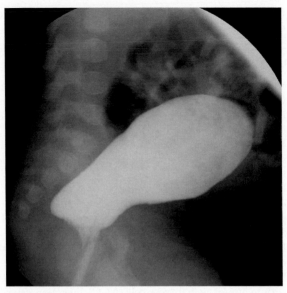

Figure 30.1 Barium enema: Rectal barium enema contrast study shows spasm of aganglionic segment and dilated normal segment—"transition zone." (Reprinted with permission from White AJ. *The Washington Manual of Pediatrics*. 2nd ed. Philadelphia, PA: Lippincott Williams & Wilkins; 2016.)

- **Gold standard**: rectal biopsy-suction biopsy in children up to age 3 years, then full thickness biopsy about 2 cm above dentate line.
- Histopathologic criteria: absent ganglia, hypertrophied nerve trunks, immunostaining for acetylcholinesterase, and loss of calretinin.[2]

MEDICAL AND SURGICAL MANAGEMENT

- First and foremost, resuscitation is paramount for intestinal obstruction, and broad-spectrum antibiotics, for enterocolitis.
- Nasogastric tube is for decompression. Rectal decompression can be performed by digital rectal stimulation or irrigations.
- In emergent cases, a diverting colostomy using normal ganglionated bowel can be performed initially and definitive treatment can be semielective.

- Sequential colonic biopsies can be performed by laparotomy, laparoscopically, or through an umbilical incision.
- **Swenson procedure** (Figure 30.2A): The patient is placed in supine position and a midline laparotomy is made.
  - The affected colon and rectum are dissected out down to the level of the internal sphincters.
  - The intra-abdominal part can also be performed laparoscopically.
  - A perineal approach is then used to create a coloanal anastomosis.
- **Soave procedure** (Figure 30.2B): Through a perineal approach (either supine or prone), the submucosa is dissected endorectally starting from 0.5 to 1 cm above the dentate line and to normal colon.
  - The normal colon is then pulled through for a coloanal anastomosis. This leaves a cuff of aganglionic muscle.
  - The intra-abdominal rectum and sigmoid can be laparoscopically dissected for a safer, more efficient technique.
- **Duhamel procedure** (Figure 30.2C): The patient is supine and through a laparotomy incision, the aganglionic colon is resected but the rectum is left.
  - The normal colon is then anastomosed to the posterior rectal wall, which is in a safe avascular space, with an endorectal stapler.
  - For long-segment disease (proximal to transverse colon), one can proceed with a straight pull through like above, colon patch, or J-pouch.
  - Colon patch has 2 types:
    - **Martin procedure**: side-to-side anastomosis of small bowel with aganglionic colon to preserve stool reservoir and water absorption function.
    - **Kimura procedure**: 2-step operation with right colon and small bowel side-to-side anastomosis that is then later on connected to the anus as a pouch.[5]

POSTOPERATIVE CARE

- Most children with pull-through procedures can be fed immediately postoperatively and discharged in 1 to 2 days.

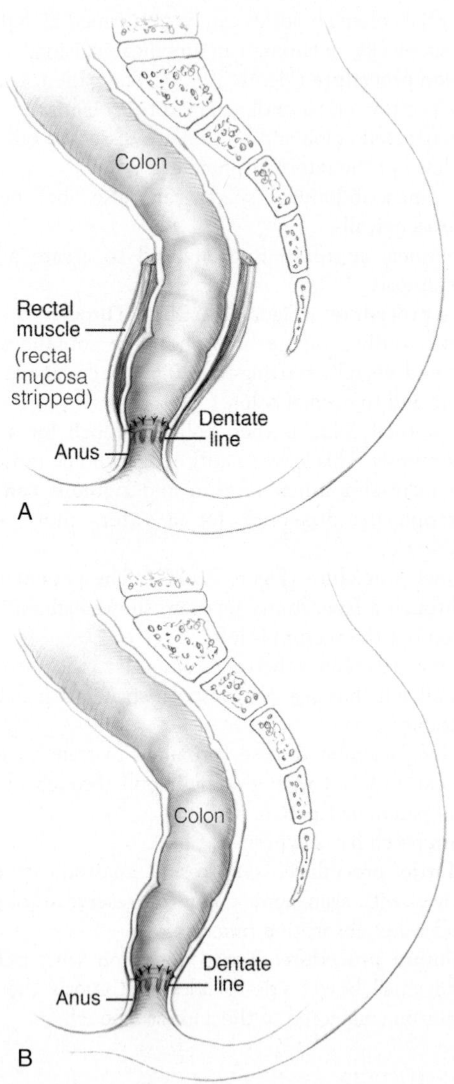

Figure 30.2 A, Soave. B, Swenson. C, Duhamel. (Reprinted with permission from Carmel J, Colwell J, Goldberg MT. *Wound, Ostomy and Continence Nurses Society® Core Curriculum: Ostomy Management.* Philadelphia, PA: Wolters Kluwer; 2016.)

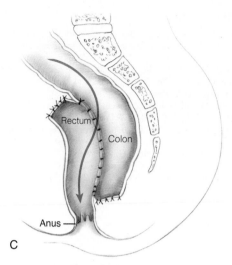

Rectum

Colon

Anus

C

Figure 30.2—cont'd

COMPLICATIONS

- Early: wound infection, intra-abdominal bleeding, anastomotic leak or stricture, intestinal perforation, bowel obstruction, enterocolitis
- Late: obstructive symptoms, soiling, and enterocolitis[5]
- Although post-op problems are common, after approximately 5 years, most children overcome these issues and have normal quality of life and function.[5]

PEARLS AND PITFALLS

- Hirschsprung disease is a failure of NCC to migrate toward the anus, leading to a distal colonic failure to relax.
- While more than 90% present in infancy with obstructing, abdominal distention, it can present later on in children with chronic constipation.
- Pull-through procedures are common for short-segment disease but less used for long-segment disease.
- Close follow-up is necessary to manage postoperative obstruction, soiling, and enterocolitis.

REFERENCES

1. Grosfeld JL. Hirschsprung's disease: a historical perspective — 1691-2005. In: *Hirschsprung's Disease and Allied Disorders.* N.p.; 2008 [Print].
2. Townsend CM, Daniel BR, Mark EB. Pediatric surgery. In: *Sabiston Textbook of Surgery: The Biological Basis of Modern Surgical Practice.* 19th ed. N.p.; 2012 [Print].
3. Kenny SE, Tam PKH, Garcia-Barcelo M. Hirschsprung's disease. *Semin Pediatr Surg.* 2010;19(3):194-200 [Web].
4. Dasgupta R, Langer JC. Evaluation and management of persistent problems after surgery for Hirschsprung disease in a child. *J Pediatr Gastroenterol Nutr.* 2008;46(1):13-19 [Web].
5. Langer JC. Hirschsprung's disease. In: Coran AG, Anthony C, Adzick NS, eds. *Pediatric Surgery.* 7th ed. N.p.; 2012 [Print].

Chapter 31

Anorectal Malformations

Paige E. Finkelstein

- One does not have to be a doctor to make the diagnosis of anorectal malformation (ARM), and thus it has been known throughout history for centuries—as early as 650 BC.[1]
- Aristotle described humans born with ARM in the third century BC, and reports of treatment via membrane incision and dilation began to appear in the second century CE.[2]
- With primitive surgery, children with low malformations tended to have greater survival than those with high malformations.[3]
- Dr Douglas Stephens in 1953 was the first pediatric surgeon who studied the pelvic anatomy in patients who died from ARM; posterior sagittal anorectoplasty (PSARP) by Dr Alberto Peña was published in 1982, which became a preferred technique for surgical management of these conditions.[4,5]

RELEVANT ANATOMY

- The anal passage may be narrow or misplaced in front of where it should be located.
- A membrane may be present over the anal opening.
- The rectum may not connect to the anus.
- The rectum may connect to part of the urinary tract or the reproductive system through a passage called a fistula, and an anal opening is not present.

EPIDEMIOLOGY AND ETIOLOGY

- **Incidence**: It is approximately 1 to 2 in 5000 live births.[6,7]
- Most common ARM in females is rectovestibular fistula, and the most frequent ARM in males is rectourethral fistula.[8]
- **Etiology**: It is unknown, but genetic factors are believed to play an important role, as evidenced by increased risk in first-degree relatives of probands, association with

chromosomal abnormalities, and reproducibility using knock-out animal models.[6,8]

- Up to 50% is estimated to be unrelated to any known syndrome.[7]
- Chromosomal abnormalities are present in 4.5% to 11% of patients.[6]
- Maternal exposure during pregnancy has been associated with increased risk of anorectal atresia, including lorazepam, and lack of folic acid, vitamin A, as well as obesity, asthma, epilepsy, and thyroid disease.[6,9]

CLINICAL PRESENTATION

- Classic presentation of ARMs can range in phenotypes from perfectly healthy infant with minor abnormalities who can be easily treated to complex with poor functional prognosis.[6,8]
- Diagnosis is made by newborn physical examination (Figure 31.1).
- 50% of ARMs are associated with genitourinary, cardiovascular, skeletal, or gastrointestinal (GI) defects.[6,8]

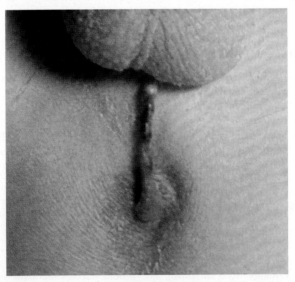

Figure 31.1 Imperforate anus without fistula. The visible meconium streak along the raphe is consistent with a low imperforate anus. (Courtesy of Kevin P. Lally, MD. Reprinted with permission from Ricci SS, Kyle T, Carman S. *Maternity and Pediatric Nursing*. 3rd ed. Philadelphia, PA: Wolters Kluwer; 2016.)

- This nonrandom coexistence of anomalies is often part of the **VACTERL** association, which includes spinal and/or vertebral defects (V), ARM (A), congenital cardiac anomalies (C), esophageal atresia/tracheoesophageal fistula (TE), renal and urinary abnormalities (R), and limb lesions (L).[10]
- Persistent cloaca represents the most severe malformation, where the rectum, vagina, and urinary tract converge into a single channel.[11]
- High malformation: Inspection of the buttocks may reveal a flat bottom with lack of midline gluteal fold or the absence of an anal dimple, indicating poor muscles of the perineum[8] (Figure 31.2A).
- Low malformation: It is characterized by the presence of meconium at the perineum, a prominent skin tag located at the anal dimple, or an anal membrane[8] (Figure 31.2B).

DIAGNOSIS

Laboratory Findings

- Complete blood count, blood typing/screening, and serum electrolytes should be measured in all children pending an operation.
- Urinalysis determines the presence of urinary fistulas.

Imaging Findings

- Ultrasound is used to evaluate for urologic anomalies, and plain radiographs, to check for spinal and sacral anomalies[8] (Figure 31.3).
- Radiographs within the first 24 hours may show final anatomy, as rectal sphincter is still collapsed.[3]
- After newborn period/colostomy creation (see below), a high-pressure distal colostography should be performed to find precise distal rectum to plan for surgical repair.[8]
- Other imaging that may be of use includes CT, MRI, lower GI series, and upper GI series to evaluate organs and look for obstructions and strictures or other problems.

MEDICAL AND SURGICAL MANAGEMENT

- Surgery is the main treatment modality for correcting ARM.
- After the baby is born, IV access should be made available for fluids and antibiotics, and nasogastric tube placed to keep stomach decompressed.[8]

A

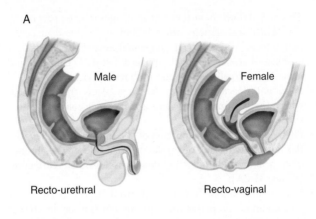

Male   Female

Recto-urethral   Recto-vaginal

B

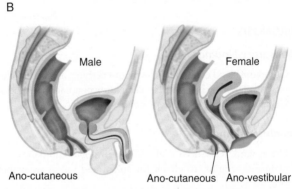

Male   Female

Ano-cutaneous   Ano-cutaneous   Ano-vestibular

Figure 31.2 Classification of anorectal malformations. Anomalies are classified as low or high depending on their relationship to the pubococcygeal line on X-ray film (broken line). Fistula tracts between the rectum and other structures are indicated by stippling. A, Low anomalies, which are usually associated with an external fistula to the vestibule (in girls) or the skin. B, High anomalies, in which fistulas are internal, usually to the posterior vagina in girls or the proximal urethra in boys. (Redrawn with permission from Stocker JT, Dehner LP, Husain AN. *Stocker and Dehner's Pediatric Pathology.* 3rd ed. Philadelphia, PA: Wolters Kluwer Health/Lippincott Williams & Wilkins; 2010.)

- Within the first 24 to 48 hours it should be decided if the infant will undergo anoplasty during the newborn period versus protective colostomy with delayed repair.
- This decision depends on the infant's physical examination, appearance of perineum, and risk of metabolic acidosis or sepsis.[8]

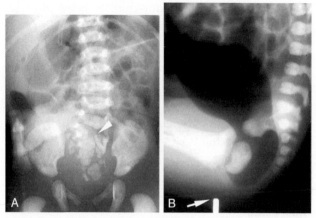

Figure 31.3 X-rays for anorectal malformation. A, A high anorectal malformation. Frontal radiograph shows multiple segmentation anomalies of the sacrum (arrowhead) and absence of gas in the distal bowel. B, A low anorectal malformation. Lateral radiograph shows air in the distal colon. Opaque marker (arrow) shows expected location of anus. (Reprinted with permission from Siegel MJ, Coley BD. *Core Curriculum: Pediatric Imaging.* Philadelphia, PA: Lippincott Williams & Wilkins; 2005.)

- Surgical repair is either performed immediately or occurs in 3 stages: (1) neonatal colostomy, (2) Peña's PSARP, and (3) colostomy closure.[5]
- The baby should be worked up for VACTERL anomalies, including cardiac echo, before surgery.

Operative Intervention

- The sex of the patient and high versus low ARM will determine the surgical pathway:
  - Male:
    - With fistula → anoplasty
    - Rectal gas present below coccyx, no associated defects → PSARP with or without colostomy
    - Rectal gas above coccyx, associated defects → colostomy
  - Female:
    - Single perineal orifice → colostomy, drain hydrocolpos, with possible urinary diversion
    - Perineal fistula → anoplasty or dilatation
    - Vestibular fistula → colostomy or primary repair

- No visible fistula, and rectum is below the coccyx → colostomy or primary repair
- No visible fistula, and rectum is above the coccyx → colostomy
- Preferred colostomy is a descending colostomy, made from the descending portion of the colon.[8]
- Laparoscopy-assisted PSARP was introduced in 2000, although PSARP is still the gold standard.[12]

Surgical Approaches

- Surgery can be performed with an open or laparoscopic approach.

Open PSARP

- Determine position of rectum preoperatively via a colostogram.
- Place Foley catheter before beginning procedure.
- Place patient prone, and usually an incision is made from coccyx to perineal body.
- Dissection is carried in midline and continued until rectal fascia is encountered.
- Rectum is opened in midline, and traction sutures, placed.
- Dissection is carried up until fistula site.
- Rectum is separated from urinary tract.
- Submucosal dissection is continued above fistula for about 2 cm.
- Fistula is then closed on urinary side with fine, absorbable suture.
- Rectum is continually dissected until there is enough length to perform an anastomosis between rectum and perineum.
- Once mobilized, the sphincters are identified via muscle stimulator.
- Anterior portion of incision is closed, and the rectum is placed within the sphincter.
- Levator muscles are closed posterior to rectum.
- Anoplasty is performed between rectum and skin with interrupted absorbable sutures.

Laparoscopic PSARP

- There are many different modifications of the technique, but most involve using 3 access ports (a camera port and 2 working ports).

- This technique includes many of the same fundamental principles as the open PSARP, but those in favor of the laparoscopic approach report better visualization and fewer wound infections.[13]
- There are also less pelvic dissection and oftentimes lack of division of the muscle complex.[13]

POSTOPERATIVE CARE

- Post-op course tends to be smooth, with little pain. Most patients are discharged 2 days after PSARP.[3]
- Anal dilations are begun 2 weeks post-op and increased in size weekly.[14]

Complications

- The major complications after surgery for ARM include wound infection, anal strictures, constipation, and difficulty urinating.
- Most patients suffer from some degree of long-term defecating disorder.[3]

PEARLS AND PITFALLS

- Patients born with ARM need to be evaluated for other congenital abnormalities, specifically VACTERL.
- Surgical decisions must be made within the first 24 to 48 hours of life.
- Colostography should be performed to predict rectum position before surgery.
- Posterior sagittal anorectoplasty is the classical repair method of choice.
- Most patients do well post-op but will end up suffering from some sort of long-term defecation disorder.

REFERENCES

1. Peña A, Bischoff A. *Surgical Treatment of Colorectal Problems in Children.* Springer International Publishing; 2015:1-16. doi:10.1007/978-3-319-14989-9_1.
2. Herman RS, Teitelbaum DH. Anorectal malformations. *Clin Perinatol.* 2012;39:403-422.

3. Holcomb III, George W, Murphy JD, Ostlie DJ. *Ashcraft's Pediatric Surgery*. Elsevier Health Sciences; 2014.

4. Zaiem M, Zaiem F. Muscle complex saving posterior sagittal anorectoplasty. *J Pediatr Surg*. 2016. doi:10.1016/j.jpedsurg.2016.12.013.

5. Menon P, Rao KLN, Sinha AK, et al. Anorectal malformations in males: pros and cons of neonatal versus staged reconstruction for high and intermediate varieties. *J Indian Assoc Pediatr Surg*. 2017;22;83-86.

6. Wang C, Li L, Cheng W. Anorectal malformation: the etiological factors. *Pediatr Surg Int*. 2015;31;795-804.

7. Schramm C, Draaken M, Tewes G, et al. Autosomal-dominant non-syndromic anal atresia: sequencing of candidate genes, array-based molecular karyotyping, and review of the literature. *Eur J Pediatr*. 2011;170:741-746.

8. Levitt MA, Peña A. Anorectal malformations. *Orphanet J Rare Dis*. 2007;2:33.

9. Bonnot O, Vollset SE, Godet PF, D'Amato T, Robert E. Maternal exposure to lorazepam and anal atresia in newborns: results from a hypothesis-generating study of benzodiazepines and malformations. *J Clin Psychopharmacol*. 2001;21:456-458.

10. England RJ, Eradi B, Murthi GV, Sutcliffe J. Improving the rigour of VACTERL screening for neonates with anorectal malformations. *Pediatr Surg Int*. 2017:1-8. doi:10.1007/s00383-017-4094-3.

11. Peiro JL, Scorletti F, Sbragia L. Prenatal diagnosis of cloacal malformation. *Semin Pediatr Surg*. 2016;25:71-75.

12. De Vos C, Arnold M, Sidler D, Moore SW. A comparison of laparoscopic-assisted (LAARP) and posterior sagittal (PSARP) anorectoplasty in the outcome of intermediate and high anorectal malformations. *S Afr J Surg*. 2011;49:39-43.

13. Gurusamy R, Raj S, Maniam R, Regunadan S. Laparoscopic-assisted anorectoplasty: a single-center experience. *J Indian Assoc Pediatr Surg*. 2017;22:114-118.

14. Peña A, Grasshoff S, Levitt M. Reoperations in anorectal malformations. *J Pediatr Surg*. 2007;42:318-325.

Chapter 32

Tracheoesophageal Fistula

Michael A. Lopez

- Esophageal atresia (EA) and tracheoesophageal fistula (TEF) are congenital malformations that occur approximately in 1:3500 live-born infants.[1]
- It is defined as an interruption in the continuity of the esophagus.
- TEFs may or may not be present in patients with EA.
- This abnormality is usually due to improper separation of the trachea and esophagus during the 4th week of gestation when the primitive foregut is developed.[1]
- The first successful primary repair of EA was accomplished in 1941 by Cameron Haight.
- The high mortality rates associated with EA and TEFs have decreased, thanks to early diagnosis, preoperative management/preparation, and clever surgical techniques.

EPIDEMIOLOGY AND ETIOLOGY

- Most cases are sporadic.
- 35% to 60% of infants with EA will also have other congenital abnormalities.[2]
- ~25% of patients trisomy 18 will be born with EA/TEF.[2]
- Once the diagnosis is made, a thorough physical examination must be performed to determine if any other abnormalities are present.
- Approximately 10% to 20% occur with VACTERL or CHARGE (although not criteria for diagnosis).[9]
- Associated abnormalities:[2]
  - Cardiovascular (ventricular septal defect, atrial septal defect, tetralogy of fallot) → 20% to 30%
  - Gastrointestinal (GI) (imperforate anus, duodenal atresia, Meckel diverticulum) → 15% to 25%
  - Genitourinary → 10% to 20%
  - Musculoskeletal → 10% to 15%
  - Craniofacial/Central nervous system → 5% to 10%
  - Chromosomal abnormalities → 3% to 5%

CLINICAL PRESENTATION

- EA may be suspected when absence of gastric bubble, poly-hydramnios (earliest symptom, found during second half of pregnancy), and distension of upper esophagus are seen on prenatal ultrasound.
- Fetal MRI can confirm diagnosis of atresia or TEF when suspected.[5]
- After birth, the child may present with excessive salivation with choking and cyanotic spells.

DIAGNOSIS

- If clinical presentation suggests EA, the diagnosis can be made inserting 10- or 12-F Replogle into the esophagus.
- Inability to advance tube further than 10 cm is highly suggestive of EA.
- The tube can then be left in place to aspirate secretions, preventing aspiration.
- Once the tube is in place, AP and lateral chest radiographs are performed while injecting a small amount of air into the tube.
- This will provide the exact location of the atretic esophagus and demonstrate whether or not a TEF is present (Figure 32.1).
- If abdominal gas is seen, it is very likely that a distal or H-type TEF is present.[6]
- No air in the GI tract suggests pure atresia.
- Injecting barium into the Replogle tube can be performed to confirm diagnosis but is rarely needed.[8]
- The most commonly used systems to classify this disease process are described by Gross (Figure 32.2).
- The most frequent type of EA is the blind-ending esophageal pouch with a fistula between the trachea and lower esophagus, classified as C (Gross).
- Approximately 85% of patients diagnosed with EA will fall under this classification.[7]
- Type A, pure atresia with TEF, is seen in approximately 7% of cases.
- Type B, EA with a TEF between the trachea and upper esophageal pouch, is seen in approximately 2% of cases.
- Type D, where both upper and lower esophageal segments communicate with the trachea, is seen in approximately 3% of cases.
- Type E, also known as H-type TEF, is a different entity because no EA is present (Figure 32.3).

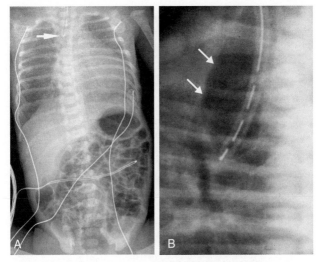

Figure 32.1 Esophageal atresia with distal tracheoesophageal fistula. A, Frontal radiograph of the chest and abdomen demonstrates a nasogastric tube within the upper esophageal pouch (arrow). The air in the bowel indicates a distal tracheoesophageal communication. B, Lateral view in another patient shows a dilated upper esophageal pouch (arrows) containing a nasogastric tube. (Reprinted with permission from Siegel MJ, Coley BD. *Core Curriculum: Pediatric Imaging.* Philadelphia, PA: Lippincott Williams & Wilkins; 2005.)

MEDICAL AND SURGICAL MANAGEMENT

- If no other life-threatening issues are present, surgery should not be delayed.
- Although placement of the Replogle tube minimizes secretions, these patients are still at high risk for aspiration.
- In premature infants with respiratory distress, early operative intervention is still preferred, as it can be difficult to adequately aerate noncompliant lungs when a majority of air will enter the esophagus in those with TEFs.[3]
- Bronchoscopy should be performed on all infants suspected to have pure EA.
- The management for these patients is typically a feeding gastrostomy tube followed by a primary esophageal anastomosis after 2 to 3 months.[6]
- The importance of bronchoscopy in this subset of patients is because there has been a reported 10% to 15% of undiagnosed proximal TEF when pure EA was determined by lack of abdominal gas.

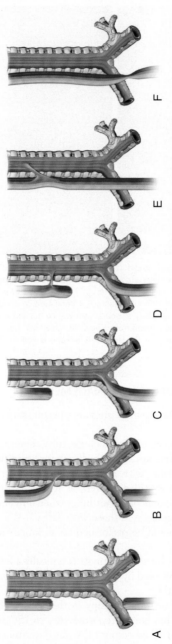

Figure 32.2 Gross classification of TEF. A, Esophageal atresia with distal tracheoesophageal fistula. B, Esophageal atresia without tracheoesophageal fistula. C, Tracheoesophageal fistula without esophageal atresia. D, Esophageal atresia with proximal tracheoesophageal fistula. E, Esophageal atresia with both proximal and distal tracheoesophageal fistulas. F, Esophageal stenosis. (Reprinted with permission from LoCicero J, Feins RH, Colson YL, Rocco G, eds. *Shields' General Thoracic Surgery.* 8th ed. Philadelphia, PA: Wolters Kluwer; 2019.)

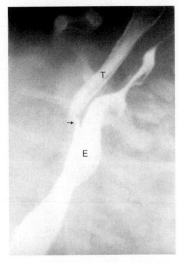

Figure 32.3 A barium esophagram on a baby with recurrent pneumonia shows a connection between the esophagus (E) and the trachea (T), a so-called H-type or N-type tracheoesophageal fistula (arrow). This abnormality can sometimes be extremely difficult to detect. (Reprinted with permission from Smith WL. *Radiology 101*. 4th ed. Philadelphia, PA: Wolters Kluwer Health/Lippincott Williams & Wilkins; 2014.)

- Failure to recognize this will result in recurrent aspiration and pneumonia during the 2- to 3-month waiting period.
- Preoperative management should include comprehensive laboratories and crossmatch.
- It may also be wise to obtain an echocardiogram to evaluate cardiac function and determine the location of the aortic arch in relation to the atretic esophagus, which can influence operative planning.
- Once the patient is intubated, a rigid bronchoscope can be used to rule out undiagnosed fistulas (most commonly missed proximal TEF) and ensure that the endotracheal tube is secured distal to the TEF.[6]

Repair of EA With Proximal, Distal, or Proximal and Distal TEFs

- Standard approach for esophageal repair (Figure 32.4) in these patients is a right laterodorsal thoracotomy, unless preoperative workup showed a right-sided aortic arch.[4]
- A slightly curved incision is made 1 cm below the tip of the scapula from midaxillary line to angle of the scapula.

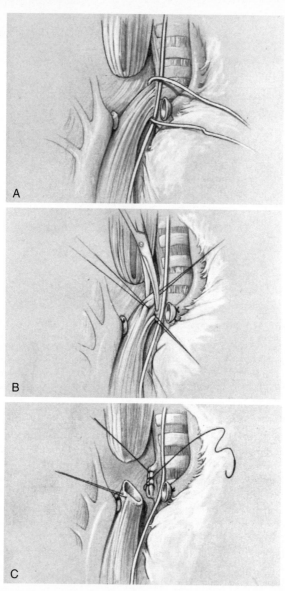

Figure 32.4 Surgical repair of type C TEF. A, The tracheoesophageal fistula site is mobilized circumferentially distal to the fistula, and the area is encircled with a vessel loop. B, Traction sutures are placed, with great care taken not to encroach on the lumen of the trachea, which can result in narrowing with closure. Division of the fistula is then performed using tenotomy scissors. C, The tracheal end is closed with a 5-0 continuous or interrupted suture. The closure is tested with positive-pressure ventilation to rule out a leak. The tracheal suture line is covered with mediastinal pleura to reduce the risk of recurrent tracheoesophageal fistula should an anastomotic leak occur. (Reprinted with permission from Fischer JE, Bland KI, Callery MP, et al, eds. *Fischer's Mastery of Surgery*. 7th ed. Philadelphia, PA: Wolters Kluwer; 2018.)

- This incision allows the opportunity to enter the thoracic cavity without dividing any muscle layers.
- The latissimus dorsi is released and mobilized posteriorly.
- The serratus anterior can then be released from its attachments and mobilized superiorly with the scapula.
- The intercostal muscles are then divided off the superior border of the fifth rib.
- Once the parietal pleura is encountered, gentle blunt dissection can free the pleura off the chest wall and allow for an extrathoracic approach.
- A rib spreader can then be inserted, as the extrapleural dissection is taken toward that posterior mediastinum.
- Once the dissection to the mediastinum is complete, the azygos vein is divided and the right vagus nerve is identified.
- This should provide adequate exposure of the proximal and distal esophageal segments.
- The distal esophageal segment is typically weak and hypoplastic.
- Mobilization must be performed with extreme care, as damage to vagal fibers can result in motility disorders and severe reflux in the future.
- Take down of the distal TEF begins with mobilization of the distal esophagus from the trachea by creating traction with a vessel loop.
- Stay sutures are then placed on tracheal and esophageal ends of the fistula.[6]
- The communication is then divided as close the trachea as possible, and the tracheotomy is closed with running or interrupted 6-0 monofilament suture.
- An air-water leak test can be performed to evaluate the tracheal closure by filling the chest with warm saline and forcefully ventilating after the ET has been moved proximal to the repair.[3]
- The upper pouch, which is often retracted cephalad, can be found by asking the anesthesiologist to push the Replogle tube until the proximal pouch is in the field.
- Careful sharp dissection of the proximal pouch from the esophagus is then performed to gain adequate length for the repair.
- If a proximal fistula is encountered, it is taken down in the same fashion as described earlier.
- Because of the excellent blood supply of the proximal esophagus, dissection can be taken all the way to the thoracic inlet if necessary.

- Mobilization should be carried out until a tension-free anastomosis can be achieved.
- To preserve as much length as possible, a horizontal incision is made on the proximal pouch at the tip of the Replogle tube.
- An end-to-end anastomosis is then accomplished with interrupted 6-0 absorbable suture, starting with full thickness bites on each side.
- The back wall is brought together first.
- The Replogle tube is then exchanged for a 5-F nasogastric tube, and the anterior wall is then closed over the tube.
- The NG tube is left in place for gastric decompression and early enteral feeding.

Additional Surgical Tips

- If it is felt that the anastomosis is under too much tension despite complete mobilization, length can be achieved with a circular myotomy on the upper pouch.
- This is done prior to the anastomosis by replacing the Replogle tube with an 8-F balloon catheter.
- Once inflated, the muscular layers are easily seen.
- While providing caudal countertension on the proximal pouch, the muscle layer is divided 1 cm proximal to future anastomosis.
- This myotomy can be performed in circular or spiral fashion.
- This technique can provide 5 to 10 mm of extra length before creating the anastomosis.[6]
- Another alternative technique to creating a tension-free anastomosis is to mobilize the stomach through the hiatus or elongate the lower esophagus by performing a Collis gastroplasty.

Repair of Pure Esophageal Atresia

- For patients with pure EA and no TEF, surgical repair can be challenging because of the distance between esophageal segments.
- The decision is then whether to attempt to preserve the patient's esophagus or replace it.
- When attempting to preserve the esophagus in the children, 3 different approaches have been described.
  - First is to allow time for spontaneous growth of the proximal pouch as historically, waiting 8 to 12 weeks has shown to allow adequate time for the proximal pouch to lengthen enough for a tension-free anastomosis.
  - The second option is to promote elongation of the proximal pouch by regular longitudinal stretching.

- Last, in addition to stretching the proximal segment, a dilator can be inserted via gastrostomy to lengthen the distal segment as well.
- Twice a day for 3 to 5 minutes, a radio opaque instrument is gently advanced into the upper and lower esophageal segments under fluoroscopic guidance until it is determined that an end-to-end anastomosis can be achieved with minimal tension.[7]

Repair of H-Type Tracheoesophageal Fistula

- Patients with H-type TEF can present with different symptoms than those with pure EA.
- Presentation of symptoms is often delayed, sometimes over a year.
- Classic symptoms are choking episodes while eating with cyanotic spells. Diagnosis can be made with contrast esophagram or bronchoscopy.
- During preoperative bronchoscopy, a ureteric catheter is advanced through the fistula to help aid the future dissection.[7]
- Surgical repair is often accomplished through a cervical incision, 1 cm above the medial third of the right clavicle.
- Dissection is taken down medial to the carotid artery, until the catheter can be palpated posterior to the thyroid.
- Care must be taken to identify the recurrent laryngeal nerve.
- Once the fistula is identified, traction sutures are placed, the catheter is removed, and the fistula is transected.
- Absorbable 6-0 monofilament suture is used to close the tracheal and esophageal defects.[7]

POSTOPERATIVE CARE

- Postoperative management begins with careful NICU monitoring until the child is extubated and stable.
- The child should have an extrapleural chest tube, set to water seal, and daily output should be closely monitored.
- Parenteral nutrition is usually started at this time, and enteral feeds are slowly started through the nasogastric tube as soon as possible.
- If the patient is stable after 5 to 7 days, a contrast esophagram and upper GI series are performed to determine if the anastomosis is patent and ensure no leak is present.
- These studies also allow the surgeon to evaluate the swallowing reflex and esophageal motility. It is not unusual for early images to show a narrow anastomosis and a dilated upper pouch, as long as contrast passes through the anastomosis with ease.

- Next, it is important to evaluate the flow of contrast into the stomach to evaluate the presence of gastroesophageal reflux and ensure adequate gastric emptying.[6]
- Once all these examinations confirm a well functioning GI tract, feeding can be initiated.
- The patient will likely have difficulty tolerating a sufficient PO diet, so they are usually discharged with the NG tube to supplement enteral feeds.
- The child should also be discharged with H2 blockers for the expected reflux.[6]
- Family must understand that the expected scaring at the anastomotic site will prevent normal distension of the esophagus, and the child should therefore only be fed pureed food for 1 year and minced meals until around 5 years of age, when the patient learns to completely chew meals.
- They must also be aware that swallowing larger pieces of food may result in foreign body impaction at the anastomotic site.[6]

COMPLICATIONS

- Anastomotic leak
- Anastomotic dehiscence
- Recurrent fistulas
- Swallowing difficulty/poor suck
- Tracheomalacia
- Gastroesophageal reflux
- Recurrent pneumonia
- Failure to thrive

PEARLS AND PITFALLS

- Diagnosis of TEF and EA can be made prenatally.
- After birth, diagnosis can be made by passing a Replogle tube and injecting air into the tube.
- Bronchoscopy can assist with diagnosis.
- Surgery should not be delayed if the infant is stable.
- Posterolateral thoracotomy with an extrapleural dissection provides best outcomes.
- Lengthening procedures may be necessary if unable to create a tension-free repair.
- H-type fistulas approached through cervical incision.

REFERENCES

1. De Jong EM, Felix JF, de Klein A, Tibboel D. Etiology of esophageal atresia and tracheoesophageal fistula: "Mind the Gap". *Curr Gastroenterol Rep*. 2010;12(3):215-222. doi:10.1007/s11894-010-0108-1.
2. Felix JF, Tibboel D, de Klein A. Chromosomal anomalies in the aetiology of oesophageal atresia and tracheo-oesophageal fistula. *Eur J Med Genet*. 2007;50:163-175.
3. Holcomb GW, Rothenberg SS, Bax KMA, et al. Thoracoscopic repair of esophageal atresia and tracheoesophageal fistula: a multi-institutional analysis. *Ann Surg*. 2005;242(3):422-430. doi:10.1097/01.sla.0000179649.15576.db.
4. Ke M, Wu X, Zeng J. The treatment strategy for tracheoesophageal fistula. *J Thorac Dis*. 2015;7(suppl 4):S389-S397. doi:10.3978/j.issn.2072-1439.2015.12.11.
5. Langer JC, Hussain H, Khan A, et al. Prenatal diagnosis of esophageal atresia using sonography and magnetic resonance imaging. *J Pediatr Surg*. 2001;36:804-807.
6. Laberge JM. Congenital diaphragmatic hernia. In: Mattei P, ed. *Fundamentals of Pediatric Surgery*. New York: Springer; 2011:223-232.
7. Hollwarth ME, Zaupa P. Oesphageal atresia. In: Schroder G, ed. *Pediatric Surgery*. Heidelberg, Germany; 2006:29-48.
8. Scott DA. Esophageal atresia/tracheoesophageal fistula overview. In: Adam MP, Ardinger HH, Pagon RA, et al, eds. *GeneReviews® [Internet]*. Seattle, WA: University of Washington; March 12, 2009 [Updated June 12, 2012]:1993-2018.
9. Vissers LE, van Ravenswaaij CM, Admiraal R, et al. Mutations in a new member of the chromodomain gene family cause CHARGE syndrome. *Nat Genet*. 2004;36:955-957.

Chapter 33

Foreign Body Ingestion

Nadine Najjar

- Young children are instinctively curious about their environment, and their exploration can result in ingestion of a variety of foreign bodies.
- Anything can be ingested—commonly ingested foreign bodies include toys, fish bones from food, button batteries (Figure 33.1), coins, safety pins, magnets, food boluses, and much more.
- Most cases occur by accident in children, and they are often asymptomatic. However, complications can carry significant morbidity and mortality.

RELEVANT ANATOMY

- Ingested foreign bodies tend to lodge in areas of *physiologic narrowing*:
  - Upper esophagus at the level of the cricopharyngeus muscle
  - Midesophagus at the level of the aortic arch
  - Lower esophagus at the level of the gastroesophageal junction
- If the foreign body has passed the cricopharyngeus muscle, there is a much greater chance that it will pass into the stomach without consequence because this is the area of greatest narrowing.

EPIDEMIOLOGY

- More than 100 000 cases are reported each year, and 80% of these cases are in children.[1]
- Foreign body ingestion is common in children, particularly aged 6 months to 4 years.[2]
- A vast majority of ingested foreign bodies pass uneventfully through the gastrointestinal tract. However, the most common areas of impaction are the upper esophagus at the level of the cricopharyngeus muscle (~70% of all cases), midesophagus at the level of the aortic arch (10%-15%), and gastroesophageal junction (5%-10%).[3]

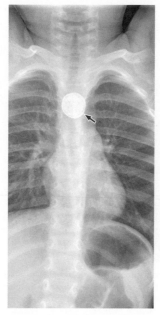

Figure 33.1 A 3-year-old boy with ingested button battery complicated by tracheoesophageal fistula (TEF). Frontal radiograph shows a foreign body projecting over the upper chest with a circle within a circle appearance (arrow), consistent with an ingested button battery. (Reprinted with permission from Lee EY. *Pediatric Radiology: Practical Imaging Evaluation of Infants and Children.* Philadelphia, PA: Wolters Kluwer; 2018.)

CLINICAL PRESENTATION

- Symptoms depend on the size of the object in relation to the patient, location, and duration.
- More often than not, patients are asymptomatic.
- However, if the object lodges in the esophagus (Figure 33.2), children can present with sudden onset of coughing, chest pain, poor feeding, and drooling.
- Esophageal symptoms can cause inflammation of the surrounding areas, resulting in respiratory symptoms such as wheezing, coughing, and stridor.
- If the lodgment results in significant impaction resulting in esophageal dilation, this can compromise the airway.
- In the case of ingestion of a battery, symptoms may result due to caustic injury, electrical discharge, and toxin release resulting in tissue necrosis—causing fistulas, burns, perforation, stricture, and death.[4]

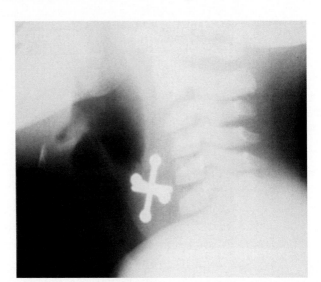

Figure 33.2 Radiograph of a 4-year-old child with a jack in cervical esophagus; lateral view of the neck shows the position of the pointed projections and the resulting tracheal compression. (Reprinted with permission from Stedman TL, ed. *Stedman's Medical Dictionary*. 28th ed. Philadelphia, PA: Lippincott Williams & Wilkins; 2006.)

DIAGNOSIS

- Because aspiration of foreign bodies in children often goes unwitnessed, if there is any suspicion, imaging is essential.
- Radiographic examination includes anteroposterior and lateral views of the neck and chest to determine the location of the foreign body[4] (Figure 33.3).
- If suspicion is high, with or without radiographic confirmation, endoscopic evaluation may be performed to minimize complications due to a delayed diagnosis.

MANAGEMENT

- 80% to 90% of foreign bodies pass without consequence, while 10% to 20% must be removed endoscopically, and less than 1% require surgical intervention.[5]
- However, clinicians should have a high index of suspicion and a low threshold to recommend endoscopic evaluation after aspiration of a foreign body.
- Urgent intervention is recommended when the ingested object is

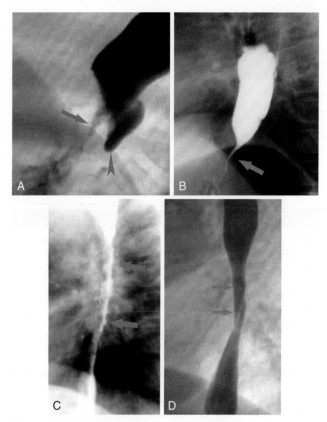

Figure 33.3 Esophageal stricture. A, Contrast esophagram shows a stricture (arrow) with a posterior pseudodiverticulum (arrowhead) that was caused by a retained plastic foreign body lodged in the distal esophagus. B, The beaklike narrowing (arrow) of the distal esophagus in a different child was caused by gastroesophageal reflux. The stricture mimics achalasia. C, The long-segment, irregular configuration of the stricture in this child (arrows) is characteristic of caustic ingestion. This stricture was the result of lye ingestion. D, A long concentric stricture (arrows) in a child with epidermolysis bullosa. (Reprinted with permission from Brant WE, Helms C. *Fundamentals of Diagnostic Radiology*. 4th ed. Philadelphia, PA: Wolters Kluwer/Lippincott Williams & Wilkins Health; 2012.)

- Sharp
- Long (>5 cm)
- A superabsorbent polymer
- Located in the esophagus
- A magnet
- A disc battery in the esophagus specifically

- Additionally, urgent intervention is necessary when there is evidence of airway, esophageal, or intestinal obstruction or inflammation.
- Multiple methods for retrieval of foreign bodies have been reported in the literature, including Foley catheter extraction, bouginage, and endoscopic retrieval.[3]
- For example, in 1 study of 1625 cases at a single institution, 41% of coins and 95% of sharp objects were lodged at sites suitable for removal by direct laryngoscopy with high success rates.[5]
- Generally, rigid endoscopy has higher success rates in dislodging and retrieving the foreign body than other methods.[4]

PEARLS AND PITFALLS

- The vast majority of ingested foreign bodies pass without consequence.
- The most common location where foreign bodies lodge is in the upper esophagus at the level of the cricopharyngeus muscle.
- Foreign body ingestion often presents asymptomatically but can progress to respiratory or feeding issues.
- While endoscopic evaluation is not always necessary, clinicians should have a low threshold for electing to perform one.

REFERENCES

1. Kay M, Wyllie R. Pediatric foreign bodies and their management. *Curr Gastroenterol Rep*. 2005;2007:212-218.
2. Hutson JM, O'Brien M, et al. Foreign Bodies. *Jones' Clinical Paediatric Surgery: Diagnosis and Management*. 6th ed. Blackwell; 2009.
3. Uyemura MC. Foreign body ingestion in children. *Am Fam Physician*. 2005;72(2).
4. Lelli JL. Chapter 11: Foreign bodies. *Ashcraft's Pediatric Surgery*. N.p.: Elsevier Health Sciences; 2014:8-9 [Print].
5. Cheng W, Tam PKH. Foreign-body ingestion in children: experience with 1,265 cases. *J Pediatr Surg*. 1999;34(10):1472-1476.

Chapter 34

Congenital Chest Wall Disorders

Marcus E. Eby

- Chest wall deformities can be divided into 2 main categories:
  - **Congenital** versus acquired
- Pediatric congenital chest wall deformities present anytime between birth and adolescence and can subdivided into 2 main groups:
  - Depression or protrusion of the sternum
    - (eg, pectus excavatum [PE] or pectus carinatum [PC])
  - Aplasia or dysplasia of the chest wall
    - (eg, thoracic ectopia cordis, sternal clefts, Poland syndrome)
- The most common chest wall deformities are congenital PE (88%) and PC (5%).[1]

Pectus Excavatum

BACKGROUND

- PE is a congenital deformity of the anterior thoracic wall in which the sternum and rib cage grow abnormally to produce a "caved-in" appearance of the chest (also known as **funnel chest**) (Figure 34.1).
  - PE is the **most common** congenital chest wall deformity.
  - **Epidemiology**: It occurs in 1 in 400 births (0.25%); ~95% of cases are Caucasian patients, boys > girls (5:1 ratio).[2]

ETIOLOGY

- The exact cause of PE development has yet to be established although studies have confirmed a strong genetic predisposition to have PE (~40% of PE cases have a family member with an associated chest wall deformity).
  - Commonly proposed mechanism is an abnormal posterior tethering of the sternum to the diaphragm during development, causing the "caved-in" appearance.
    - **Clinical note:** The theory is supported by ~1 out of 3 patients acquiring PE after repair of a posterolateral congenital diaphragmatic (Bochdalek) hernia.[3]

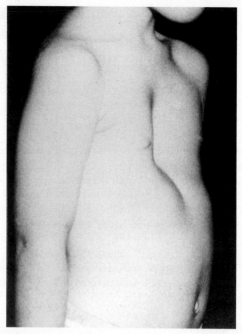

Figure 34.1 Pectus excavatum. Photograph of a 4.5-year-old girl with a symmetric pectus excavatum deformity. Note that the depression extends to the sternal notch. (Reprinted with permission from Shamberger RC. Chest wall deformities. In: Shields TW, ed. *General Thoracic Surgery.* 4th ed. Baltimore, MD: Williams & Wilkins; 1994:529-557.)

SYMPTOMS

- Most common complaints include **exercise intolerance, lack of endurance, and shortness of breath on exertion** (usually asymptomatic during childhood; may become symptomatic during more active teenage years).
  - Suspected pathophysiology of easy fatigability: Decreased chest wall motion during respirations at the area of the pectus defect results in less efficient mechanism of breathing during strenuous exercise.

MANAGEMENT

- Surgical correction of PE is offered to symptomatic patients who are interested in attempting to improve exercise tolerance. This can be performed either as a minimally invasive or open approach depending on surgeon preference.[1]

OPEN REPAIR OF PECTUS EXCAVATUM: (RAVITCH PROCEDURE)

- The open surgical repair of PE involves various modifications of the original procedure described by Brown and modified by Ravitch.
  - A transverse thoracic incision is made in the inframammary crease.
  - Electrocautery is used to create cutaneous flaps, and the pectoralis muscle is elevated to expose the depressed sternum and costal cartilages.
  - The perichondrium is scored longitudinally, and the deformed cartilages are resected either partially or completely with preservation of the perichondrial sheaths.
  - The xiphoid may require division from the sternum if it is expected to protrude after correction.[5]
  - An anterior table, wedge-shaped, sternal osteotomy is performed at the cephalad transition from the normal to the depressed sternum near the level of the insertion of the second or third costal cartilages.
  - The posterior aspect of the sternum is dissected free, elevated, and fractured by upward traction. The osteotomy is closed with nonabsorbable sutures.
  - A drain is positioned below the muscle flaps. The muscle flaps are sutured back into position, and the incisions are closed.[5,6]
- **NOTE**: Open repair in younger children is discouraged owing to risk of interference with the growth plates and subsequent development of acquired thoracic chondrodystrophy.

MINIMALLY INVASIVE REPAIR OF PECTUS EXCAVATUM: (NUSS PROCEDURE)

- This repair is performed with arms abducted approximately ~70° from the thorax and ~90° at the elbow to prevent excess traction on the brachial plexus.
- The chest is measured transversely from bilateral points located medial to the anterior axillary line.
- The bar length selected is 1″ less than this measurement to account for the shorter course the bar takes as it traverses the chest wall.
- The optimal shape is different for each patient, but a slight bend on the ends of the bar with an approximately 2-cm flat section in the middle to support the sternum is recommended.[4]

- Lateral incisions are made, and tunnels are created to the planned entrance and exit sites, which are medial to the greatest apex.
- All this is carried out under direct thoracoscopic visualization. Using an umbilical tape, the bar that has previously been measured and bent is then passed and flipped. In older patients or those with stiff, asymmetric, or saucer-shaped defects, 2 bars are frequently required.
- The bar is then secured with a stabilizer and pericostal sutures.
- The incisions are closed, and a chest radiograph is acquired to ensure there is no unrecognized pneumothorax or bar shift. The bar is maintained for 2 to 3 years to decrease recurrence rates.[4]

Pectus Carinatum

BACKGROUND

- PC is a congenital deformity of the anterior thoracic wall in which the sternum and rib cage grow abnormally to produce a "protruding" appearance of the chest (also known as **pigeon chest** or **pyramidal chest**) (Figure 34.2).

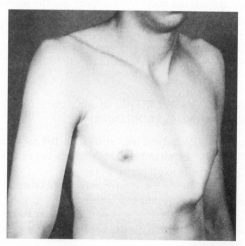

Figure 34.2 Pectus carinatum. Photograph of chondrogladiolar pectus carinatum in a 19-year-old man. (Reprinted with permission from Shamberger RC. Chest wall deformities. In: Shields TW, ed. *General Thoracic Surgery*. 4th ed. Baltimore, MD: Williams & Wilkins; 1994:529-557.)

- PC is the **second most common** congenital chest wall deformity.
- **Epidemiology**: It is more commonly seen in South American countries (eg, PC occurs in ~55% of all congenital chest wall deformities in Argentina), but PC is 5× less common in North America than PE, boys > girls (4:1 ratio).[7]

ETIOLOGY

- Similar to PE, studies have confirmed a strong genetic predisposition to developing PC (~25% of PC cases have a family member with an associated chest wall deformity); however, the exact cause of PC development has yet to be established.

SYMPTOMS

- Most children with PC are asymptomatic. Most common complaints with PC include the following:
  - **Tenderness when lying prone,** musculoskeletal pain of the chest, and psychological distress (secondary to negative body image).

MANAGEMENT

- First-line therapy is **orthotic bracing** (best when patient is <18 years old with a malleable chest).
  - Correction of PC with orthotic bracing alone has been shown to have success rates up to 80%.[8]
    - **Clinical note:** The number one reason bracing fails to correct PC is poor patient compliance with brace.
  - If bracing fails to adequately correct PC, the surgical management is similar to the open operative procedure used to correct PE (ie, **the Ravitch procedure**)—*see above.*

Other Congenital Sternal Defects

- Compared with PE and PC, other sternal defects are extremely rare and often **associated with additional congenital abnormalities and high mortality rate.** Such sternal defects include the following.

ECTOPIA CORDIS

Thoracic Ectopia Cordis (The "Naked Heart")

- Thoracic ectopia cordis is the exposure of the heart with no overlying structures; often associated intrinsic cardiac defects are common; survival is rare.
- Repair requires grafting over the exposed heart; must avoid posterior compression of the heart into a limited thoracic space (successful only in absence of intrinsic cardiac anomalies noncompatible with life).[9]

Cervical Ectopia Cordis

- Cervical ectopia cordis is the fusion between the apex of the heart and the mouth and is associated with severe craniofacial anomalies; no survivors have been reported.

STERNAL CLEFT (AKA BIFID STERNUM)

- Sternal cleft is a gap in the midline of the anterior chest between the 2 halves of the sternum.
- It is the **least severe anomaly of the sternum**, usually asymptomatic, and **rarely associated cardiac defects**.[11]
  - It may be a partial or complete gap (most are partial with an intact lower sternum and xiphoid creating a classic "V- shape").

Presentation

- The heart can be seen beating directly under the skin on physical examination at birth.

Management

- Sternal clefts should be repaired in the neonatal period when the chest wall is most compliant to provide bony protection of the heart and improve respiratory dynamics.

Surgical Repair of Sternal Clefts

- A midline longitudinal incision is made directly over the sternal defect, and the sternal cleft edges are dissected free.
- If an incomplete sternal cleft is encountered, the inferior bridging cartilage is resected to make it complete.

- The edges are then reapproximated primarily with interrupted sutures.[10]
- **Clinical note**: It is important to assess the hemodynamic status during approximation of the sternal plates to ensure that the now completely closed thoracic cavity remains large enough to allow adequate cardiac output.

PEARLS AND PITFALLS

- PE is the **most common** congenital chest wall deformity.
- First-line approach to repair symptomatic PE is the **nuss procedure** (minimally invasive repair with similar results but less morbidity compared with the Ravitch procedure).
- First-line approach to repair symptomatic PC is **orthotic bracing**.
- The least severe sternal anomaly is **sternal cleft** (usually asymptomatic, rarely associated cardiac defects).

REFERENCES

1. Obermeyer RJ, Goretsky MJ. Chest wall deformities in pediatric surgery. *Surg Clin N Am.* 2012;92:669-684.
2. Fonkalsrud EW. Current management of pectus excavatum. *World J Surg.* 2003;27(5):502-508.
3. Nobuhara KK, Lund DP, Mitchell J, et al. Long-term outlook for survivors of congenital diaphragmatic hernia. *Clin Perinatol.* 1996;23:873-887.
4. Croitoru DP, Kelly RE, Goretsky MJ, et al. Experience and modification update for the minimally invasive Nuss technique for pectus excavatum repair in 303 patients. *J Pediatr Surg.* 2002;37(3):437-445.
5. Ravitch M. The operative treatment of pectus excavatum. *Ann Surg.* 1949;129(4):429-444.
6. Brown AL. Pectus excavatum (funnel chest): anatomic basis, surgical treatment of the incipient stage in infancy, and correction of the deformity in the fully developed stage. *J Thorac Surg.* 1939;9:164-184.
7. Westphal FL, Lima LC, Lima Neto JC, et al. Prevalence of pectus carinatum and pectus excavatum in students in the city of Manaus, Brazil. *J Bras Pneumol.* 2009;35(3):221-226.
8. Martinez-Ferro M, Fraire C, Bernard S. Dynamic compression system for the correction of pectus carinatum. *Semin Pediatr Surg.* 2008;17(3):194-200.
9. Dobell AR, Williams H, Long R. Staged repair of ectopia cordis. *J Pediatr Surg.* 1982;17:353-358.
10. Acastello E, Majluf R, Garrido P, et al. Sternal cleft: a surgical opportunity. *J Pediatr Surg.* 2003;38(2):178-183.
11. Shamberger R, Welch KJ. Sternal defects. *Pediatr Surg Int.* 1990;5:156-164.

Chapter 35

Pulmonary Sequestration

David Rubay

- Pulmonary sequestration is a mass of nonfunctioning lung tissue with no communication with the tracheobronchial tree (Figure 35.1).
- This sequestered mass of lung tissue receives its blood supply anomalously from the systemic circulation.
- Pulmonary sequestration appears to result from abnormal budding of the primitive foregut.[1]
- The tissue in this accessory lung bud migrates with the developing lung but does not communicate with it.
- It receives its blood supply from vessels that connect to the aorta or one of its side branches.
- The arterial supply is derived in most cases from the thoracic aorta (75%) or the abdominal aorta (20%).[1]
- In some cases (15%), 2 different arteries supply the blood.

EPIDEMIOLOGY AND ETIOLOGY

Incidence: Pulmonary sequestration represents approximately 6% of all congenital pulmonary malformations.

- Types:
  - Intrapulmonary sequestrations are the most common form, and 60% of these are found in the posterior basal segment of the left lower lobe.
    - Overall, 98% occur in the lower lobes.
    - Bilateral involvement is uncommon.
    - About 10% of cases may be associated with other congenital anomalies.
  - Extrapulmonary sequestrations occur on the left in 95% of cases.[1-3]
    - Of these, 75% are found in the costophrenic sulcus on the left side.
    - They may also be found in the mediastinum, pericardium, and within or below the diaphragm.

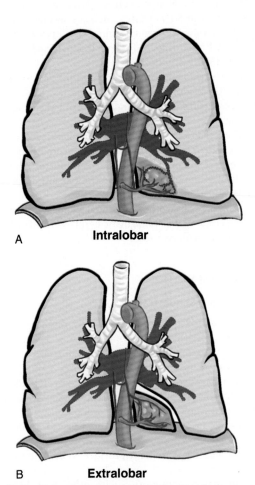

Figure 35.1   Diagrammatic representation of 2 types of pulmonary seques-tration. A, Intralobar pulmonary sequestrations are lesions mostly confined to the lower lobes, intimately connected with the adjacent lung, usually hav-ing venous drainage through the pulmonary veins and no separate pleural covering. B, Extralobar pulmonary sequestrations are accessory lobes with separate pleural covering and have an anomalous venous drainage through a systemic vein. (Reprinted with permission from Lee EY. *Pediatric Radiology: Practical Imaging Evaluation of Infants and Children.* Philadelphia, PA: Wolters Kluwer; 2018.)

- They are associated with other congenital malformations in more than 50% of cases, such as congenital diaphragmatic hernias, congenital pulmonary airway malformation (CPAM) type II (hybrid lesions), and congenital heart disease.[1,4-6]
- Sex: In the extrapulmonary form, males are affected approximately 4 times more often than females.[7]
- Incidence is equal in males and females in the intrapulmonary type.
- Age: More than one half of intrapulmonary sequestrations are diagnosed in later childhood or even in adulthood.[7]
- Neonates and infants are usually asymptomatic. More than one half of extrapulmonary sequestrations are diagnosed in patients younger than 1 year.
- Often, this is because other congenital anomalies are present, including congenital diaphragmatic hernia, cardiac malformations, and GI malformations.[7,8]

CLINICAL PRESENTATION

Intrapulmonary Sequestration

- Intrapulmonary sequestration is usually diagnosed later in childhood or adolescence; symptoms may begin early in childhood with multiple episodes of pneumonia.
- A chronic or recurrent cough is common.
- Intrapulmonary sequestration shares the visceral pleura that covers the adjacent lung tissue and is usually located in the posterobasal segment of the lower lobes.
- The thoracic or abdominal aorta often provides the arterial blood supply.
- Venous drainage is commonly provided to the left atrium via the pulmonary veins.
- An elemental communication with other bronchi or lung parenchyma may be present, allowing infection to occur.
- Rarely, an esophageal bronchus may be present.
- Resolution of infection is usually slow and incomplete because of inadequate bronchial drainage.
- Over distension of the cystic mass with air can result in compression of normal lung tissue with impairment of cardiorespiratory function.
- Aeration probably occurs through the pores of Kohn.
- Other congenital anomalies may appear in 10% of cases.[1,8]

Extrapulmonary Sequestration

- Many patients present in infancy with respiratory distress and chronic cough. Lesions are commonly diagnosed coincidentally during investigation of, or surgery for, an associated congenital anomaly.[1,7-9]
- Therefore, clinical symptoms may be absent or minor.
- Extrapulmonary sequestration may manifest as GI symptoms if communication with the GI tract is present.[8]
- As a result, infants may have feeding difficulties.
- Extrapulmonary sequestration may manifest as recurrent lung infection, as for the intrapulmonary form.
- This type of sequestration does not contain air unless communication with the foregut is present.[3]

DIAGNOSIS

Imaging Studies

- Chest radiography findings vary depending on the size of the sequestered lung tissue and whether infection is present.[1,3]
- If no communication between sequestration and normal lung tissue is present, radiography usually reveals a dense opacity in the posterior basal segment of the lower lobe (Figure 35.2).

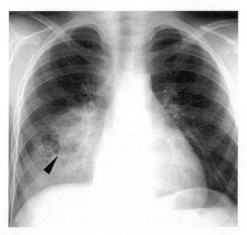

Figure 35.2 Pulmonary sequestration in a boy with recurrent pneumonia. Frontal radiograph demonstrates right lower lobe opacity with air-fluid levels (arrowhead). (Reprinted with permission from Siegel MJ, Coley BD. *Pediatric Imaging*. Philadelphia, PA: Lippincott Williams & Wilkins; 2006.)

- A cystic appearance may also be observed.
- Intrapulmonary lesions tend to be heterogeneous and are not well defined.
- Extrapulmonary masses are usually observed as solid, well defined, and retrocardiac.
- CT scanning with contrast or magnetic resonance angiography (MRA) has been very useful.[3]
- The arterial supply and venous drainage both should be outlined because of the unpredictability of vascular connections.
- CT angiography is helpful in identifying aberrant systemic arterial supply, and the 3-dimensional rendering of multidetector row CT scanning can reveal venous drainage (Figure 35.3).

MEDICAL AND SURGICAL MANAGEMENT

- Management of an asymptomatic pulmonary sequestration with no connection to the surrounding lung is controversial.[1,10]
- Most advocate resection of these lesions because of the likelihood of recurrent lung infection, the need for larger resection if the sequestration becomes chronically infected, and the possibility of hemorrhage from arteriovenous anastomoses.
- Surgical resection is the treatment of choice for patients who present with infection or symptoms resulting from compression of normal lung tissue.
- Extrapulmonary lesions can usually be excised without loss of normal lung tissue.
- Intrapulmonary lesions often require lobectomy because the margins of the sequestration may not be clearly defined.[10]
- Complete thoracoscopic resection of pulmonary lobes in infants and children has been described with low mortality and morbidity.

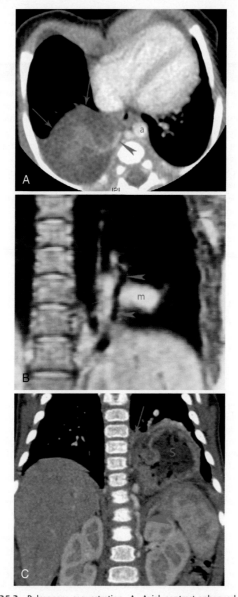

Figure 35.3 Pulmonary sequestration. A, Axial contrast-enhanced CT of a child shows a right lower lobe mass (arrows) with a feeding vessel (arrowhead) that extends to the aorta (a), indicating a pulmonary sequestration. B, Coronal T2-weighted MR image of another child shows a left lower lobe sequestration as a high-signal-intensity mass (m) associated with a large abnormal vessel (arrowheads). C, Coronal reformatted CT of a 10-month-old with a Bochdalek diaphragmatic hernia containing the stomach (S) and a partially seen pulmonary sequestration (arrow). An abnormal vessel arising from the abdominal aorta (arrowhead) is the feeding vessel to the pulmonary sequestration. (Reprinted with permission from Brant WE, Helms C. *Fundamentals of Diagnostic Radiology*. 4th ed. Philadelphia, PA: Wolters Kluwer/Lippincott Williams & Wilkins Health; 2012.)

PEARLS AND PITFALLS

- Pulmonary sequestration is a mass of nonfunctioning lung tissue with no communication with the tracheobronchial tree of lung tissue that receives its blood supply anomalously from the systemic circulation.
- There are 2 major types, intra- and extrapulmonary sequestration.
- Clinical presentation and timing depend largely on the type, and both types cause recurrent lung infection.
- Surgical resection is the best treatment for the symptomatic pulmonary sequestration.
- The treatment for the asymptomatic patient is still controversial.

REFERENCES

1. Holcomb G, Murphy J. *Ashcraft's Pediatric Surgery*. 5th ed. Saunders; 2009.
2. Pikwer A, Gyllstedt E, Lillo-Gil R, et al. Pulmonary sequestration–a review of 8 cases treated with lobectomy. *Scand J Surg.* 2006;95(3):190-194.
3. Khan AN. *Pulmonary Sequestration Imaging*. Medscape Reference; November 24, 2015.
4. Dong J, Cai Y, Chen, et al. A case report and a short literature review of pulmonary sequestration showing elevated serum levels of carbohydrate antigen 19-9. *J Nippon Med Sch.* 2015;82(4):211-215.
5. Brown EG, Marr C, Farmer DL. Extralobar pulmonary sequestration: the importance of intraoperative vigilance. *J Pediatr Surg Case Rep.* 2013;1(4):74-76.
6. Mason. *Murray & Nadel's Textbook of Respiratory Medicine*. 4th ed. Saunders; 2005.
7. Abuhamad AZ, Bass T, Katz ME, Heyl PS. Familial recurrence of pulmonary sequestration. *Obstet Gynecol.* 1996;87(5 Pt 2):843-845.
8. Becker J, Hernandez A, Dipietro M, Coran AG. Identical twins concordant for pulmonary sequestration communicating with the esophagus and discordant for the VACTERL association. *Pediatric Surg Int.* 2005;21(7):541-546.
9. Kliegman. Chapter 392-Congenital disorders of the lung. In: Finder JD, Michelson PH, eds. *Nelson Textbook of Pediatrics*. 18th ed. Saunders; 2007;
10. Townsend. *Sabaston Textbook of Surgery*. 18th ed. Saunders; 2007.

Chapter 36

Congenital Diaphragmatic Hernia

Michael A. Lopez

- Congenital diaphragmatic hernias (CDHs) occur in approximately 1 in every 2000 to 5000 live births.[1]
- There are many forms of CDHs, named for the location of the defect, and each has different physiologic effects on the patient. The 2 most common are the following:
  - Bochdalek hernias
  - Morgagni hernias
- Other less commons forms of CDH include anterior hernias associated with pentalogy of Cantrell (which includes defects in the supraumbilical midline abdominal wall, lower sternum, diaphragmatic pericardium, and heart) and central hernias (rare diaphragm defect involving the central tendinous [eg, amuscular] portion of the diaphragm) (Figure 36.1).[2]
- The size of the hernia can range from only a few centimeters to involving most of the hemidiaphragm.
- CDH is more frequently being diagnosed because of improved prenatal ultrasound monitoring.
- Early diagnosis is crucial in the management of these patients because all have the potential to clinically deteriorate after birth.
- Pulmonary hypoplasia and pulmonary hypertension are the clinical manifestations of CDH that cause significant morbidity and mortality.
- Approximately 5% to 10% of patients with CDH will not present with symptoms in the neonatal period but rather present with respiratory distress or gastrointestinal distress later in infancy.[2]

EPIDEMIOLOGY AND ETIOLOGY

- Etiology is not completely understood, but it is thought to be due to error in mesenchymal cell differentiation between the 4th and 10th weeks of gestation, when pleuroperitoneal folds usually develop.[1]

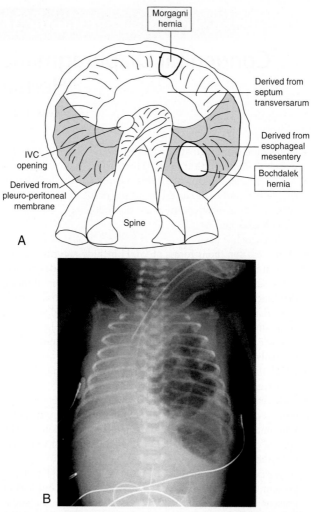

Figure 36.1 Development of the diaphragm and congenital diaphragmatic hernia. A, Abdominal surface of the diaphragm and the derivation of the components during development. The pleuroperitoneal membranes, the septum transversum, and the esophageal mesentery form the diaphragm. A Bochdalek hernia forms when there is a posterolateral defect. Morgagni hernias are less common and are present anteriorly. B, Chest radiograph of a child with a congenital posterolateral (Bochdalek) diaphragmatic hernia on the left. The mediastinum is displaced to the right by the intestinal loops present in the left chest. IVC, Inferior vena cava (Reprinted with permission from Yamada T, Alpers DH, Kaplowitz N, et al. *Textbook of Gastroenterology*. 4th ed. Philadelphia, PA: Lippincott Williams & Wilkins; 2003.)

- CDH can be associated with cardiac, gastrointestinal, and genitourinary anomalies or with chromosomal aneuploidy such as trisomies.
  - 10% of patients will also have chromosomal abnormalities (trisomy 18 or 13).
- Environmental exposures and nutritional deficiencies have also been linked to the development of CDH.[3]
  - Evidence suggests that retinoic acid and vitamin A play an important role in the development of the human diaphragm.[3]
- CDH is occasionally associated with syndromes such as Apert, Beckwith-Wiedemann, or colomba, heart anomaly, choanal atresia, retardation of growth, genitourinary issues, ear abnormalities.

Bochdalek Hernia

- Bochdalek hernia is the most common form of CDH.
- It is a posterolateral defect in the diaphragm (foramen of Bochdalek).
- About 85% of these hernias occur on the left side, about 10% occur on the right, and approximately 5% are bilateral.
- Almost all patients will have an intestinal nonrotation or malrotation because the bowel is stuck in the thoracic cavity; however, incidence of volvulus and intestinal atresia is low.

Morgagni Hernia

- Morgagni hernia is an anterior retrosternal or parasternal defect in the diaphragm.
- It is usually on the right side and can result in the herniation of liver or intestines into the chest cavity.
- Small, asymptomatic Morgagni hernias can be observed if incidentally found later in life.
- These hernias make up approximately 10% of all CDHs.[2]
- Morgagni hernias are generally accompanied by a hernia sac.
- They are less likely to cause devastating pulmonary derangements than Bochdalek hernias.

DIAGNOSIS

Prenatal Diagnosis and Care

- CDH is often ultrasonographically diagnosed before birth.
- Lung growth is measured as a proportion of head growth; a lung-to-head ratio (LHR) has some prognostic value because when it is below 1, survival is compromised.[2]

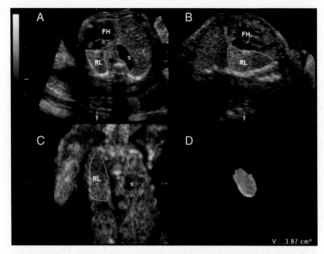

Figure 36.2 Three-dimensional multiplanar imaging of the fetal thorax and measurement of the contralateral (right) lung volume at 23 gestational weeks in a case of left congenital diaphragmatic hernia. A, Transverse plane. B, Sagittal plane. C, Coronal plane. D, 3D rendering of the right lung, the volume of which is 3.87 cm³. FH, fetal heart; RL, right lung; s, stomach. (From Ruano R, Aubry MC, Barthe B, et al. Three-dimensional sonographic measurement of contralateral lung volume in fetuses with isolated congenital diaphragmatic hernia. *J Clin Ultrasound.* 2008;36(5):273-278. Copyright © 2007 Wiley Periodicals, Inc. Reprinted by permission of John Wiley & Sons, Inc.)

- A LHR of >1.4 is generally associated with an improved chance of survival.
- Other options for prenatal evaluation include lung/thorax (L/T) transverse area ratio or volumetry by MRI (Figure 36.2).[2]
- In cases where the liver is herniated into the thorax (liver-up), prognosis is usually poor because these patients will likely require extracorporeal membrane oxygenation (ECMO).[4]
- Timing of delivery is controversial, but recent data suggest that a later gestational age is associated with fewer preterm labor complications and therefore increased survival.[5]

Postnatal Diagnosis

- Chest X-ray is used to confirm the diagnosis of CDH, evaluate the extent of bowel distension, and assess lung volume.

- Echocardiogram is performed to measure pulmonary artery pressures and determine if any cardiac abnormalities are present.

MEDICAL MANAGEMENT

- Early medical management is vital in infants diagnosed with CDH.
- Infants should be taken to a well-equipped NICU, where continuous cardiac monitoring, nasogastric decompression, bladder catheterization, and placement of umbilical artery and vein cannulas are immediately performed.[1]
- Continuous monitoring of oxygen saturation is crucial.
- Pulmonary hypoplasia is the result of the viscera occupying space in the chest.
- Respiratory therapy, mechanical ventilation, and exogenous surfactant (in the premature infants) are used to support the patient while the lung matures.
- Pulmonary hypoplasia is typically a self-limited disease, although it can take up to 8 years for complete maturation.
- Pulmonary hypertension is more difficult to manage and is often unresponsive to medical therapy.
  - Progression to late or chronic phase is a poor predictor of survival.[6]
- Severity of disease can vary widely from patient to patient.
- Care must be taken while managing these patients because barotrauma, volutrauma, and oxygen toxicity are common consequences of aggressive attempts to oxygenate the infant.
- Taking into account all these factors, mainstay of medical management includes the following:
  - Gentle ventilation, allowing for permissive hypercapnia.
    - $PaCO_2$ 60 to 65 mm Hg and even up to 70 mm Hg, as long as pH >7.20.[1]
    - Ventilator should be set on intermittent mandatory ventilation mode, with a rate of 40/min (can go up to 80/min if necessary), I:E ratio of 1:2, positive and expiratory pressure of 3 to 5 cm H_2O, tidal volume around 5 to 6 mL/kg (just enough to create movement of the thoracic cavity), and FiO_2 at 100% initially.[1]
    - Inappropriate response prompts high-frequency mechanical ventilation.[1]

- If pH remains below 7.20 or $PaCO_2$ >60 to 65 mm Hg on HFOV, initiation of ECMO needs to be considered.[6]
  - Inhaled nitric oxide, a pulmonary vasodilator, is the first agent used for treatment of pulmonary hypertension in infants >34 weeks' gestation.[7]
- Delay surgical repair until the infant is hemodynamically stable for at least 24 hours.
- ECMO has proven to be a useful adjunct for management of patients with CDH, especially in those with large defects, left-sided defects, and liver-up deformities.
- ECMO can be achieved via cannulation of the carotid artery and internal jugular vein or through the femoral veins for venovenous ECMO.
- The use of ECMO provides continued gas exchange, which can be critical while managing ventilation settings in attempts to prevent lung injury.

SURGICAL APPROACH

- Surgical correction of CDH is only considered once the patient is stable.
- A discussion between all physicians involved in preoperative management will help determine the optimal time for intervention, which can take days to weeks.
- The medical consequences must be addressed; surgery will not correct pulmonary hypertension or hypoplasia.[1]
- Open surgical approach is typically through a transverse subcostal incision.
- The bowel can be eviscerated, and the contents of the hernia can be reduced.
- The defect should be closed with interrupted permanent sutures.
- If there is too much tension for a primary repair, prosthetic mesh can be used to create a tension-free repair.
  - These repairs are associated with a higher rate of recurrence because these are typically larger defects and durable tissue can be difficult to incorporate into the repair.[8]
- If the posterior rim of the diaphragm is absent, a periosteal or pericostal suture can be placed on the lower ribs.
- Another option for a tension-free repair would be to use an abdominal wall or latissimus dorsi flap, but these are not tolerated in the critically ill patient.[8]

- If possible, avoid placement of chest tubes after the repair has been performed.
  - This will help avoid barotrauma, as the chest tube will increase transpulmonary pressure gradient.
- Thoracoscopic and laparoscopic approaches are both acceptable modalities to repair diaphragmatic hernias; however, the patient's condition may prohibit minimally invasive techniques.[1]

POSTOPERATIVE CARE

- Patients with CDH must receive continued medical care for long-term complications of conditions associated with CDH and those secondary to treatment[9] (Figure 36.3).
  - Respiratory complications: They include chronic lung disease, bronchospasm, pulmonary hypertension, aspiration, pneumonia, and pulmonary hypoplasia.
  - Neurodevelopmental delays: Patients with large defects or required ECMO had a significantly increased risk of developing neurocognitive deficits.
  - Hernia recurrence: (8%-50%).
    - The most important determinants of recurrence are large defect and the use of mesh.
  - Orthopedic deformities: Pectus deformities and progressive asymmetry of the chest wall are seen in patients with CDH.
  - Scoliosis is appreciated in 10% to 27% of patients with CDH (Figure 36.4).

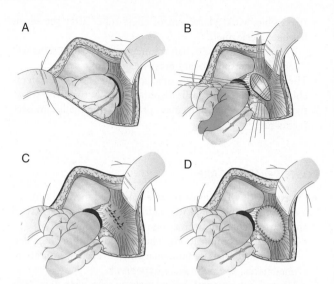

Figure 36.3 Repair of congenital diaphragmatic hernia. A, Operative appearance of congenital diaphragmatic hernia. B, Placement of sutures for repair of typical left posterolateral diaphragmatic defect. C, Completed repair. D, Prosthetic material may be used for large defects to avoid tension. (Reprinted with permission from Mulholland MW, Lillemoe KD, Doherty GM, et al. *Greenfield's Surgery: Scientific Principles and Practice*. 6th ed. Philadelphia, PA: Wolters Kluwer; 2017. Originally adapted from Stollar CJH. Congenital diaphragmatic hernia. In: Spitz L, Coran AG, eds. *Rob and Smith's Operative Surgery: Pediatric Surgery*. 5th ed. London: Chapman and Hall; 1995.)

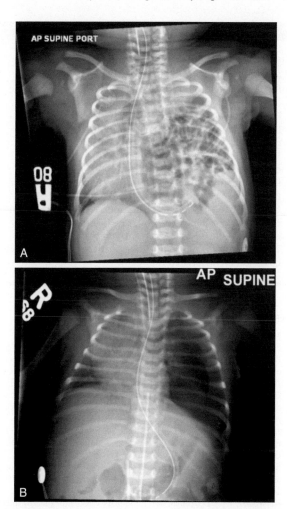

Figure 36.4 Before and after surgery for congenital diaphragmatic hernia (CDH). A, Chest radiograph of a newborn with a left CHD. Mediastinal structures are shifted to the right. Abdominal viscera occupy the left hemithorax. The nasogastric tube locates the stomach. The child underwent repair of the CHD after treatment and resolution of pulmonary hypertension. B, Immediate postoperative photograph demonstrates hypoplastic lung, flattening of diaphragm, and return of abdominal viscera to normal position. (Reprinted with permission from Mulholland MW, Lillemoe KD, Doherty GM, et al. *Greenfield's Surgery: Scientific Principles and Practice.* 6th ed. Philadelphia, PA: Wolters Kluwer; 2017.)

PEARLS AND PITFALLS

- There are 2 classic forms of CHD, Bochdalek and Morgagni, which differ in location and severity of symptoms.
- Prenatal diagnosis and possible intervention has allowed the opportunity to manage these critically ill infants efficiently, increasing likelihood of survival.
- Medical management, including permissive hypercapnia, gentle high-frequency ventilation, and ECMO, is crucial for stabilizing the patient, giving them the opportunity for a corrective surgery.
- It is important to evaluate for possible congenital abnormalities that may be associated with CDH.
- Once the patient is stable, the goal of surgery is to reduce the contents of the thorax and repair the defect either primarily or with a synthetic graft versus rotational flap.
- These patients require long-term management of the medical complications associated with CDH.

REFERENCES

1. Mattei P. Congenital diaphragmatic hernia. In: Mattei P, ed. *Fundamentals of Pediatric Surgery*. New York: Springer; 2011:535-541.
2. Pober BR, Russell MK, Ackerman KG. Congenital diaphragmatic hernia overview. In: Adam MP, Ardinger HH, Pagon RA, et al, eds. *GeneReviews® [Internet]*. Seattle, WA: University of Washington; 2006:1993-2018.
3. Golzio C, Martinovic-Bouriel J, Thomas S, et al. Matthew-Wood syndrome is caused by truncating mutations in the retinol-binding protein receptor gene STRA6. *Am J Hum Genet*. 2007;80:1179-1187.
4. Jani JC, Nicolaides KH, Gratacós E, et al. Severe diaphragmatic hernia treated by fetal endoscopic tracheal occlusion. *Ultrasound Obstet Gynecol*. 2009;34:304-310.
5. Sengupta S, Carrion V, Shelton J, et al. Adverse neonatal outcomes associated with early-term birth. *JAMA Pediatr*. 2013;167(11):1053-1059. doi:10.1001/jamapediatrics.2013.258.
6. Kinsella JP, Ivy DD, Abman SH. Pulmonary vasodilator therapy in congenital diaphragmatic hernia: acute, late, and chronic pulmonary hypertension. *Semin Perinatol*. 2005;29:123-128.
7. Chandrasekharan PK, Rawat M, Madappa R, Rothstein DH, Lakshminrusimha S. Congenital diaphragmatic hernia – a review. *Matern Health Neonatol Perinatol*. 2017;3:6. doi:10.1186/s40748-017-0045-1.
8. Puri P. Congenital diaphragmatic hernia and eventration. In: Schroder G, ed. *Pediatric Surgery*. Heidelberg: Germany; 2006:115-124.
9. Lally KP, Engle W, American Academy of Pediatrics Section on Surgery, American Academy of Pediatrics Committee on Fetus and Newborn. Postdischarge follow-up of infants with congenital diaphragmatic hernia. *Pediatrics*. 2008;121(3):627-632. doi:10.1542/peds.2007-3282.

Chapter 37

Torticollis

Olga Zhadan

- "Torticollis" is the term for twisted or rotated neck, derived from Latin, "tortus"—"twisted" and "collum"—"neck."

PATHOPHYSIOLOGY

- Torticollis can be congenital or acquired.
- **Congenital**—postural deformity of the neck, most common type, results from fibrosis (deposition of collagen and fibroblasts around individual muscle fibers that undergo atrophy) and shortening in sternocleidomastoid muscle, which pulls the head and neck to the side of lesion.
- Three types of congenital torticollis, in order of increasing severity:
  - **Postural**—babies have postural preference but no muscle tightness or restriction to passive range of motion.
  - **Muscular**—tightness of the sternocleidomastoid muscle and limitation of passive range of motion.
  - **Sternocleidomastoid muscle mass** (also called fibromatosis colli)—thickening (palpable fibrous tissue) of the sternocleidomastoid muscle and limitation of passive range of motion are developed.
- Association with breech presentations and other abnormal obstetric positions supports both the tumor etiology and the injury (due to difficult extraction), although torticollis is also found in the babies delivered by cesarean section. No single explanation of torticollis etiology exists.
- **Acquired** torticollis develops at any age secondary to cervical hemivertebra and imbalance of the ocular muscles, otolaryngologic infection, and gastroesophageal reflux (Sandifer syndrome).
- Other causes of torticollis: Klippel-Feil anomaly (congenital fusion of any 2 of the 7 cervical vertebrae), different neurologic disorders.[1]

CLINICAL PRESENTATION AND DIAGNOSIS

- In 66% of cases, torticollis presents as "tumor" in the muscle, and in 34%, as fibrosis.
- Usually the mass is not found in the neonatal period and first noted at the "well-baby" checkup 6 weeks after birth.
- The babies have characteristic posture: face and chin rotated away from the affected side and the head tilted toward the ipsilateral shoulder.[2,3]
- Facial and cranial asymmetry and flattening of the facial structures on the side of the lesion develop with time. The symptoms may become irreversible by the age of 12 years.[4]

TREATMENT

- Goals of congenital muscular torticollis treatment:
  - Achievement of midline head position, symmetric posture, and gross motor skills
  - Prevention/improvement of craniofacial asymmetry
  - Elimination of restricted cervical range of motion ($<5°$ limitation in active and passive cervical rotation and lateral flexion)
- 80% to 97% of infants do not require surgery.
- The key to successful treatment is early recognition and physical therapy.
- Physical therapy includes early range-of-motion and stretching exercises and positional changes with the infant in the crib multiple times a day.[5]
- Botulinum toxin is **not recommended**, as sufficient data regarding comparative effectiveness of botulinum toxin injection are lacking and studies are necessary to assess rare adverse effects of botulinum toxin in infants.

Operative Treatment

- Indicated in children of 6 to 12 months of age who continue to have:
  - Limited range of motion of the neck (ie, deficit in rotation of $>15°$)
  - Clinically significant plagiocephaly (asymmetrical flattening of one side of the skull) or facial hemihypoplasia

Surgical Procedures

- Simple myotomy
- Bipolar release of sternocleidomastoid muscle

- Open unipolar release with partial resection of sternocleido-mastoid muscle
- Myoplasties, combined subperiosteal lengthening of the sternocleidomastoid muscle at its mastoid insertion with division of the fibrotic band, or radical resections

Operative Technique

- Lateral collar incision, transection of the muscle in the middle third is the simplest and provides the most aesthetically acceptable scar.
- Fascia colli can also be divided anteriorly from the midline and posteriorly to the anterior border of the trapezius.[6]
- Postoperative physiotherapy should be started as early as possible.

PEARLS AND PITFALLS

■ Congenital muscular torticollis is postural deformity characterized by lateral neck flexion (head tilted to one side) and neck rotation (chin pointed to the opposite side); it is noticeable at 4 to 6 weeks of age.

■ The earlier the treatment is initiated, the more effective and shorter in duration it will be.

■ The majority of cases resolve with first-line interventions.

REFERENCES

1. Acierno S, Waldhausen J. Torticollis. In: *Ashcraft's Pediatric Surgery*. 5th ed. Philadelphia: Elsevier Saunders; 2010:1006-1007.
2. Cheng JC, Tang SP, Chen TM, et al. The clinical presentation and outcome of treatment of congenital muscular torticollis in infants–a study of 1,086 cases. *J Pediatr Surg*. 2000;35:1091.
3. Wei JL, Schwartz KM, Weaver AL, Orvidas LJ. Pseudotumor of infancy and congenital muscular torticollis: 170 cases. *Laryngoscope*. 2001;111:688.
4. Boere-Boonekamp MM, van der Linden-Kuiper LT. Positional preference: prevalence in infants and follow-up after two years. *Pediatrics*. 2001;107:339.
5. Kaplan SL, Coulter C, Fetters L. Physical therapy management of congenital muscular torticollis: an evidence-based clinical practice guideline: from the Section on Pediatrics of the American Physical Therapy Association. *Pediatr Phys Ther*. 2013;25:348.
6. Stassen LF, Kerawala CJ. New surgical technique for the correction of congenital muscular torticollis (wry neck). *Br J Oral Maxillofac Surg*. 2000;38:142.

Chapter 38

Thyroglossal Duct Cysts and Branchial Cleft Cysts

Jessica L. Buicko and Adam Michael Kravietz

- Head and neck masses are common in children.
- Location of the mass is key to diagnosis.
- Also it is important to determine if the lesion is solid or cystic.

DIFFERENTIAL DIAGNOSIS OF HEAD AND NECK MASSES IN CHILDREN (FIGURE 38.1)

- Thyroglossal duct cyst
- Branchial cleft cyst
- Lymphatic malformation
- Cervical bronchogenic cyst
- Ectopic thyroid
- Dermoid cyst

Thyroglossal Duct Cyst

RELEVANT ANATOMY AND EMBRYOLOGY (FIGURE 38.2)

- Most thyroglossal duct cysts are located close to the hyoid bone.
- The thyroid gland derives from endoderm originating from the junction of the anterior two-thirds and posterior one-third of the tongue (foramen cecum).
- The developing thyroid then descends through the developing hyoid bone and ultimately is located anterior to the third to firth tracheal cartilage.[1]
- A thyroglossal duct cyst is due to incomplete obliteration of the thyroglossal duct.
- It is rarely seen off the midline.

EPIDEMIOLOGY

- Most common midline surgical mass in childhood[1]
- Same occurrence in males and females

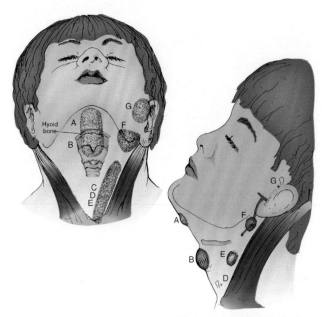

Figure 38.1 Head and neck congenital lesions seen in children in frontal and lateral views. The shaded areas denote the distribution in which a given lesion may be found: (A) dermoid cyst; (B) thyroglossal duct cyst; (C) second branchial cleft appendage; (D) second branchial cleft sinus; (E) second branchial cleft cyst; (F) first branchial pouch defect; and (G) preauricular sinus or appendage. (Reprinted with permission from Shaw KN, Bachur RG, eds. *Fleisher & Ludwig's Textbook of Pediatric Emergency Medicine*. 7th ed. Philadelphia, PA: Wolters Kluwer; 2016.)

CLINICAL PRESENTATION

- Usually a firm midline swelling/mass in the anterior neck in the midline, sometimes present after precedent upper respiratory infection (Figure 38.3)
- May present with an acute infection, most commonly due to *H. influenzae* or *S. aureus*[1]
- May also present as a draining sinus
- May move upward with swallowing and tongue protrusion because of its connection with the foramen cecum of the tongue (would not be seen with dermoid cysts or lymph nodes)

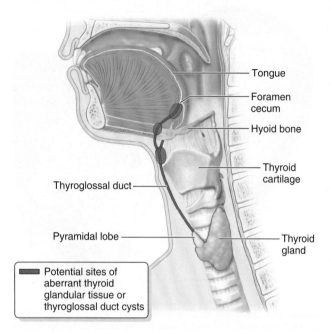

Tongue

Foramen cecum

Hyoid bone

Thyroid cartilage

Thyroglossal duct

Pyramidal lobe

Thyroid gland

Potential sites of aberrant thyroid glandular tissue or thyroglossal duct cysts

Figure 38.2 Thyroglossal duct vestiges. (Reprinted with permission from Moore KL, Dalley AF, Agur AMR. *Clinically Oriented Anatomy.* 8th ed. Philadelphia, PA: Wolters Kluwer; 2017.)

DIAGNOSIS

- Diagnosis is primarily by history and physical examination.
- Ultrasound can be used as adjunct to identify normal thyroid gland and confirm cystic lesion (Figure 38.4).
- Radioisotope scanning is useful only if unable to see normal thyroid gland and suspect lingual thyroid.

SURGICAL MANAGEMENT

- It is known as Sistrunk procedure.
  - This is usually performed under general anesthesia.
  - The neck is then hyperextended with a roll under shoulders.
  - A small horizontal skin incision is made over the cyst, and the cyst is dissected free from surrounding tissue.

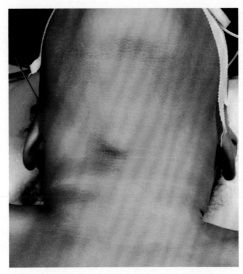

Figure 38.3 A child with thyroglossal duct cyst. (Reprinted with permission from Mulholland MW, Lillemoe KD, Doherty GM, Upchurch GR, Alam HB, Pawlik TM. *Greenfield's Surgery: Scientific Principles and Practice.* 6th ed. Philadelphia, PA: Wolters Kluwer; 2017.)

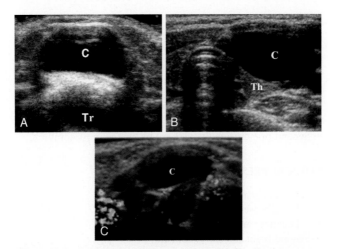

Figure 38.4 Thyroglossal duct cyst. A, Suprahyoid cyst. Transverse sonogram of an 8-year-old girl beneath the chin shows a midline cystic mass (C) just anterior to the trachea (Tr). B, Subhyoid cyst. Transverse sonogram of a 15-year-old girl shows an off-midline well-defined cystic mass (C) anterior to the left lobe of the thyroid gland (Th). C, Longitudinal color Doppler imaging demonstrates no internal flow, typical of a cyst (C). (Reprinted with permission from Siegel MJ. *Pediatric Sonography.* 4th ed. Philadelphia, PA: Wolters Kluwer Health/Lippincott Williams & Wilkins; 2011.)

- The central part of hyoid bone is identified and excised (usually with Mayo scissors) along with the cyst.
- If the cyst extends posterior to hyoid, it is followed and divided close to the base of the tongue.
- If the floor of the mouth is entered, the mucosa is closed with suture.[2]
- If patients present with an infected cyst, they are usually treated with course of antibiotics.
  - Incision and drainage is avoided initially because it may lead to a persistent sinus with increased recurrence risk after definitive surgical intervention.

POSTOPERATIVE CARE

- Usually patients discharged home the same day after surgery.
- If only simple excision is performed, the risk of recurrence is 38% to 70% rather than 2.6% to 5% as with Sistrunk procedure.[2]

Branchial Cleft Cysts

RELEVANT ANATOMY AND EMBRYOLOGY

- During weeks 4 to 8 of gestation, 4 pairs of branchial arches and intervening clefts and pouches are formed.
- Branchial cleft cysts are remnants of these structures.[3]

EPIDEMIOLOGY

- Branchial cleft cysts can account for up to one-third of cystic neck masses in children.[1]
- Second branchial cleft cysts are by far the most common.[1]

CLINICAL PRESENTATION

- First branchial cleft remnant
  - Usually present with infection
  - Location: anterior to tragus
- Second branchial cleft remnant
  - Usually family describes a small opening that occasionally drains clear fluid along the middle to upper third of the anterior border of the sternocleidomastoid muscle
  - Usually nontender but can present with infection
  - Deep lesions can cause stridor or odynophagia

- Third and fourth branchial cleft remnants (pyriform sinus fistula)
  - More common on the left side
  - Usually present as neck mass or recurrent abscess

DIAGNOSIS

- Usually history and physical examination are helpful.
- For first branchial cleft remnants, one should also examine external canal by otoscopy and occasionally need CT to evaluate relation of sinus tract to facial nerve.
- For second branchial cleft remnants, usually history and physical examination are sufficient to diagnosis.
- For third and fourth branchial cleft remnants, ultrasound can be a helpful adjunct. If still unclear, CT can be considered (gas pocket near upper pole of the left thyroid lobe is very suggestive) (Figure 38.5).

SURGICAL MANAGEMENT

- If present with infection, first-line treatment is antibiotics.
- If antibiotics fail, needle aspiration can be considered.

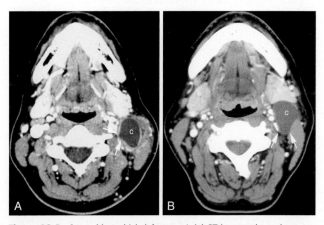

Figure 38.5 Second branchial cleft cysts. Axial CT images show characteristic location of the cysts (c) between the sternocleidomastoid muscle and the submandibular gland and characteristic pointing (arrows) of the cysts medially (A) and posteriorly (B). Sometimes, these lesions extend medially between the internal and external carotid arteries to the pharyngeal mucosa. (Reprinted with permission from Barkovich AJ, Raybaud C. *Pediatric Neuroimaging*. 5th ed. Philadelphia, PA: Wolters Kluwer/Lippincott Williams & Wilkins; 2012.)

- Incision and drainage is usually avoided because it can complicate definitive excision later.
- Ultimately, treatment is surgical excision after any infection subsides.

PEARLS AND PITFALLS

- Thyroglossal duct cysts are midline, whereas branchial cleft cysts are lateral.
- First-line treatment when patients present with infection is antibiotics.
- Sistrunk procedure, removal of cyst and portion of the hyoid bone, is a classic procedure for thyroglossal duct cyst excision.

REFERENCES

1. Olutoye OO. Cystic neck masses. In: Mattei P, ed. *Fundamentals of Pediatric Surgery*. 1st ed. Philadelphia: Springer International Publishing; 2011.
2. Höllwarth ME. Thyroglossal duct cyst. In: Puri P, Hollwarth M, eds. *Pediatric Surgery*. 1st ed. Germany: Springer; 2006.
3. Höllwarth ME. Branchial cysts and sinus. In: Puri P, Hollwarth M, eds. *Pediatric Surgery*. 1st ed. Germany: Springer; 2006.

Chapter 39

Thyroid and Parathyroid Disease

Adam Michael Kravietz and Jessica L. Buicko

- Although the Romans observed "goitres" among the peoples of the Alpine regions during their conquests, the term "thyroid," Latin for "shield shaped," dates to the 1500s.[1]
- Parathyroid gland was identified by Ivar Sandström in 1880, but the role of the gland was not elucidated until the link between the gland and hypocalcemic tetany following thyroidectomy was made in the early 1900s by William MacCallum and William Halsted.[2]
- Early thyroid and parathyroid surgery had high mortality rates due to air embolism, sepsis, asphyxiation, and hemorrhage.
- Descriptions of recurrent laryngeal nerve (RLN) damage during surgery date back to the sixth century AD.
- Improvements in antiseptic technique and anesthesia in the mid-1800s drastically reduced mortality.[1,2]
- Kocher won the Nobel Prize in 1909 for his thyroidectomy surgery, and Lahey published his technique to dramatically reduce RLN palsies by ligating the inferior thyroid artery in 1938.[1]

RELEVANT ANATOMY

- Thyroid gland begins developing at about week 4 of gestation, then descends from the base of the tongue to its final location inferior to the thyroid cartilage by the week 7 of gestation.
- Thyroid gland begins producing thyroid hormone at about week 11.
- The thyroid has 2 lateral lobes with a connecting isthmus across the midline, an anterior suspensory ligament tethering the gland to the thyroid and cricoid cartilages, and a posterior suspensory ligament tethering the gland to the cricoid cartilage and first 2 tracheal rings.
- Covering the thyroid gland anteriorly are the sternohyoid and sternothyroid muscles.

- *Blood supply* is received from the superior thyroid artery (branch of the external carotid) and the inferior thyroid artery (branch of the thyrocervical trunk).
- *Venous drainage* is via the superior, middle, and inferior thyroid veins, which drain into the innominate or internal jugular vein.
- Beginning in week 5 of gestation, 2 parathyroid glands develop from the fourth brachial pouch and 2 glands develop from the third brachial pouch, then descend to a position inferior to the fourth pouch's glands (superior and inferior parathyroid glands, respectively).
- Final parathyroid position is on the posterior aspect of the thyroid gland.
- Parathyroid blood supply usually comes from the inferior thyroid artery.
- The RLN lies in a triangle between the carotid artery laterally, the trachea medially, and the thyroid superiorly and typically follows the course of the inferior thyroid artery (Figure 39.1).[3,4]

EPIDEMIOLOGY AND ETIOLOGY

Epidemiology

- Two billion people in the world are at risk for iodine deficiency–induced goiter.
- Iodine supplementation has decreased the incidence of iodine-deficiency goiter in the United States, Canada, and Western Europe; however, countries in Africa still require further efforts to provide iodine supplementation.
- 20% of thyroid nodules in children contain cancer, higher than in adults, although the rate is decreasing owing to less common use of neck irradiation.
- Risk of thyroid dysfunction is 25% in patients receiving >25 Gy of neck irradiation.
- There is a risk of hyperparathyroidism and medullary thyroid cancer in multiple endocrine neoplasia subtypes.
- 1/200 000 have ectopic thyroid due to failure of descent; 90% are lingual thyroid.[5,6]

Etiologies of Thyroid and Parathyroid Disease

- **Congenital hypothyroidism**: inborn errors of thyroid hormone production, thyroid agenesis, maternal ingestion of antithyroid medications or goitrogens (lithium, kelp, and expectorants), transplacental passage of thyroid-blocking or stimulating antibodies, immature pituitary-thyroid axis due to prematurity, maternal iodine deficiency

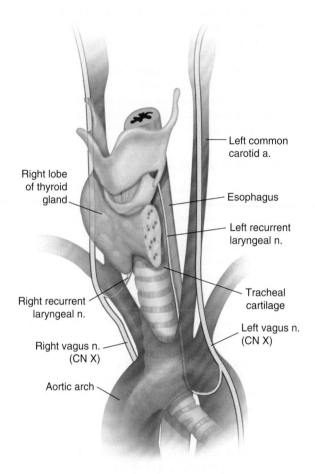

Figure 39.1 Thyroid gland and neck anatomy. (Reprinted with permission from Myers E, Ferris R. *Master Techniques in Otolaryngology - Head and Neck Surgery*. Vol 2. Philadelphia, PA: Lippincott Williams & Wilkins; 2013.)

- **Congenital hyperthyroidism**: transplacental passage of thyroid-stimulating antibodies (maternal Graves disease), activating mutations in the thyroid-stimulating hormone (TSH)-receptor
- **Acquired hypothyroidism**: iodine deficiency, Hashimoto thyroiditis, radiation exposure, liver hemangiomas, ingestion of goitrogens
- **Acquired hyperthyroidism**: functional thyroid adenoma, subacute thyroiditis, acute suppurative thyroiditis, Graves disease, toxic goiter

- **Other**: thyroid cyst, thyroid teratoma, thyroid carcinoma, infiltrative disease
- **Hyperparathyroidism**: functional parathyroid adenoma or carcinoma, multiple endocrine neoplasia (MEN) types 2A and 2B, chronic kidney disease secondary to congenital or acquired renal defects, PTHrP secretion from mesoblastic nephroma, rhabdomyosarcoma, neuroblastoma
- **Hypoparathyroidism**: DiGeorge syndrome, iatrogenic following thyroid surgery[4]

CLINICAL PRESENTATION

- Benign or malignant disease may present as an incidentally discovered thyroid nodule or palpable cervical lymph node on physical examination.
- Frank goiter occurs secondary to thyroid overstimulation or underproduction of thyroid hormone and, based on the size, may cause obstructive symptoms such as dysphagia, hoarseness, Horner syndrome, vocal cord palsy, and breathing difficulty.
- Hypothyroidism presents with galactorrhea, precocious puberty or gynecomastia in males, and classical findings of weight gain, cold intolerance, and hypoactive deep tendon reflexes.
- Hyperthyroidism
  - Graves disease presents with nervousness, emotional lability, declining performance in school, and classical signs such as weight loss, heat intolerance, and diaphoresis; exophthalmos is uncommon.
  - Subacute thyroiditis presents with a tender thyroid gland after upper respiratory tract infection and with possible symptoms of thyrotoxicosis such as arrhythmias.
  - Acute suppurative thyroiditis presents with an erythematous and tender thyroid, systemic signs, and possible fluctuance.
- Hyperparathyroidism presents with an incidental finding of elevated serum calcium or symptoms of hypercalcemia such as bone pain, nephrocalcinosis, abdominal pain, and psychiatric disturbances.
  - Neonatal presentation: respiratory distress, failure to thrive, and hypotonia.
- Hypoparathyroidism presents with symptoms of hypocalcemia such as perioral numbness, hyperactive deep tendon reflexes, paresthesias, Chvostek and Trousseau signs.[3-7]

DIAGNOSIS

Thyroid Disease

- Neonatal screening: TSH and free T4
  - Low TSH and low T4 suggests secondary (central) hypothyroidism → confirmatory thyrotropin-releasing hormone stimulation test
  - High TSH and low T4 suggests primary hypothyroidism → measure urinary iodine excretion, test for thyroid autoantibodies, obtain thyroid ultrasound or thyroid radioiodine uptake scan to evaluate for ectopic thyroid or thyroid agenesis
  - Normal TSH and low T4 in premature neonates suggests immature pituitary-thyroid axis → recheck thyroid studies at 2 and 4 weeks of age
  - Low TSH and high T4 suggests primary hyperthyroidism → measure thyroid autoantibodies, obtain thyroid ultrasound[4-7]
- Routine thyroid hormone screening in infants, children, and adolescents → follows the same workup as described for neonates[4-7]
- Goiter
  - Measure TSH and free T4 to determine whether it is due to thyroid overstimulation or underproduction of thyroid hormone
  - Low TSH and high free T4 warrants measurement of thyroid autoantibodies and a radioiodine uptake scan to determine whether the cause is Graves disease (diffuse increase), multinodular goiter (multifocal uptake), toxic adenoma (focal uptake), or acute thyroiditis (decreased uptake)
  - Normal or high TSH warrants measurement of thyroid peroxidase antibodies (thyroid-blocking antibodies) and an ultrasound[4-7]
- For children, American Thyroid Association (ATA) guidelines stipulate fine needle aspiration (FNA) of nodules that are >1 cm, enlarging, or <1 cm with concerning features by ultrasound → 22% who meet criteria have malignancy
  - Concerning features for malignancy on ultrasound are hypoechoic, microcalcifications, central vascularity, and irregular margins
  - ATA risk of malignancy
    - Low risk → cancer is confined to thyroid, <1 cm, no metastases or micrometastases to central compartment lymph nodes

- Intermediate risk → extensive central compartment lymph node involvement but no lateral compartment involvement
- High risk → regionally extensive disease, with lateral compartment involvement or extracapsular spread
- Chest X-ray if evidence of malignancy in cervical lymph nodes to assess for pulmonary metastases
- Thyroid teratoma will show calcifications, best evaluated with a CT neck (soft tissue) or MRI[5-7]

Parathyroid Disease

- Measure parathyroid hormone (PTH), serum calcium, and serum phosphorous
- Hypocalcemia
  - Low PTH suggests DiGeorge syndrome, other genetic syndromes, gland agenesis, mitochondrial disorders, or acquired causes such as postoperative damage, and copper or iron deposition → genetic testing and ultrasound
  - High PTH suggests vitamin D deficiency, liver or kidney disease, medications that activate the cytochrome p450 enzyme, or genetic end-organ resistance
  - Measure serum magnesium level
  - Chest X-ray to look for absence of thymic shadow in context of hypocalcemia and hypoparathyroidism suggests DiGeorge syndrome[4,8,9]
- Hypercalcemia
  - High PTH suggests autonomous gland function → ultrasound and sestamibi scan to assess for functional adenoma or hyperplasia, renal function tests, and urinary calcium
    - Low urinary calcium suggests familial hypocalciuric hypercalcemia
  - Low PTH suggests possible PTHrP secretion from a neoplasm[4,8,9]

SURGICAL MANAGEMENT

- Medical management of hyperthyroidism includes antithyroid medications such as propylthiouracil (PTU) or methimazole, with addition of propranolol[4-6]
- Medical management of hypothyroidism includes levothyroxine supplementation[4-6]

Surgical Considerations

- **Thyroid teratoma**: resection
- **Ectopic thyroid**: because patients are typically hypothyroid requiring levothyroxine even before surgery, and there is risk of malignant degeneration, complete removal is advocated
- **Goiter**: removal if compressive symptoms, otherwise medical management of underlying hyperthyroidism or hypothyroidism
- **Graves disease**: medical management is first line, radioactive iodine ablation (RAI) is indicated for refractory disease; however, if contraindications to RAI, then thyroidectomy is indicated[4-6,10]
- **Thyroid nodule**
  - If FNA shows indeterminate findings, repeat FNA, but if suspicion for malignancy or follicular atypical cells, then perform thyroid lobectomy
  - Papillary cancer tends to be bilateral or multifocal → total thyroidectomy indicated
  - Medullary thyroid carcinoma → total thyroidectomy
    - Prophylactic total thyroidectomy by age 1 year in MEN2B, by age 5 years in MEN2A
  - Evidence of regional lymph node involvement requires lymph node dissection
  - Evidence of extracapsular and local spread requires extensive local excision[4-7,10]
- Hyperparathyroidism
  - **Familial hypocalciuric hypercalcemia:** does not require surgery
  - Surgery indicated if symptomatic hypercalcemia such as nephrolithiasis or nephrocalcinosis, serum calcium >1.0 mg/dL above the upper limit of normal, GFR <60 mL/min, osteoporosis, 24-hour urinary calcium >400 mg/day, age <50 years[8,9]

Surgical Approach

- **Preoperative management of hyperthyroidism**: PTU or methimazole, propranolol then Lugol solution 5 to 10 drops per day for 4 to 7 days before surgery to reduce thyroid vascularity, and vitamin D with calcium supplementation to reduce risk of hungry bone syndrome postoperatively[3,4]
- **Technique**: neck hyperextension, skin incision 3 to 5 cm wide 2 cm above the clavicular head, divide platysma, isolate the RLN, retract the strap muscles laterally from the midline, expose the thyroid gland (Figure 39.2)

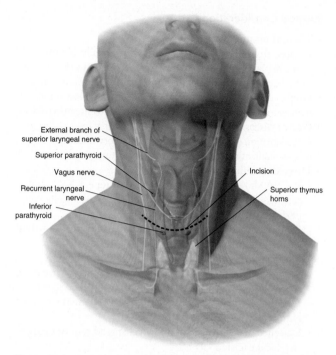

External branch of
superior laryngeal nerve

Superior parathyroid

Vagus nerve

Recurrent laryngeal
nerve

Inferior
parathyroid

Incision

Superior thymus
horns

Figure 39.2 Surgical anatomy of the thyroid gland and neck: surgical incision for appropriate isolation of thyroid and parathyroid glands. (Reprinted with permission from Myers E, Ferris R. *Master Techniques in Otolaryngology - Head and Neck Surgery*. Vol 2. Philadelphia, PA: Lippincott Williams & Wilkins; 2013.)

- **Parathyroidectomy**: see the abovementioned technique, then ligate the middle thyroid vein to rotate the thyroid medially to isolate the parathyroid glands
  - **Adenoma**: isolate the affected gland using preoperative sestamibi scan, then resect
  - **Hyperplasia**: resect $3\frac{1}{2}$ glands, or if evidence of parathyroid devascularization, then perform total resection with autotransplant of 1 gland into the sternocleidomastoid muscle or nondominant forearm
  - If cannot isolate all 4 glands, first explore the carotid sheath, then retroesophageal/retropharyngeal space, superior mediastinum with thymectomy, thyroid lobectomy, then lastly sternotomy
  - Bilateral surgical exploration of all 4 parathyroid glands is indicated for bilateral foci of disease or inability to localize adenoma

- Measure baseline PTH then repeat measurements at 5 and 10 minutes after removal of presumptive abnormal gland → >50% decrease in PTH at 10 minutes signifies successful removal[3,4,8,9]
- **Thyroidectomy**: each thyroid lobe is dissected anteriorly from medial to lateral position, ligate the middle thyroid vein to isolate the tracheoesophageal groove, identify and ligate the superior pole, then inferior pole vessels, and then the posterior suspensory ligament
  - For lobectomy cross-clamp the thyroid, divide bluntly at the midline, and suture the stump
  - For medullary thyroid cancer and papillary thyroid cancer with extracapsular extension or size >4 cm → level VI lymphadenectomy[3,4]

POSTOPERATIVE CARE

- For thyroidectomy, total or lobular, and parathyroidectomy, there is risk of transient hypocalcemia, thyrotoxicosis, transient or permanent RLN injury, tracheal stenosis, and Horner syndrome → measurement of calcium, phosphorous, and thyroid hormone and cranial nerve assessment are required
  - Laryngoscopy to assess for vocal cord fixation due to RLN injury → transient injury can take 10 weeks to resolve
  - ECG to assess for QT changes secondary to electrolyte abnormalities[3-6,8,9]
- **Parathyroidectomy**: for postoperative asymptomatic hypocalcemia, treat with short course of vitamin D and calcium carbonate supplementation until the remaining half gland or autotransplant assumes full function
  - Cure is defined as normocalcemia for minimum of 6 months[3,4,8,9]
- For total thyroidectomy: thyroid scintigraphy 6 weeks later with RAI if there is residual thyroid issue
- **Thyroid malignancy**: measure thyroglobulin levels, but most sensitive if thyroidectomy with postoperative RAI
  - If ATA guideline classification intermediate or high risk, should get postoperative thyroid scintigraphy with measurement of thyroglobulin and RAI
  - Supplementation with thyroid hormone suppresses TSH to prevent recurrence → Goal TSH level is 0.5 to 1 mIU/L for low risk, 0.1 to 0.5 mIU/L for intermediate risk, and <0.1 mIU/L for high risk[3-6,8-10]

PEARLS AND PITFALLS

- In children, the presenting sign of hypothyroidism may be galactorrhea, gynecomastia, or precocious puberty, while the presenting sign of hyperthyroidism may be nervousness, emotional lability, and declining performance in school.
- FNA for thyroid nodules >1 cm, enlarging, or <1 cm with concerning ultrasound features.
- Medical management is key for preoperative management of hyperthyroidism.
- Isolation of the RLN, with dissection or neuromonitoring.
- Thyroglobulin is a sensitive marker of thyroid malignancy recurrence in patients who received thyroidectomy with postoperative radioactive iodine ablation.

REFERENCES

1. Giddings AEB. The history of thyroidectomy. *J R Soc Med.* 1998;91(33):3-6.
2. Hackett DA, Kauffman GL Jr. Historical perspective of parathyroid disease. *Otolaryngol Clin North Am.* 2004;37(4):689-700.
3. Bliss RD, Gauger PG, Delbridge LW. Surgeon's approach to the thyroid gland: surgical anatomy and the importance of technique. *World J Surg.* 2000;24(8):891-897.
4. Ashcraft K, Whitfield Holcomb G, Murphy JP, eds. *Ashcraft's Pediatric Surgery.* 5th ed. Philadelphia: Elsevier; 2010.
5. Wells SA Jr, Asa SL, Dralle H, et al. Revised American Thyroid Association guidelines for the management of medullary thyroid carcinoma. *Thyroid.* 2015;25:567-610.
6. Francis GL, Waguespack SG, Bauer A, et al. Management guidelines for children with thyroid nodules and differentiated thyroid cancer. *Thyroid.* 2015;25(7):716-759.
7. Gupta A, Ly S, Castroneves LA, et al. A standardized assessment of thyroid nodules in children confirms higher cancer prevalence than in adults. *J Clin Endocrinol Metab.* 2013;98(8):3238-3245.
8. Wilhelm SM, Wang TS, Ruan DT, et al. The American Association of Endocrine Surgeons guidelines for definitive management of primary hyperparathyroidism. *JAMA Surg.* 2016;151(10):959-968.
9. Bilezikian JP, Brandi ML, Eastell R, et al. Guidelines for the management of asymptomatic primary hyperparathyroidism: summary statement from the Fourth International Workshop. *J Clin Endocrinol Metab.* 2014;99(10):3561-3569.
10. Rivkees SA, Mazzaferri EL, Verburg FA, et al. The treatment of differentiated thyroid cancer in children: emphasis on surgical approach and radioactive iodine therapy. *Endocr Rev.* 2011;32:798-826.

Chapter 40

Cleft Lip and Palate

Stephanie Scurci

- The earliest documented history of cleft lip (CL) and cleft palate (CP) was described by the Romans and Spartans and was thought to be evidence of evil spirits in the affected child.
- The first CL surgery was performed in 390 BC by a Chinese physician named Wey Young-Chi on an 18-year-old.
- CW Tennison in 1953 and Peter Randall in 1958 made important modifications of the triangular flap repair.
- In 1955, Peter Millard introduced the rotation-advancement flap, which remains the most commonly used technique for unilateral repair.[1]

RELEVANT ANATOMY (FIGURE 40.1)

- Closure of the lip requires fusion of the lateral nasal, medial nasal, and maxillary process at 35 days postconception.
- Failure of closure of any 1 or all of the above 3 processes may produce unilateral or bilateral lip clefting, which may extend into the palate.
- Conversely, isolated CP results from failure of primary fusion of the palates, which may occur after closure of the lip because palatal fusion occurs 56 days postconception.

ETIOLOGY AND EPIDEMIOLOGY

- The most common craniofacial defect is the cleft lip with or without cleft palate (CL/P) and isolated CP.
- These 2 defects vary in etiology, epidemiology, and genetic predisposition.

Incidence: In the United States for all orofacial clefts is 1 of 690; about one-third of those have CP alone and two-thirds have CL/P.[2]

- Rates of CP alone are consistent across races. CL/P is most highly associated with Asian populations. Caucasian and

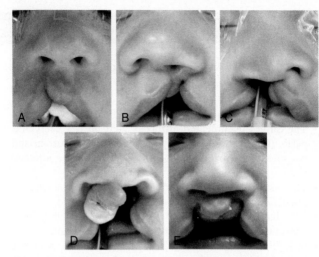

Figure 40.1 The spectrum of cleft lip deformities. A, Microform cleft lip. B, Unilateral incomplete cleft lip. C, Unilateral complete cleft lip. D, Bilateral complete cleft lip. E, Bilateral incomplete cleft lip. (Reprinted with permission from Thorne CH, Grabb WC, Smith JW, eds. *Grabb and Smith's Plastic Surgery*. 6th ed. Philadelphia, PA: Wolters Kluwer Health/Lippincott Williams & Wilkins; 2007.)

Hispanics have an intermediate risk, and the lowest rates are among African Americans.
- About 50% of CP and 30% of CL/P are associated with syndromes.[2]
- The male to female ratio for CL/P is 2:1 and 1:2 for CP.

Etiology: CL and CP have different etiologies; genetic and environmental factors affect the development of CP more than CL.

- Phenytoin, smoking in the first trimester, folate deficiency, and maternal age <20 or >39 years are associated with CL/P.
- There is a 3% to 5% chance that an affected parent will have a child with CL/P.

CLINICAL PRESENTATION

- CL and CP may present with obvious craniofacial deformity; however, some cases of isolated CP may be more occult (Figure 40.2).
- Signs and symptoms of CL and/or CP include difficulty with feedings, difficulty swallowing with possibility of liquids to come out the nose, nasal voice, and chronic ear infections.

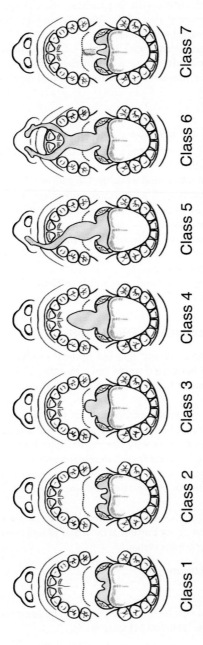

Figure 40.2 Classification of cleft lip and cleft palate. Class 1: Cleft of the tip of the uvula; Class 2: cleft of the uvula (bifid uvula); Class 3: cleft of the soft palate; Class 4: cleft of the soft and hard palates; Class 5: cleft of the soft and hard palates that continues through the alveolar ridge on one side of the premaxilla, usually associated with cleft lip of the same side; Class 6: cleft of the soft and hard palates that continues through the alveolar ridge on both sides, leaving a free premaxilla, usually associated with bilateral cleft lip; Class 7: submucous cleft in which the muscle union is imperfect across the soft palate. The palate is short, the uvula is often bifid, a groove is situated at the midline of the soft palate, and the closure to the pharynx is incompetent. (Reprinted with permission from Wilkins EM. *Clinical Practice of the Dental Hygienist.* 12th ed. Philadelphia, PA: Wolters Kluwer; 2016.)

Class 1 Class 2 Class 3 Class 4 Class 5 Class 6 Class 7

- The incidence of otitis media in patients with CP is 97%, likely due to abnormal eustachian tube anatomy and insertion of the pharyngeal musculature.[2]
- Regarding feeding, infants with isolated CL can usually be fed by breast or bottle. Those with CP have difficulty creating adequate suction and benefit from modified nipples.

DIAGNOSIS

- CL and CP can be diagnosed with fetal ultrasound in the second trimester, at which time the soft tissues of the face can be well visualized.
- The sensitivity of ultrasound when the CL and/or CP is highest when associated with a syndrome and other anatomic abnormalities. The isolated CP is the most difficult to diagnose on ultrasound alone.
- Fetuses found to have orofacial clefts should be offered amniocentesis for karyotype due to the high rate of associated chromosomal defects.
- Some commonly associated syndromes include Treacher Collins, DiGeorge, and oral-facial-digital syndrome.

MEDICAL AND SURGICAL MANAGEMENT

- CL repair can occur at any age, but optimal results occur with early repair between 6 weeks and 6 months.
- Palatal repair usually follows about 6 months after primary lip repair.
- Optimal timing remains controversial, because speech and hearing outcomes are best with early palate repair and facial growth outcomes are best with late repair. Most favor early closure (<1 y) to facilitate speech development.[6]
- Speech and hearing outcomes are best with early palate repair. Facial growth and maturation are best with late repair.
- Intrauterine surgery has been modeled by MH Hedrick in the fetal lamb but is not current standard of practice owing to risks including preterm labor.[3]

Operative Intervention

Cleft Lip Repair

- The choice of surgical technique depends on the presence of unilateral or bilateral defects (Figure 40.3).

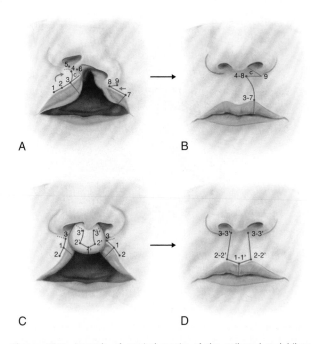

Figure 40.3 Example of surgical repairs of the unilateral and bilateral cleft lip deformities. A, Preoperative markings for the unilateral lip repair. B, Postoperative result for unilateral lip repair. C, Preoperative markings for the bilateral lip repair. D, Postoperative result for bilateral lip repair. (Reprinted with permission from Brown DL, Borschel GH, Levi B. *Michigan Manual of Plastic Surgery*. 2nd ed. Philadelphia, PA: Lippincott Williams & Wilkins, a Wolters Kluwer Business; 2014.)

- Many techniques exist for CL repair, and the most common performed today is the Millard rotation-advancement repair.
- The Millard rotation-advancement repair essentially rotates a medial lip flap downward and fills the resultant defect with lateral lip.
- The scar is well concealed within the new philtrum.[4]
- Three flaps are created after the initial incision.
- The C flap or columnar flap is a small triangle of skin below the nares, the medial (M) rotational flap off the medial lip element, and the lateral (L) advancement flap off the lateral lip element.
- The medial flap is rotated inferiorly, and the lateral flap is advanced medially to close the defect[7] (Figure 40.4).

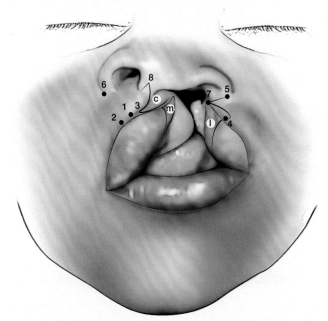

Figure 40.4 Skin markings and landmarks for a Millard advancement–rotation flap repair of a unilateral cleft lip. m, medial mucosal flap; l, lateral mucosal flap; c, central cutaneous flap. (Reprinted with permission from Larrabee WF, Ridgway J, Patel S. *Master Techniques in Otolaryngology - Head and Neck Surgery: Facial Plastic Surgery.* Philadelphia, PA: Wolters Kluwer; 2018.)

Cleft Palate Repair

Soft Palate Repair

Double opposing Z-plasty: Two Z-plasties consisting of the nasal and oral mucosal surfaces are created.

- Flaps are mobilized off the hard palate and the defect is closed by transposing the flaps across the space.
- No relaxing incisions are required in this repair (Figure 40.5).

Hard Palate Repair

Von Langenbeck technique: Bilateral, bipedicled, mucoperiosteal flaps are elevated by creating incisions along the oral side of the cleft edges (Figure 40.6).

- The flaps are mobilized medially and sutured in the midline.

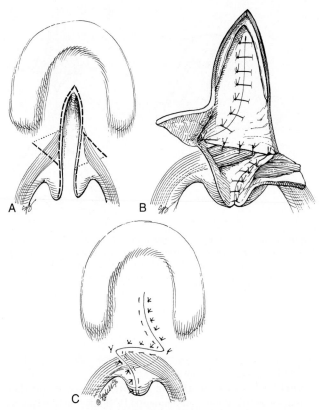

Figure 40.5 Double opposing Z-plasty closure of an isolated cleft palate. A, Design of the incisions. B, Muscle included in the posteriorly based flap. C, Final result with recreation of the levator sling. (Reprinted with permission from Thorne CH, Grabb WC, Smith JW, eds. *Grabb and Smith's Plastic Surgery.* 6th ed. Philadelphia, PA: Wolters Kluwer Health/Lippincott Williams & Wilkins; 2007.)

Veau-Wardill-Kilner V-Y pushback palatoplasty: Bilateral mucoperiosteal flaps are elevated and closed in V-Y fashion.

• Lateral relaxing incisions are required.

POSTOPERATIVE CARE

• Postoperative care is similar after CL and/or CP repair.
• Immediately postoperatively, airway monitoring with continuous pulse oximetry is necessary.

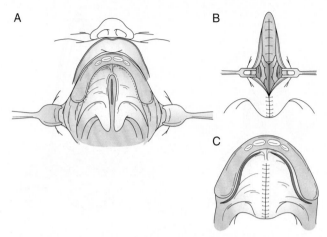

Figure 40.6 A, Von Langenbeck palatoplasty. B, Nasal mucosa and levator muscles approximated. C, Layered closure of oral mucosa and lateral relaxing incisions. (Adapted with permission from Jurkiewicz MJ, Krizek TJ, Mathes SJ, et al. *Plastic Surgery: Principles and Practice.* Vol 1. St. Louis: Mosby; 1990:91.)

- Some surgeons use elbow immobilizers to reduce the risk of accidental orofacial injury.
- Oral intake is encouraged shortly after surgery. A soft diet may be initiated with supplemental IV fluids if intake is poor initially.
- Patients may be discharged once tolerating oral intake with adequate analgesia, which is usually postoperative day 1.

COMPLICATIONS

- The acute complications after CL repair are whistling deformity (can be corrected by V-Y advancement), short lip (can be corrected with rerotation), widened lip scar, and lip landmark abnormalities.[5]
- The acute complications after CP repair are airway compromise, hemorrhage, dehiscence, and dehydration. More chronic complications after CP repair are palatal fistula, velopharyngeal dysfunction, and maxillary hypoplasia.[6]

PEARLS AND PITFALLS

- CL/P and isolated CP differ in etiologies, genetic predisposition, and epidemiology.
- Associated syndromes are more commonly associated with isolated CP.
- Diagnosis by prenatal ultrasound is possible in the second trimester, and affected patients should undergo karyotype testing.
- Surgical repair of CLs and CPs vary depending on the characteristics of the defect.
- Optimal management of CLs and CPs include a multidisciplinary team.

REFERENCES

1. Battacharya S, Khanna V, Kohli R. Cleft lip: the historical perspective. *Indian J Plast Surg.* 2009;42(12)S4-S8.
2. Shi M, Wehby GL, Murray JC. Review on genetic variants and maternal smoking in the etiology of oral clefts and other birth defects. *Birth Defects Res C Embryo Today.* 2008;84(1):16.
3. Dhillon R. The middle ear in cleft palate children pre and post palatal closure. *J Roy Soc Med.* 1988;81(4):710-713.
4. Hedrick MH, Rice HE, Vander Wall KJ, et al. Delayed in utero repair of surgically created fetal cleft lip and palate. *Plast Reconstr Surg.* 1996;97(5):900-905.
5. Harrison B. Chapter 24: Cleft lip. In: Janis JE, ed. *Essentials of Plastic Surgery.* 2nd ed. Boca Raton: CRC Press; 2014:264-274.
6. Czerwinski M, Gosman A. Chapter 25: Cleft palate. In: Janis JE, ed. *Essentials of Plastic Surgery.* 2nd ed. Boca Raton: CRC Press; 2014:275-287.
7. Millard DR. Closure of bilateral cleft lip and elongation of columella by two operations in infancy. *Plast Reconstr Surg.* 1971;47(10):324-331.

Chapter 41

Breast Disorders and Gynecomastia

Alison M. Moody and Jessica L. Buicko

EMBRYOLOGY

- At the 5th or 6th week of fetal development, 2 mammary ridges (bands of thickened ectoderm) form. These extend form the axilla to the inguinal region bilaterally. Paired breasts develop along these ridges.[1]
- Breasts develop when an ingrowth of ectoderm forms a primary tissue bud in the mesenchyme.[1]
- At birth, breasts are identical in males and females.[1]

RELEVANT ANATOMY

- Breasts are composed of 15 to 20 lobes, each of which is composed of several lobules. Each lobe of the breast terminates in a major (lactiferous) duct (2-4 mm in diameter), which opens through a constricted orifice (0.4-0.7 mm in diameter) into the ampulla of the nipple.[1]
- Cooper suspensory ligaments are fibrous bands of connective tissue that travel through the breast and insert perpendicularly into the dermis to provide structural support.[1]
- The epidermis of the nipple-areola complex is pigmented and variably corrugated. The areola contains sebaceous glands, sweat glands, and accessory glands. The dermal papilla at the tip of the nipple contains numerous sensory nerve endings.[1]

EPIDEMIOLOGY AND ETIOLOGY

Incidence: Gynecomastia affects up to 65% to 70% of adolescent males.[2]

- Three different age groups experience gynecomastia: neonates (secondary to transplacental transfer of maternal estrogen), pubertal males, and senescent males.[3]

- This chapter will focus on pubertal gynecomastia. Onset occurs between ages 10 and 12 years with peak pathology occurring between ages 13 and 14 years. Gynecomastia develops at least 6 months after the development of secondary sexual characteristics, when Tanner stages 3 to 5 in sexual development are reached.[3] (Figure 41.1).

- At the onset of puberty, the pituitary gland stimulates the testes to secrete testosterone only at night. As puberty advances, testosterone begins to be secreted during the day.

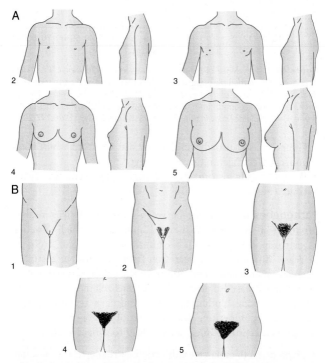

Figure 41.1 Female Tanner stages. Female breast development. Sex maturity rating 1 (not shown): prepubertal; elevation of papilla only. Sex maturity rating 2: breast buds appear; areola is slightly widened and projects as small mound. Sex maturity rating 3: enlargement of the entire breast with no protrusion of the papilla or the nipple. Sex maturity rating 4: enlargement of the breast and projection of areola and papilla as a secondary mound. Sex maturity rating 5: adult configuration of the breast with protrusion of the nipple; areola no longer projects separately from the remainder of the breast. (Reprinted with permission from Silbert-Flagg J, Pilliterri A. *Maternal and Child Health Nursing.* 8th ed. Philadelphia, PA: Wolters Kluwer; 2018.)

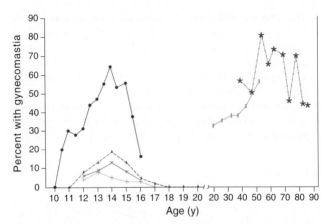

Figure 41.2 Prevalence of gynecomastia at various chronologic ages. Data were derived from multiple population studies. (Reprinted with permission from Harris JR, ed. *Diseases of the Breast*. 5th ed. Philadelphia, PA: Wolters Kluwer; 2014. Originally adapted from Braunstein GD. Pubertal gynecomastia. In: Lifshitz F, ed. *Pediatric Endocrinology*. New York: Marcel Dekker; 1996:197-205.)

Gynecomastia usually resolves by age 17 years when adult androgen/estrogen ratios are achieved.[3]

- Positive family history of gynecomastia is present 50% of the time[2] (Figure 41.2).

Pathogenesis: imbalance between estrogens that stimulate proliferation of breast tissue and androgens, which function as estrogen antagonists.[2] This imbalance can occur from an increase in free estrogen secretion (from adrenals or testes), a decrease in androgen secretion from the testes, altered metabolism, or increased binding of androgens relative to estrogens by sex hormone–binding globulin. Androgen receptor abnormalities and competitive displacement of androgens from their receptors by certain drugs can also lead to gynecomastia.[3]

- Hyperprolactinemia can indirectly contribute to the development of gynecomastia because high prolactin levels induce a hypogonadal state and may lead to secondary testicular failure.[3]
- Leptin may play a role in development of gynecomastia.[2]

Etiology: Broadly defined, gynecomastia can be caused by endocrine disorders, systemic illnesses, and medications, or defined as an idiopathic condition.[2]

- Endocrine causes of gynecomastia include the following:
  - **Hypogonadism:** primary testicular failure or secondary gonadal insufficiency can occur secondary to hypothalamic-pituitary disease[3]

- **Klinefelter syndrome**: testosterone levels are low and luteinizing hormone (LH) levels are subsequently increased secondary to loss of testosterone inhibition[3]
- **Defects in testosterone synthesis or action**[3]
- **Hermaphroditism**: both ovarian and testicular tissue are present[3]
- **Adrenal disorders**: Adrenocorticotropic hormone deficiency (results in lack of corticosteroid feedback and upregulation of LH), congenital adrenal hyperplasia (results in increased production of androstenedione, which is aromatized to estrogen)[3]
- **Hyperthyroidism**: leads to an increase in bound testosterone and decrease in free testosterone[3]
- **Tumors**: pituitary tumors, such as prolactinomas; adrenal (produce androstenedione) or testicular tumors (can secrete estrogen or human chorionic gonadotropin [hCG]); hepatocellular carcinomas; brain, chest, and abdominal cell tumors that produce hCG, which causes an increase in estradiol secretion by the testes.[3]
- Chronic disease leading to malnutrition (ie, AIDS, cystic fibrosis, ulcerative colitis, liver disease, renal failure) can result in gynecomastia.[2] Sex hormone production is decreased in starvation.[3]
- Drugs implicated in gynecomastia include finasteride, ketoconazole, spironolactone, metoclopramide, amiodarone, ACE inhibitors, calcium channel blockers, digoxin, ketoconazole, metronidazole, diazepam, tricyclic antidepressants, haloperidol, atypical antipsychotics, antiretrovirals, acid-suppressing medications, and numerous anticancer medications, among others.[2]
- Drugs of abuse, such as alcohol, amphetamines, marijuana, and opiates, can lead to gynecomastia.[2]
- Hormones implicated in gynecomastia include anabolic androgenic steroids, estrogens, testosterone, and chorionic gonadotropin.[2]

CLINICAL PRESENTATION

Classic presentation: On breast palpation, the examiner will feel a firm or rubbery, mobile, disklike (fibroglandular) mound of tissue arising concentrically from beneath the nipple and areolar region[2] (Figure 41.3).

- Glandular tissue is usually less than 4 cm[3].
- Bilateral in two-thirds of patients.[2]
- Patients will often complain of breast tenderness.[4]
- Tissue enlargement normally regresses within 1 to 3 years.[2]

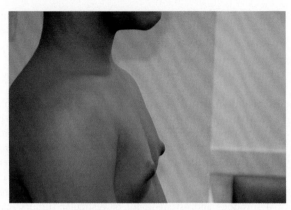

Figure 41.3 Gynecomastia. Thirteen-year-old boy with gynecomastia Tanner stage 2 breasts. (Reprinted with permission from Chung EK, Atkinson-McEvoy LR, Lai N, Terry M. *Visual Diagnosis and Treatment in Pediatrics*. 3rd ed. Philadelphia, PA: Wolters Kluwer; 2014.)

DIAGNOSIS

- Gynecomastia is a clinical diagnosis. Diagnosis starts with a thorough history and physical examination. The examiner should attempt to identify or rule out cause(s) of gynecomastia, such as hyperthyroidism, hypogonadism, malnutrition, cirrhosis, and medication use.[3]
- Additional workup should be undertaken in patients with "warning signs" that indicate the presence of more serious pathology. This includes patients with prepubertal "gynecomastia," individuals without adequate development of sexual organs, those with rapid growth of breast tissues, or individuals with a concomitant testicular mass. On physical examination, warning signs include hard breast tissue, eccentric masses outside of the nipple-areolar complex, and overlying skin changes.[2]
- Further workup should also be undertaken if gynecomastia persists beyond 18 months[2]
- Initial laboratory tests include testosterone, estradiol, hCG, luteinizing hormone, and thyroid function tests.[2]
- Pending results of initial laboratory work, additional tests to consider include karyotyping, liver and renal function studies, DHEA, and prolactin.[2]
- Any patient with a testicular mass should have a testicular ultrasound.[2]
- If a pituitary tumor or adrenal tumor is on the differential diagnosis, workup should also include brain and adrenal imaging.[2]

SURGICAL MANAGEMENT

- Gynecomastia is normally NOT a surgical disease. Patients should be monitored clinically for up to 2 years with follow-up occurring every 3 to 6 months.[2]
- Patients and their families should be reassured of the benign course of gynecomastia.[2]
- Medical treatment with tamoxifen is a noninvasive treatment option for patients with persistent disease[5]; however, it is not an FDA-approved treatment. Other medications that have been tried include raloxifene, danazol, testolactone, and anastrazole. Medications are only effective in early gynecomastia (active proliferation phase) and none is FDA-approved.[3]
- Surgery is indicated for individuals with persistent and severe breast enlargement, fibrotic alterations in breast tissue, pain,[5] or if breast enlargement is having psychological consequences that cannot be addressed in another way.[2]
- Surgical treatment of gynecomastia involves subcutaneous mastectomy or subcutaneous mastectomy with liposuction[5] (Figure 41.4).
- Mastectomy is performed by making a semiareolar incision from 3 to 9 o'clock. Cooper ligaments are transected. The hypertrophic glandular tissue is removed en block. The surgeon must be careful to leave enough tissue beneath the nipple-areolar complex to allow for sufficient perfusion of the nipple to prevent loss of sensation and fibrotic scarring.[5]
- When liposuction is also undertaken, a stab incision is made in the skin laterally and medially in the submammary fold. Tumescence solution (containing sodium bicarbonate, mepivacaine, and epinephrine) is instilled. After an exposure time of 30 minutes, liposuction was performed with a 4-mm cannula. Afterward a 3-mm cannula was used to contour the breast tissue and retract overlying skin.[5]

POSTOPERATIVE CARE

- Some authors advocate for the placement of suction drains for the first 2 postoperative days.[5]
- After operation, the patient should wear a compressive strap or bra over the breasts for 4 to 6 weeks.[5]
- Potential complications following surgical intervention include hematoma formation (early complication), hypertrophic scar formation, nipple retraction, loss of nipple sensation, wound infection, and recurrence.[5]

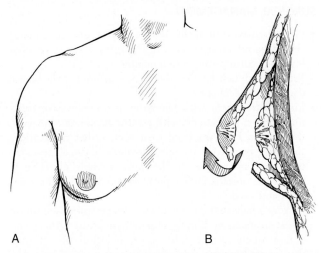

Figure 41.4 A, Periareolar incision. Medial and lateral extensions are used only if needed. B, Resection of gynecomastia through periareolar incision. Note the cuff of tissue left under areola. (Reprinted with permission from Grabb WC, Beasley RW, Thorne CH, Aston SJ, Gurtner GC, Spear SL. *Grabb and Smith's Plastic Surgery*. 6th ed. Philadelphia, PA: Lippincott Williams & Wilkins; 2006.)

BREAST MASSES

- Breast masses in pediatric patients are almost always benign.[2]
- Incidence of primary and secondary breast cancers in girls age 15 to 19 years during 2007 to 2009 was 0.2 per 100 000.[2]
- Biopsies of breast masses in adolescents most commonly show fibroadenoma (67%), fibrocystic change (15%), and abscess (3%).[2]

Fibroadenomas

- Most common breast mass in adolescent girls[2]
- Composed of glandular and fibrous tissue[2]
- Seen predominantly in younger women, age 15 to 25 years[2]
- Clinical presentation: nontender, rubbery, smooth, well-circumscribed mass in the upper outer quadrant of the breast[2]; average size = 1 to 2 cm.[1]
- Some patients will have multiple and even bilateral lesions[2]

Diagnosis

- Ultrasound with or without core needle biopsy
- Management: Patients may be managed with observation, surgical excision, or cryoablation

- Fibroadenomas are benign, and patient and clinician preference dictates treatment.[1] Patients with masses larger than 5 cm or overlying skin changes should be referred to a breast specialist[2] (Figure 41.5)

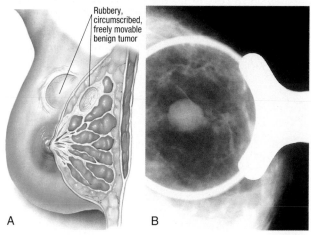

A   B

Figure 41.5 A, Fibroadenoma. B, Spot compression view of a smoothly marinated mass proven to represent a fibroadenoma. Ultrasonography demonstrated a solid mass. (Reprinted with permission from Ricci SS, Kyle T, Carman S. *Maternity and Pediatric Nursing.* 2nd ed. Philadelphia, PA: Wolters Kluwer Health/Lippincott Williams & Wilkins; 2012.)

PEARLS AND PITFALLS

- Gynecomastia is a benign condition.
- History and physical examination are the cornerstone of the patient workup
- Most patients can be managed with observation.
- Surgery is reserved for patients with persistent and severe breast enlargement, fibrotic alterations in breast tissue, pain, or if breast enlargement is having psychological consequences that cannot be addressed in another way.
- Surgical treatment includes mastectomy with or without liposuction.
- Breast malignancy in adolescents is incredibly rare.
- Ultrasound is the best test to investigate breast masses in adolescents.

REFERENCES

1. Brunicardi FC. *Chapter 17: The breast*. In: *Schwartz's Principles of Surgery*. McGraw-Hill Education; 2015.
2. Hay William W. *Chapter 4: Adolescence. Current Diagnosis and Treatment: Pediatrics*. Lange Medical Books; 2009.
3. Lazala C, Saenger P. Pubertal gynecomastia. *J Pediatr Endocinol Metab*. 2002;15(5):553-560.
4. Ferraro GA, De Francesco F, Romano T, et al. Clinical and surgical management of unilateral prepubertal gynecomastia. *Int J Surg Case Rep*. 2014;5(12):1158-1161.
5. Fischer S, Hirsch T, Hirche C, et al. Surgical treatment of primary gynecomastia in children and adolescents. *Pediatr Surg Int*. 2014;30(6):641-647.

Chapter 42

Testicular Torsion

Lauren P. Shapiro

- Torsion was first described in 1840 by Delasiauve, yet it was not discussed as a problem until 1907 when Rigby and Russell published work on the subject in *Lancet*.
- Later, Colt reported torsion of the appendix testis in 1922.
- Testicular torsion, twisting of the testis and spermatic cord, is an acute and serious diagnosis affecting the scrotum and its contents, which can result in the loss of a child's testicle.
- The loss of the testicle is due to complete obstruction of the testicular vasculature resulting in infarction.

RELEVANT ANATOMY

- The testicle is covered by the tunica vaginalis, which is encased by a capsule termed the "tunica albuginea."
- The tunica vaginalis attaches to the posterolateral surface of the testis, allowing for restriction of mobility of the testicle within the scrotum.
- The 2 types of testicular torsion, extravaginal and intravaginal, involve the spermatic cord but differ at their proximity to the tunica vaginalis (Figure 42.1).
- The testicle is secured to the scrotum by the gubernaculum distally.

EPIDEMIOLOGY AND ETIOLOGY

- There are 2 types of testicular torsion: extravaginal and intravaginal.
- The extravaginal type is seen more often in neonates, which is caused by torsion of the spermatic cord proximal to the tunica vaginalis attachment at the level of the external inguinal ring.[1,2]
- The intravaginal type is overall more common in children and adolescents and is secondary to a deformity termed the "bell clapper."[1-3]
- The "bell clapper" deformity involves the tunica vaginalis, which joins proximal on the spermatic cord, allowing the testicle to twist freely in the scrotum.

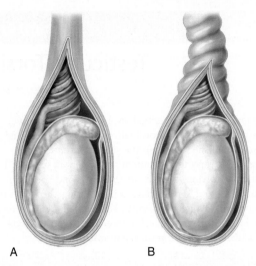

A   B

Figure 42.1 Types of testicular torsion. A, Schematic illustration of intravaginal testicular torsion. B, Schematic illustration of extravaginal testicular torsion. (Reprinted with permission from Kawamura DM, Nolan TD, eds. *Diagnostic Medical Sonography: Abdomen and Superficial Structures.* 4th ed. Philadelphia, PA: Wolters Kluwer; 2018).

- The cord twists inside the tunica vaginalis.
- The abnormal fixation of the testis within the tunica vaginalis has an incidence as high as 12%.[3]
- Testicular torsion affects 3.8 per 100 000 males younger than 18 years each year and accounts for 10% to 15% of acute scrotal disease in children.[4]

CLINICAL PRESENTATION

Classic presentation: an otherwise healthy baby or adolescent who presents with sudden onset of acute, unilateral pain in the scrotum or testicle with associated erythema and swelling (Figure 42.2).

- This pain may present as inguinal or lower abdominal pain with or without radiation to the scrotum with the affected testis being very tender to palpation.
- The symptoms are often accompanied by nausea and vomiting.
- If episodes of intermittent testicular pain are present, this may suggest occurrences of torsion and spontaneous detorsion.
- Physical examination may reveal a testicle riding high in the groin with an absent cremasteric reflex.

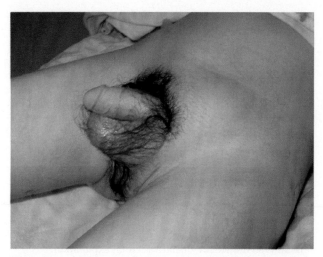

Figure 42.2 Adolescent with clinical findings of testicular torsion. (Reprinted with permission from Chung EK, Atkinson-McEvoy LR, Lai NL, Terry M, eds. *Visual Diagnosis and Treatment in Pediatrics.* 3rd ed. Philadelphia, PA: Wolters Kluwer Health; 2015).

DIAGNOSIS

Laboratory Findings

- Diagnosis of testicular torsion is performed via mostly clinical presentation with additional imaging.

Imaging Findings

- Imaging modality of choice for the diagnosis of testicular torsion is a scrotal ultrasound, which is performed using grayscale and color Doppler.[1]
- A definitive diagnosis is made when the color Doppler depicts blood flow on the normal scrotum and absence of blood flow on the torsed side.
- **Key ultrasound findings** that are suggestive of testicular torsion: when the color Doppler depicts blood flow on the normal scrotum and absence of blood flow on the torsed side.
- In the scenario of incomplete torsion, ultrasound may show persisting blood flow.
- Other radiologic findings on ultrasound include twisting of the spermatic cord, reactive hydrocele, and edema of the scrotal wall.[1]

- Ultrasound should only be used if the diagnosis is not certain because imaging will only delay an operation to treat the torsion.[3]
- Although torsion is usually diagnosed clinically or with ultrasound, other diagnostic studies, such as urinalysis, may be used.
- Pyuria and bacteriuria, although more indicative of infectious epididymitis and orchitis, can be found in testicular torsion[3] (Figure 42.3).

SURGICAL MANAGEMENT

- Surgery for testicular torsion is an emergency, and it is **paramount to salvage the testicle**.
- If testicular torsion is expected, the gold standard of treatment is an immediate operative scrotal exploration.[2,3]
- The salvage of the testicle is dependent on how rapidly the torsion is diagnosed and treated (Table 42.1).
- If detorsion is performed within 6 hours after onset of symptoms, the salvage rate is up to 97%; however, if it is delayed more than 24 hours, the salvage rate is less than 10%.[2,4]
- There is about a 4- to 8-hour window after the onset of symptoms before any significant damage occurs but significantly declines after 6 hours.[3,4]
- The only prognostic factor of testicular viability is the time between the onset of symptoms and explorative surgery.
- Manual detorsion may be attempted before surgery, and studies have confirmed that manual detorsion is associated with improved surgical salvage in cases of testicular torsion.[5]

Operative Intervention
Approach

- The surgery is initiated by performing a median raphe scrotal incision.[3]
- After detorsion of the affected spermatic cord, the testicular viability must be assessed.
- The operation corrects the torsion and fixes the gonad to the hemiscrotum in 3 places.[2]

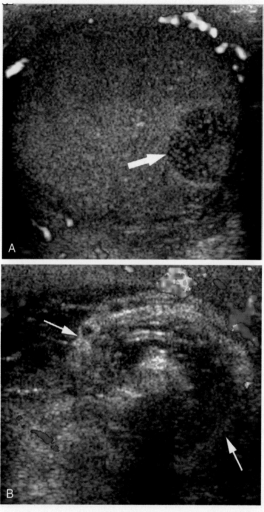

Figure 42.3 Testicular torsion. A, Acute torsion is accompanied by decreased echogenicity of the testis and absence of intratesticular flow with color Doppler. Note the area of central necrosis (arrow). B, The spiral appearance of the spermatic cord indicates torsion (arrows). (Courtesy of T. Ernesto Figueroa, MD, FAAP, FACS. Reprinted with permission from Brant WE, Helms C. *Fundamentals of Diagnostic Radiology*. 4th ed. Philadelphia, PA: Wolters Kluwer/Lippincott Williams & Wilkins Health; 2012).

TABLE 42.1	
Duration of Torsion and Testicular Salvage Rates	
Duration of Torsion (h)	**Testicular Salvage (%)**
<6	85-97
6-12	55-85
12-24	20-80
>24	<10

Data from Smith-Harrison L, Koontz WW Jr. Torsion of the testis: changing concepts. In: Ball TP Jr, Novicki DE, Barrett DM, et al, eds. *AUA Update Series, Vol. 9 (Lesson 32)*. Houston: American Urological Association Office of Education; 1990.

- Owing to the increased risk for torsion of the paired testicle, a contralateral orchiopexy is performed regardless of the viability of the affected testicle.[4]
- The bilateral fixation reduces the risk of torsion in the future.[3]
- An orchiectomy is performed if grossly necrotic tissue is present resulting in a nonviable testicle.
- Orchiectomy rates widely vary between 39% and 71%.[4]
- Most neonatal testicular torsions result in orchiectomy (85%), whereas most adolescent testicular torsions result in detorsion and orchiopexy (65%).[6]
- These findings are due to presentation, ability to vocalize symptoms in a timely manner, and need of pediatric specialty surgeons.

POSTOPERATIVE CARE

- Even if the surgeons are able to salvage the testicle, testicular morphology and fertility may be affected from ischemic damage.[3]
- There is a 6.4% association of torsion with testicular cancer.[7]

PEARLS AND PITFALLS

- Always consider testicular torsion in an acutely erythematous and painful testicle in baby and adolescent boys.
- Gold standard of treatment is an immediate operative scrotal exploration.
- Ultrasound is the best imaging modality for diagnosis in this patients.
- Testicular torsion is **A SURGICAL EMERGENCY.**

REFERENCES

1. Speer M, Mahlmann M, Caero J, Morani AC. Pediatric radiology. In: Elsayes KM, Oldham SA, eds. *Introduction to Diagnostic Radiology*. New York, NY: McGraw-Hill; 2015. http://accessmedicine.mhmedical.com. ezproxy.fau.edu/content.aspx?bookid=1562&Sectionid=95879884. Accessed November 16, 2016.

2. Wall J, Albanese CT. Pediatric surgery. In: Doherty GM, ed. *CURRENT Diagnosis & Treatment: Surgery*. 14th ed. New York, NY: McGraw-Hill; 2015. http://accessmedicine.mhmedical.com.ezproxy.fau.edu/content. aspx?bookid=1202&Sectionid=71529153. Accessed November 16, 2016.

3. Koontz KS, Wulkan ML. Chapter 52: The acute scrotum. *Ashcraft's Pediatric Surgery*. N. p.: Elsevier Health Sciences; 2014:702-704.

4. Sharp VJ, Kieran K, Arlen AM. Testicular torsion: diagnosis, evaluation, and management. *Am Fam Physician*. 2013;88(12):835-840.

5. Filho AC, Rodrigues O, Riccetto CL, Oliveira PG. Improving organ salvage in testicular torsion: comparative study between patients submitted or not to preoperative manual detorsion. *J Urol*. 2016. doi:10.1016/j. juro.2016.

6. Sood A, Li H, Susan K, et al. Treatment patterns, testicular loss and disparities in inpatient surgical management of testicular torsion in boys: a population-based study 1998-2010. *BJU Int*. 2016;118(6):969-979.

7. Uquz S, Yilmaz S, Guragac A, Topuz B, Aydur E. Association of torsion with testicular cancer: a retrospective study. *Clin Genitourin Cancer*. 2016;14(1):55-57.

SUGGESTED READING

Data from Smith-Harrison L, Koontz WW Jr. Torsion of the testis: changing concepts. In: Ball TP Jr, Novicki DE, Barrett DM, et al, eds. *AUA Update Series, Vol. 9 (Lesson 32)*. Houston: American Urological Association Office of Education; 1990.

Chapter 43

Undescended Testicle

Tyler Montgomery and Bradley Roche

- Although it has been known since ancient times that the testicles originated in the abdomen before migrating to the scrotum, John Hunter in the 1750s was one of the first to dissect human fetuses to analyze this process.
- Hunter named the structure attached to the fetal testes the "gubernaculum" (rudder), as he believed it was responsible for mediating testicular descent.[1]
- Until the 19th century, undescended testicles (UDTs) were generally treated with castration.
- James Adams attempted the first surgical correction of a UDT in 1871 at the London Hospital. He was successful, but the patient died on postoperative day 3 of a wound infection. Thomas Annandale performed the first successful orchiopexy 6 years later.
- In 1916, Daniel Eisendrath suggested at the American Urological Society that surgical correction be performed in all patients within the first 2 years of life.[2]

RELEVANT ANATOMY

- In utero, the testes form from the gonadal ridges in the abdomen.
- The testes travel to the scrotum through the inguinal canal during normal development from an unclear mechanism, possibly mediated by the developing gubernaculum, a structure that attaches to the fetal testes (Figure 43.1).
- Normally, the testes migrate through the inguinal canal at week 28 and are located in the scrotum by week 33.[3]
- The inguinal canal carries the spermatic cord and the ilioinguinal nerve from the abdomen to the scrotum (Figure 43.2).
- The spermatic cord contains the genital branch of the genitofemoral nerve, vas deferens, pampiniform plexus, lymphatics, and arteries.
- The deep ring of the inguinal canal is through the transversalis fascia; the superficial ring is through the aponeurosis of the external oblique muscle.

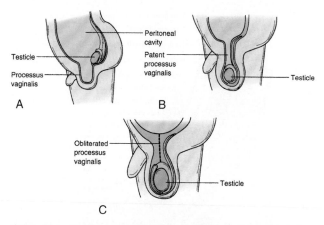

Figure 43.1 The process of testicular descent. A, The testicles originate from the posterior abdomen and begin to descend around 2 months. B, The testicles arrive in the scrotum before birth via a patent processus vaginalis. C, After birth, the processus vaginalis becomes obliterated. (Reprinted with permission from Lawrence PF, Bell RM, Dayton MT, Herbert JC. *Essentials of General Surgery.* 5th ed. Philadelphia, PA: Wolters Kluwer Health/Lippincott Williams & Wilkins; 2012).

EPIDEMIOLOGY AND ETIOLOGY

Incidence: Up to 30% of preterm and 3% of full-term infants are born with an undescended testis, but descent usually completes within the first few weeks of like. The incidence at 9 months is <1%.[4]

Etiology: Multifactorial but anatomic and hormonal factors have been implicated. The gubernaculum, which connects the inferior pole of the testis to the scrotum, is thought to guide the descent from the retroperitoneum to the scrotum. Hormonal factors, including insulinlike factor 3 and testosterone, are involved in initiating the descent.[5]

- Decreased intra-abdominal pressure due to congenital wall defects (floppy belly syndrome, gastroschisis, omphalocele) has been implicated as well.[6]

CLINICAL PRESENTATION

Classic presentation: an otherwise healthy baby who presents with a nonpalpable testis.

- It is paramount to distinguish this from retractile testis, which is a variant of normal anatomy where a hyperactive cremaster

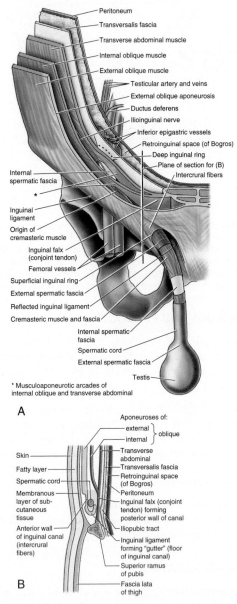

A

* Musculoaponeurotic arcades of
internal oblique and transverse abdominal

B

Figure 43.2 Inguinal canal anatomy. A, Anterior view. B, Schematic sagittal section of inguinal canal. (Reprinted with permission from Moore K, Dalley A, Agur A. *Clinically Oriented Anatomy.* 6th ed. Philadelphia, PA: Lippincott Williams & Wilkins; 2010:204).

muscle pulls the testis superiorly, through the external inguinal ring into the inguinal canal. Unlike UDTs, the testis can be permanently manipulated back into the scrotum.

- The classic physical examination finding in UDT is an empty hemiscrotum.[7]

DIAGNOSIS

Physical Examination Findings

- **Physical examination is the gold standard for identifying UDTs.**
- The patient should be examined in the supine or frog-legged position.
- Starting near the iliac spine, abdominal contents should be milked toward the scrotum along the inguinal canal, attempting to manipulate a UDT into the scrotum. Unlike retractile testis, a UDT will not remain in the scrotum once the maneuver is stopped.
- Applied abdominal pressure may also help a UDT temporarily descend into the scrotum.
- The scrotum should be touched last to avoid activating a cremasteric reflex, retracting the testis even further.[5]
- **This examination should also be performed under general anesthesia before surgical intervention, as palpating a previously nonpalpable testis is possible.**

Laboratory Findings

- Laboratory studies are not routinely indicated in UDTs.
- In cases of nonpalpable bilateral testes, anorchia, androgen insensitivity, and chromosome abnormalities should be considered and evaluated with endocrine laboratory tests: follicle-stimulating hormone, luteinizing hormone, and human chorionic gonadotropin stimulation test of testosterone levels.[5]

Imaging Findings

- Imaging is not routinely indicated in UDT, as it is mainly a clinical diagnosis. If nonpalpable, testicular position is determined laparoscopically during repair.[8]
- In cases of nonpalpable bilateral testes, MRI with contrast may be useful in locating intra-abdominal UDTs.
- **Ultrasound has a sensitivity of 45% for UDTs, does not alter clinical decision making, and should be avoided.[9]**

SURGICAL MANAGEMENT

- Surgery is recommended between 12 and 18 months of age. After 2 years of age, UDT irreversibly affects fertility.
- **Correction of UDT is paramount in managing future malignancy risk.** A 2007 retrospective study of nearly 17 000 Swedish men found that early surgical intervention before puberty dropped the relative risk of testicular malignancy from 5.40 to 2.23.[10]
- Correction allows for future monitoring with routine testicular examinations.
- The type of surgical intervention is determined by whether the UDT is palpable or nonpalpable, irrespective of a unilateral or bilateral presentation.
- No matter the approach, the goal is to deliver the testicle to the scrotum without tension on the gonadal vessels.

OPERATIVE INTERVENTION

- The classic surgical procedure for UDT is a 1-stage or 2-stage **orchiopexy**, depending on the location of the testis and the length of its vascular supply.
- In cases of nonpalpable or intra-abdominal UDTs, **exploratory laparoscopy** is indicated as well. This aids in determining the location or presence of a UDT, as well as whether a 1-stage or 2-stage orchiopexy is indicated.

Palpable UDT Orchiopexy

- If the UDT is palpable, a 1-stage orchiopexy (Figure 43.3) is performed through an incision over the internal inguinal ring, parallel to the inguinal ligament.
- The external oblique is incised, and the testicle and spermatic cord are located.
- Once freed from the canal and gubernacular adhesions, the tunica vaginalis is dissected and amputated from the vas deferens and spermatic vessels.
- At this point, the testicle is ready to be delivered to the scrotum.
- If more length is needed, retroperitoneal dissection through the internal ring may be performed.
- A finger is then inserted to dissect a pathway to the scrotum, and an incision is made in the scrotum, overlying the finger.
- A subdartos pouch is made by blunt dissection with a hemostat.
- Once formed, the hemostat is pushed superiorly through the pouch, up to the inguinal incision.

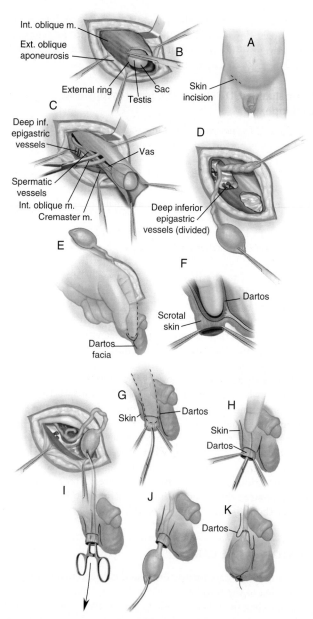

Figure 43.3 Standard inguinal orchiopexy approach. (Reprinted with permission from Lee JJ, Dairiki Shortliffe LM. Chapter 51: Undescended testes and testicular tumors. In: Holcomb GW, Murphy JD, Ostlie DJ, eds. *Ashcraft's Pediatric Surgery*. 6th ed. New York, NY: Saunders; 2014:694).

- The tissue surrounding the testicle is clamped and the testicle is brought down into the subdartos pouch, into the scrotum.
- To prevent future retraction of the testicle, a suture is placed in the dartos to narrow the opening.[5]

Nonpalpable UDT Diagnostic Laparoscopy and Orchiopexy

- If the UDT is nonpalpable or intra-abdominal, diagnostic laparoscopy is performed, with a subsequent 1-stage or 2-stage orchiopexy.
- The gonadal vessels are located and are traced back to find the UDT.
- If the vessels enter the internal inguinal ring, exploration of the inguinal canal is advised.
- Once the UDT is located, the length of the gonadal vessels determines whether a 1-stage or 2-stage orchiopexy is needed.
- UDTs distal to the iliac vessels are usually long enough to be delivered to the scrotum via a 1-stage procedure, as described earlier.
- UDTs with gonadal vessels that are too short should be dissected toward their origin, to increase length.
- At this point, they may be long enough to be delivered to the scrotum.
- Otherwise, a 2-stage orchiopexy is required.
- This can be performed by tacking the testis to the distal abdomen and subsequently be brought down into the scrotum 6 to 12 months later.
- Alternatively, a 2-stage Fowler-Stephens orchiopexy can be performed (Figure 43.4), where the spermatic vessels are ligated and clipped to gain length, allowing collaterals to develop through the vas deferens and cremasteric vessels.
- The testis is then brought into the scrotum 6 months later, after the collaterals have matured.[5]

POSTOPERATIVE CARE

- Postoperative care focuses on wound care and monitoring the position of the testicle.
- Counseling should be provided on testicular examination and future monitoring for malignancy.

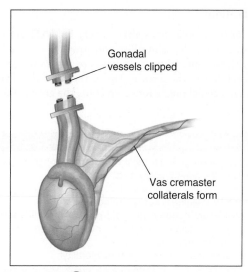

Gonadal
vessels clipped

Vas cremaster
collaterals form

(A) First procedure

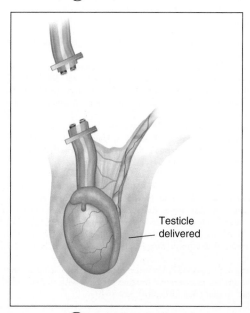

Testicle
delivered

(B) Second procedure

Figure 43.4   The major steps of a Fowler-Stephens 2-stage orchiopexy. A, The gonadal vessels (testicular artery and vein) are clipped to encourage collateral formation through the vas and cremasteric vessels. B, Once mature collaterals have formed, the testicle is then delivered to the scrotum.

Complications

- The major complications after surgery for UDT are retraction of the testicle, subfertility, and atrophy.
- The risk for subfertility or atrophy is related to the adequacy of blood flow to the testicle. The further the UDT from the internal inguinal ring before correction, the greater the risk.

PEARLS AND PITFALLS

- Cryptorchidism (UDT) is the most common congenital abnormality of the genitourinary tract.
- UDT may or may not be palpable.
- Diagnostic imaging is not recommended.
- **Physical examination is the gold standard for diagnosis.**
- Surgical correction is paramount for the management of future malignancy risk.
- Early correction reduces the risk of infertility.

REFERENCES

1. Heyns CF, Hutson JM. Historical review of theories on testicular descent. *J Urol*. 1995;153(3):754-767.
2. Tackett LD, Patel SR, Caldamone AA. A history of cryptorchidism: lessons from the eighteenth century. *J Pediatr Urol*. 2007;3(6):426-432.
3. Sadler TW. Urogenital system. In: sadler TW, Langman J, eds. *Langman's Medical Embryology*. 11th ed. Baltimore: Lippincott Williams and Wilkins; 2009.
4. Bhasin S, Jameson JL. Disorders of the testes and male reproductive system. In: Kasper D, Fauci A, Hauser S, Longo D, Jameson JL, Loscalzo J, eds. *Harrison's Principles of Internal Medicine*. 19th ed. New York, NY: McGraw-Hill; 2014.
5. Lee JJ, Dairiki Shortliffe LM. Undescended testes and testicular tumors. In: Holcomb GW, Murphy JD, Ostlie DJ, eds. *Ashcraft's Pediatric Surgery*. 6th ed. New York, NY: Saunders; 2014.
6. Koivusalo A, Taskinen S, Rintala RJ. Cryptorchidism in boys with congenital abdominal wall defects. *Pediatr Surg Int*. 1998;13(2-3):143-145.
7. Wall J, Albanese CT. Pediatric surgery. In: Doherty GM, ed. *CURRENT Diagnosis & Treatment: Surgery*. 14th ed. New York, NY: McGraw-Hill; 2014.
8. Hartigan S, Tasian GE. Unnecessary diagnostic imaging: a review of the literature on preoperative imaging for boys with undescended testes. *Transl Androl Urol*. 2014;3(4):359-364.
9. Elder JS. Ultrasonography is unnecessary in evaluating boys with a non-palpable testis. *Pediatrics*. 2002;110:748-751.
10. Pettersson A, Richiardi L, Nordenskjold A, et al. Age at surgery for undescended testis and risk of testicular cancer. *N Engl J Med*. 2007;356(18):1835-1841.

Chapter 44

Circumcision

Anne Marie Lopez, Kenan Ashouri, and Fawaz M. Ashouri

- Circumcisions have been performed for over 6000 years.
- The views on circumcision since that time have evolved based on religious beliefs, cultural backgrounds, and medical reasoning.
- Circumcision had its origins in religious sacrifices, cultural rites of passage, and as an adjunct to male hygiene.

RELEVANT ANATOMY

- The prepuce of the penis covers the glans and originates proximally to the coronal sulcus and is made up of an outer skin layer, dartos fascia, and an inner mucocutaneous layer (Figure 44.1).
- The development of the prepuce coincides with the development of the penis. Therefore, any anatomic variations or abnormalities of the penis will result in abnormal foreskin.
- Circumcision ultimately removes the inner and outer layers of the prepuce as well as dartos fascia.

EPIDEMIOLOGY

- The United States is the only country in the developed world where the majority of male newborns are circumcised for nonreligious reasons.
- It is estimated that approximately 80% of males aged 14 to 59 years are circumcised. Most of these patients underwent circumcision as newborns.[1]
- Circumcision rates in the United Sates vary depending on geographic area, race, religion, and socioeconomic status.

INDICATIONS AND BENEFITS

- The formal indications for circumcision have been debated for decades.
- Circumcision is an elective procedure, and therefore there are no current absolute medical indications.

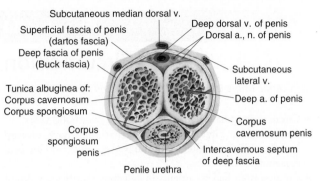

Figure 44.1 Cross-sectional anatomy of the penis. (Reprinted with permission from Anatomical Chart Company. *Male Reproductive System Anatomical Chart*. Lippincott Williams & Wilkins; 2000.)

- In the United States, 40% to 67% of parents decided to have their son circumcised for hygienic, social, and perceived medical benefits.
- Potential benefits of circumcision include lower rates of urinary tract infection (UTI), sexually transmitted infections/diseases, and penile cancer.
- In the pediatric population, decreased rates of UTI are the major benefit of circumcision.

CONTRAINDICATIONS AND RISKS

- Contraindications to neonatal circumcision include an unstable infant, prematurity, congenital penile abnormalities, blood dyscrasias, or a family history of abnormal bleeding.
- If the infant has other penile conditions that require surgical attention, circumcision should not be performed. These include hypospadias, penile curvature, dorsal hood deformity, buried penis, and webbed penis.[3]
- All circumcision procedures are delayed until at least 24 hours after birth to rule out any congenital disorders that may elevate the risk of the procedure.
- Risks of circumcision include procedure-related complications such as infection, bleeding, and problems with wound healing.
- Inadvertent (iatrogenic) amputation of the glans is a devastating but rare complication.
- In 2 major studies that included a total of over 200 000 circumcisions performed in US hospitals, the complication rate for the circumcision procedure was 0.2%.[2]

- Other disadvantages and complications from circumcision include inadequate skin removal with unsatisfactory cosmetic appearance, bleeding, infection, urethral injury, injury to the glans, and epidermal inclusion cyst.

SURGICAL MANAGEMENT

- Several techniques can be used for neonatal circumcision.
- The most commonly used method in the neonate is the Gomco clamp; however, several other clamp devices exist, including the Plastibell and Mogen clamps.
- Place the neonate in the restrictive tray and properly perform a dorsal penile nerve block.
- Ensure that the style clamp used is size-matched with all components.

Gomco Clamp (Figure 44.2)

- Dorsal slit: Place 2 hemostats at the 3- and 9-o'clock positions of the prepuce; place a straight clamp between the 2 at the dorsal midline.
- After 10 to 15 seconds, remove the clamp and complete the slit approximately 0.5 cm at the marking of the straight clamp using straight scissors.
- Next, place the bell portion under the prepuce, over the glans, ensuring that the glans is entirely covered.
- Place the baseplate over the penis by pulling the prepuce through the middle hole.
- Secure the clamp by tightening the baseplate to the bell and check the tension on the prepuce, which should be slightly loose but flat without folds.
- After leaving the clamp in place for 5 minutes, excise the foreskin with a scalpel.

Mogen Clamp

- After disrupting any adhesions between the prepuce and the glans, apply a hemostat to the dorsal midline prepuce while manually retracting the glans downward.
- With the prepuce on stretch, apply the Mogen clamp between the hemostat and glans (with the groove down), ensuring that the glans has not been incorporated.
- Remove the hemostat, and after a few minutes, excise the foreskin with a scalpel and release the clamp.

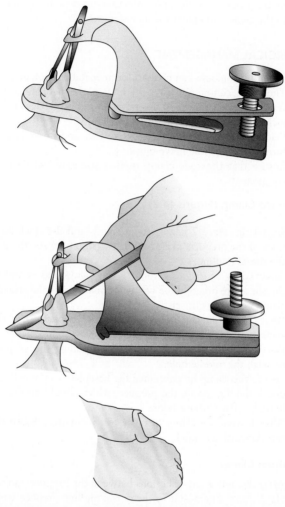

Figure 44.2 Gomco circumcision technique. The technique of performing circumcision is shown in 3 steps: circumcision clamp in place (top), the foreskin is cut (middle), and completed appearance (bottom). (LifeArt image © Lippincott Williams & Wilkins. All rights reserved.).

Sleeve Circumcision (Figure 44.3)

- Outside of the perinatal period, the sleeve technique is preferred and is performed under general anesthesia.
- With the prepuce retracted, mark out the distal margin of the future preputial edge, leaving a small rim of prepuce distal to the corona on the mucocutaneous aspect.
- This should involve the base of the frenulum.
- Make a circumferential incision on the previously marked line down to dartos fascia.
- Reduce the prepuce and mark out a corresponding incision for the outer aspect of the sleeve.
- After making your outer incision, connect the 2 and excise the skin by dividing dartos along the new distal edge of the prepuce.
- At this point, some authors advocate the use of bipolar electrocautery; however, its use should be limited to avoid unnecessary loss of penile tissue.
- Close the incision with either 5-0 chromic or vicryl in quartiles radially at 12, 6, 3, and 9 o'clock and then again splitting the distance between the original sutures.
- At our center, we prefer a nonadherent gauze dressing to reduce pain at dressing changes.

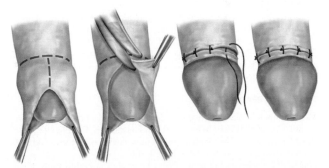

Figure 44.3 Sleeve circumcision. (Reprinted with permission from Nath JL. *Programmed Learning Approach to Medical Terminology.* 3rd ed. Philadelphia, PA: Wolters Kluwer; 2019.)

PEARLS AND PITFALLS

- Circumcision is an elective procedure with no absolute medical indications.
- The potential benefits of circumcision in the neonate include decreased rate of UTIs.
- Contraindications to circumcision include an unstable infant, prematurity, congenital penile abnormalities, bleeding disorders, or any other abnormalities of the penis that will require surgical attention.
- Be sure to carefully assess the meatus and median raphe for any congenital penile or urethral abnormalities before circumcision.
- It is absolutely crucial not to incorporate any part of the glans or urethra into the clamped portion of any of the circumcision devices.
- It is also prudent to measure and mark the desired length of foreskin before clamping.
- Postoperative infection can be treated and monitored clinically, but residual deficits in coverage should be closed primarily.
- Oral sucrose is a useful adjunct when performing circumcision under local anesthesia.

REFERENCES

1. Wiswell TE, Geschke DW. Risks from circumcision during the first month of life compared with those for uncircumcised boys. *Pediatrics.* 1989;83(6):1011-1015.
2. Morris BJ, Bailis SA, Wiswell TE. Circumcision rates in the United States: rising or falling? What effect might the new affirmative pediatric policy statement have? *Mayo Clin Proc.* 2014;89(5):677-686.
3. Palmer LS, Palmer JS. Management of abnormalities of the external genitalia in boys. *Campbell-Walsh Urology.* 11th ed. Philadelphia, PA: Elsevier; 2016.

SUGGESTED READING

McCammon KA, Zuckerman JM, Jordan GH. Surgery of the penis and urethra. *Campbell-Walsh Urology.* 11th ed. Philadelphia, PA: Elsevier; 2016.
Peleg D, Steiner A. The Gomco circumcision: common problems and solutions. *Am Fam Physician.* 1998;58:891-906.
Sinkey RG, Eschenbacher MA, Walsh PM, et al. The GoMo study: a randomized clinical trial assessing neonatal pain with Gomco vs Mogen clamp circumcision. *Am J Obstet Gynecol.* 2015;212(5):664.e1.

Chapter 45

Ovarian Torsion

Ann M. Polcari

- The ovary is a female reproductive organ suspended within the pelvis.
- It is in close proximity to the uterus and fallopian tubes by several ligaments (Figure 45.1A):
  - Directly connected to the uterus via the ovarian ligament
  - Directly connected to the pelvic wall via the suspensory, or infundibulopelvic, ligament
  - Covered by the broad ligament. As the name describes, the broad ligament consists of a wide, fibrous tissue connecting and covering the uterus, fallopian tubes, and ovaries. It is divided into 3 continuous parts: the mesometrium, mesosalpinx, and mesovarium
- The ovary has dual blood supply: from the uterine arteries, found within the broad ligament, and from the ovarian artery, found in the suspensory ligament (Figure 45.1B).
  - The uterine artery branches off of the internal iliac, whereas the ovarian artery branches directly off the descending aorta
- Venous drainage parallels the arterial supply.
- The ureters pass just posterior to the uterine artery to reach the bladder. This is a potential site of ureteral damage during pelvic surgery.

EPIDEMIOLOGY AND ETIOLOGY

Incidence: Ovarian torsion represents approximately 3% of all acute gynecologic complaints; up to 25% of these occur in children.[1,2]

- The condition is most common in women of reproductive age, particularly women in their 20s.

Etiology:

- At birth, the ovaries are positioned high in the pelvis. A surge of hormones during early puberty signals shortening of the ovarian ligaments, causing the ovaries to descend. Therefore,

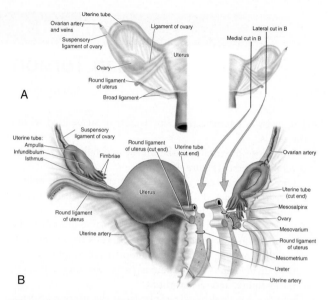

Figure 45.1 Uterus, uterine tubes, and broad ligament. A, Relationship of the broad ligament to the ovary and its ligaments (anterior view). B, Sagittal sections showing the mesentery of the uterus (mesometrium), ovary (mesovarium), and uterine tube (mesosalpinx) (anterolateral view). (Reprinted with permission from Moore KL, Agur AMR, Dalley AF, Moore KL. *Essential Clinical Anatomy*. 5th ed. Philadelphia, PA: Lippincott Williams & Wilkins, a Wolters Kluwer Business; 2015.)

prepubertal and early-pubertal girls have slack in the ovarian ligaments, a predisposition for torsion.[1]

- Torsion is more common on the right, likely because twisting of the left ovary is hindered by the sigmoid colon.[1]
- This condition is typically associated with the presence of an ovarian cyst or tumor (eg, a benign teratoma), especially if larger than 6 cm.[3]
- However, up to 33% of torsion presents in children with normal ovaries.[2]
- Ovarian torsion occurs most often owing to twisting of the broad ligament. At first, only venous obstruction occurs; owing to dual supply with high-pressured arteries, there is continued blood flow into the ovary. Maintained inflow without outflow leads to congestion and edema. Once pressure is great enough to also compress the arterial supply, hypoxia sets in, leading to a cyanotic organ (Figure 45.2).[4]

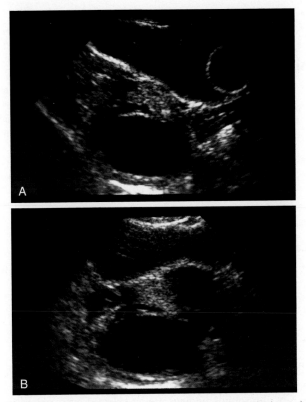

Figure 45.2 Ovarian torsion in a 15-year-old girl. A, Longitudinal transabdominal scan. B, Transverse transabdominal scans. Complex, predominantly cystic mass within the cul-de-sac and slightly to the right. Note balloon of Foley catheter within the urinary bladder. At surgery, a 6-cm blue necrotic mass compatible with torsion was found in the cul-de-sac originating from the left adnexa. (Reprinted with permission from Benrubi GI. *Handbook of Obstetric and Gynecological Emergencies.* 4th ed. Philadelphia, PA: Lippincott Williams & Wilkins, a Wolters Kluwer Business; 2010.)

CLINICAL PRESENTATION

Classic presentation: an otherwise healthy teen who presents with acute-onset unilateral lower abdominal pain, severe and sharp in nature.

- Most patients have associated nausea and vomiting.
- Pain may radiate to the flank, groin, or thigh.
- 50% to 60% of patients will have a palpable pelvic mass.[3]

- Low-grade fever at presentation suggests necrosis.
- *Note: This presentation is very similar to that of acute appendicitis, rupture of an ovarian cyst, and ectopic pregnancy.*

Special Circumstances[5]

- Ovarian torsion has been reported in infants as young as 2 months. These patients usually present with fussiness, irritability, feeding intolerance or vomiting, and abdominal distension. Usually, an ovarian mass has been previously identified on prenatal ultrasounds in these cases.
- Symptoms in premenarchal girls have also been reported to be of longer duration, with diffuse pain, fever, and a palpable mass by the time they present to a physician.

DIAGNOSIS

Laboratory Findings

- Ectopic pregnancy must be ruled out in sexually active girls with a serum beta-HCG.
- Abnormal laboratory findings are absent in most patients.
- If leukocytosis is present in a patient with suspected torsion, it can be a sign of necrosis.
- There is no single serum marker for ovarian torsion!

Imaging Findings

- The imaging modality of choice is the Doppler ultrasound.
- **Key ultrasounds findings are** an enlarged ovary or ovarian mass, raising suspicion for a source of torsion, and absence of blood flow into or out of the ovary (Figure 45.3).
- The absence of blood flow is highly predictive of torsion, but the **presence of blood flow** into a rounded and enlarged-appearing ovary **does not rule out torsion!** (Figure 45.4)
- Also on ultrasound, the twisted ligaments may look like a bull's-eye, whirlpool (Figure 45.5), or snail shell.
- Computed tomography (CT) and/or magnetic resonance imaging (MRI) are not typically required.

SURGICAL MANAGEMENT

- **Ovarian torsion is a SURGICAL EMERGENCY!**
  - Immediate operative management is vital to save the organ and maintain its functionality, which can affect a patient's future ability to reproduce.

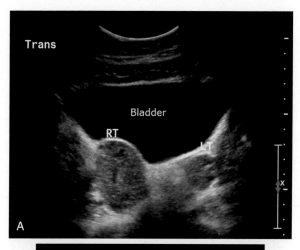

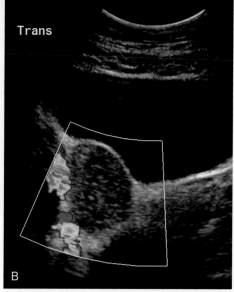

Figure 45.3 Ovarian torsion by ultrasound showing asymmetric enlargement of the ovary. A, Transverse gray-scale sonographic view of the pelvis in a 12-year-old girl shows asymmetric enlargement of the right ovary (RT) compared with the left (LT). Measured volumes were 36 and 12 cc, respectively. B, Color Doppler image of the right ovary reveals absence expected blood flow. Ovarian torsion was confirmed surgically. (Reprinted with permission from Iyer RS, Chapman T. *Pediatric Radiology: The Essentials*. Philadelphia, PA: Wolters Kluwer; 2015.)

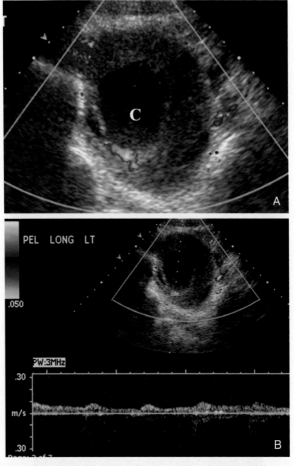

Figure 45.4 Ovarian torsion. A, Flow is noted in the cortex of the torsed left ovary, which contains a cyst (C). B, Pulsed Doppler examination shows diminished arterial flow. Venous flow is absent. (Reprinted with permission from Siegel MJ. *Pediatric Sonography*. 4th ed. Philadelphia, PA: Wolters Kluwer Health/Lippincott Williams & Wilkins; 2011.)

- Rat models have shown necrosis with torsion of just 36 hours' duration.[5]
- If one has a high suspicion of ovarian torsion, or has ultrasound results supporting the diagnosis, proceed directly to surgery.
- Definitive diagnosis is made in the operating room, via direct visualization (Figure 45.6).

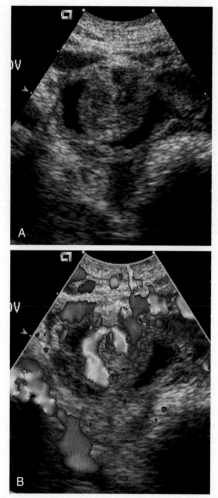

Figure 45.5 Whirlpool sign of ovarian torsion. A, Adnexal mass. B, Color Doppler reveals swirling configuration of blood vessels in the mass. At surgery, ovarian pedicle was twisted 10 to 12 times. (Reprinted with permission from Benrubi GI. *Handbook of Obstetric and Gynecological Emergencies.* 4th ed. Philadelphia, PA: Lippincott Williams & Wilkins, a Wolters Kluwer Business; 2010.)

Operative Intervention

- The operation of choice is detorsion of the ovary, with cystectomy if a benign cyst or tumor is identified.
- The laparoscopic approach is preferred.

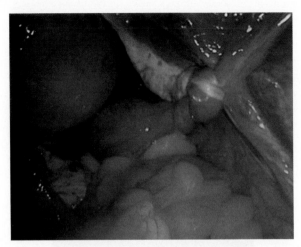

Figure 45.6 Torsion of the adnexa. (Reprinted with permission from Benrubi GI. *Handbook of Obstetric and Gynecological Emergencies*. 4th ed. Philadelphia, PA: Lippincott Williams & Wilkins, a Wolters Kluwer Business; 2010.)

- Unilateral oophorectomy or salpingo-oophorectomy is reserved only for those ovaries that are overtly necrotic—ie, the tissue appears black and the patient has systemic signs or symptoms—or on the rare occasion where a malignant lesion is suspected.
  - Studies have shown that even an ovary appearing bluish should not be removed, as it may regain function postoperatively.[4]
- Some surgeons recommend oophoropexy as a preventive measure against future torsion.
  - This can be accomplished by suturing the mesovarium or utero-ovarian ligament to either the pelvic side wall, posterior aspect of the uterus, or round ligament.[4]
  - There is little long-term evidence to prove the procedure is effective.[3]

Laparoscopic Approach

- The patient is placed supine in the Trendelenburg position.
- Three small incisions are made for laparoscopic instrument ports.
- Port placement varies by surgeon, but typically the camera goes through the umbilicus, and the other ports are placed near the anterosuperior iliac spine, above the mons pubis, or somewhere in-between these 2 sites.

- Once the camera is inserted and the torsed ovary is visualized, a determination is made to proceed with either detorsion or oophorectomy.
- Most cases require detorsion alone.
- Untwisting of the ovary is performed using a blunt probe or grasper with atraumatic teeth.
- Some surgeons have proposed intraoperative methods of determining return of ovarian perfusion after detorsion, which include making a small incision into the cortex of the ovary to observe bleeding and using IV fluorescein to directly visualize flow into the ovary under UV light.
- These methods are still considered experimental.[5,6]
- If cystectomy is required, the utero-ovarian ligament is grasped for stabilization and held by an assistant.
- Vasopressin is injected into the capsule of the ovary, just before making an incision into the capsule with either electrocautery or a knife.
- With the capsule open, dissection around the cyst is completed with blunt instruments.
- When the base of the cyst is visible, it is clamped and coagulated, and the cyst is excised.
- Cysts should be removed intact, if possible, and sent for pathology review.
- The ovarian capsule does not require closure.[6,7]
- If completing the surgery with oophoropexy, 2 to 3 interrupted sutures are used to bring together the ovarian capsule and the pelvic wall.[7]

Open Approach

- The patient is placed supine and a low-transverse abdominal incision is made.
- The procedure is performed in a similar fashion to that of the laparoscopic approach; however, untwisting can be executed manually.

Complications

- Intraoperative complications include hemorrhage and damage to the ureter as it passes under the uterine artery.
- As in most surgeries, postoperative complications include continued bleeding or infection, adhesions to the pelvic or abdominal wall, and in this case progression to necrosis of the affected ovary.
- In very rare situations, pulmonary embolism of venous clots after detorsion have occurred.

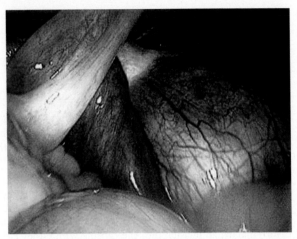

Figure 45.7 Adnexal mass with torsion. (Reprinted with permission from Berek JS. *Berek and Novak's Gynecology.* 15th ed. Philadelphia, PA: Lippincott Williams & Wilkins, a Wolters Kluwer Business; 2012.)

POSTOPERATIVE CARE

- Most ovaries regain function after detorsion and resolution of inflammation.
  - One study noted that 80% of detorsed ovaries had follicle development on follow-up ultrasound.[5]
- If the torsed ovary was blue on surgical inspection (Figure 45.7), one must be attentive to signs of sepsis and peritonitis, as either of these may signal progression to necrosis of the organ, which requires reoperation.

PEARLS AND PITFALLS

- Ovarian torsion occurs as a result of twisted ligaments compressing blood vessels.
- It can occur in pediatric patients with a benign mass or a normal-appearing ovary.
- Ultrasound is the standard imaging technique but is not always definitive.
- Ovarian torsion is **A SURGICAL EMERGENCY!**
- Operation of choice is laparoscopic detorsion, with or without oophoropexy.

REFERENCES

1. Dolan MS, Hill C, Valea FA. Benign gynecologic lesions: vulva, vagina, cervix, uterus, oviduct, ovary, ultrasound imaging of pelvic structures. In: Lobo RA, Gerhenson DM, Lentz GM, Valea FA, eds. *Comprehensive Gynecology*. Philadelphia: Saunders Elsevier; 2017:370-422.e5.

2. Veras EF, Crow JH, Robboy SJ. Non-neoplastic and tumor-like conditions of the ovary. In: Mutter GL, Prat J, eds. *Pathology of the Female Reproductive Tract*. 3rd ed. Philadelphia: Saunders Elsevier; 2014:535-563.

3. Strickland JL. Pediatric and adolescent gynecology. In: Holcomb GW, Murphy JP, Ostlie DJ, eds. *Ashcraft's Pediatric Surgery*. 6th ed. Philadelphia: Saunders Elsevier; 2010:1045-1057.

4. Hoffman BL, Schorge JO, Bradshaw KD, Halvorson LM, Schaffer JI, Corton MM. *Williams Gynecology*. 3rd ed. New York: McGraw-Hill; 2016.

5. Laufer MR. *Ovarian and Fallopian Tube Torsion. UpToDate [Internet]*. June 1, 2017. [cited 2017 Aug. 20]. Available from: https://www-uptodate-com.access.library.miami.edu/contents/ovarian-and-fallopian-tube-torsion?source=see_link&sectionName=CLINICAL%20PRESENTATION&anchor=H327710#H1.

6. Falcone T, Walters MD. Laparoscopic adnexal surgery. In: Baggish MS, Karram MM, eds. *Atlas of Pelvic and Gynecologic Surgery*. 4th ed. Philadelphia: Saunders Elsevier; 2016:1255-1262.

7. Brandt ML. Laparoscopic ovarian surgery. In: Holcomb GW, Georgeson KE, Rothenberg SS. *Atlas of Pediatric Laparoscopic and Thoracoscopy*. Philadelphia: Saunders Elsevier; 2008:149-155.

Chapter 46

Extracorporeal Membrane Oxygenation (ECMO)

Reagan Lindsay Ross

- Extracorporeal membrane oxygenation (ECMO) remains the most commonly used form of pediatric mechanical circulatory support in the United States.
- More than 3500 cases of pediatric cardiac ECMO have been registered in the Extracorporeal Life Support Organization.[1-3,5]
- ECMO is used for short-term support, significantly limiting its effectiveness as a bridge to transplantation or recovery for children, particularly in infants with unrecoverable cardiac failure who require mechanical circulatory support often die if a donor heart does not become available in a few weeks.
- As the pediatric circulatory support has increased, a greater number of devices for children have become available.
- Currently available devices include ECMO, the Bio-Pump (Medtronic Corp., Minneapolis, Minnesota), the DeBakey VAD *Child* (MicroMed Cardiovascular, Inc., Houston, Texas), the Berlin Heart VAD (Berlin Heart Inc, The Woodlands, Texas), and a number of adult devices that have been successfully used in children (Figure 46.1).[4,6]
- Each device offers certain advantages and limitations.
- This chapter will focus primarily on ECMO, specifically, the history of ECMO, the ECMO system, and indications for use (Figure 46.2).
- Additionally, the technique as well as multiorgan management during ECMO and mechanical and medical complications will be discussed.

HISTORY OF ECMO

- In 1953 JH Gibbon Jr used an artificial oxygenation and perfusion support for the first open heart surgery.[7]
- The following year, CW Lillehei developed a cross-circulation technique by using adult volunteers as live cardiopulmonary bypass apparatuses during the repair of congenital cardiac disorders.[8,9]

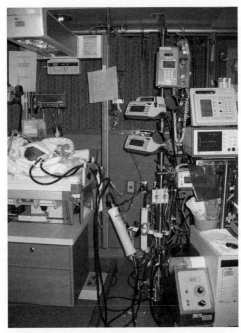

Figure 46.1 Infant on ECMO. (Reprinted with permission from Tecklin JS. *Pediatric Physical Therapy.* 5th ed. Philadelphia, PA: Lippincott Williams & Wilkins, a Wolters Kluwer business; 2014.)

- In 1965, Rashkind and colleagues were the first to use a bubble oxygenator as support in a neonate with respiratory failure.[10]
- In 1969, Dorson and coworkers reported using a membrane oxygenator for cardiopulmonary bypass in infants.[11]
- In 1970 Baffes et al reported successful use of ECMO in infants with congenital heart defects who underwent cardiac surgical intervention.[12]
- Bartlett and colleagues were the first group to successfully use ECMO in neonates with severe respiratory distress in 1975[13].

EXTRACORPOREAL MEMBRANE OXYGENATION SYSTEM

Indications for ECMO

- Neonates with a diagnosis of primary pulmonary hypertension of the newborn (PPHN), meconium aspiration

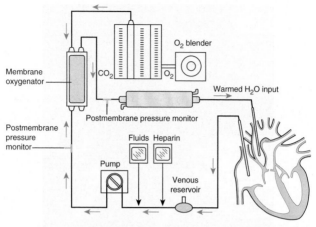

Figure 46.2   ECMO setup. Extracorporeal membrane oxygenation (ECMO) is managed by either a critical care nurse or respiratory therapist with special training in its operation. Illustrated and described here is a typical ECMO setup: arterial filter—removes air bubbles and clots from the blood as it travels through the ECMO circuit; cannula—catheter through which blood travels to and from the patient; control desk module—continuously monitors pressure throughout the circuit and regulates blood flow rate as needed in response to changing pressures in the system; heater—generates heat needed to keep blood at a constant temperature; heat exchanger—uses heat generated by a heater to maintain the temperature of the blood as it is oxygenated; Hemochron—monitors blood clotting; IV pump—allows injection of medications, such as antibiotics, into the cannula of the ECMO circuit; membrane oxygenator—serves as the artificial lung supplying oxygen to the blood; and transonic blood flowmeter—measures the amount of blood flowing through the cannula at various places along the ECMO circuit. (Reprinted with permission from *Nurse's 5-minute Clinical Consult: Treatments*. Philadelphia, PA: Lippincott Williams & Wilkins, a Wolters Kluwer Business; 2007.)

syndrome, respiratory distress syndrome, group B streptococcal sepsis, and asphyxia require the use of ECMO.

- Additionally, congenital diaphragmatic hernia may require the use of ECMO.
- Patient selection criteria may include a gestational age of 34 weeks or more, a birth weight of 2000 g or more, and no significant coagulopathy or major intracranial hemorrhage (grade 1).
- Mechanical ventilation for 10 to 14 days or less, reversible lung injury, and no major untreatable cardiac malformations are also included in the neonatal criteria.
- There should be no lethal malformations, and the neonate should have failed maximal medical therapy before instituting ECMO.

- ECMO is initiated when the infant has reached maximal ventilatory support with 100% FiO_2 with peak inspiratory pressures as high as 35 cm water.
- Additionally, qualifying patient criteria include the following:
  1. Alveolar-arterial gradient of 600 to 624 mm Hg for 4 to 12 hours at sea level
  2. The oxygenation index greater than 40 in 3 of 5 postductal gas samples obtained 30 to 60 minutes apart
  3. Acute deterioration with evidence of PaO_2 of 30 to 40 mm Hg or less for 2 hours, pH of 7.25 or less for 2 hours, and/or intractable hypotension
- ECMO is also indicated in low cardiac output resulting from right, left, and biventricular failure following repair of a congenital heart defect and pulmonary vasoreactive crisis following congenital heart defect repair with resultant severe hypoxemia, low cardiac output, or both.
- In those patients with multiorgan failure secondary to low cardiac output from congenital heart disease and requiring a bridge to cardiac surgery, ECMO may be instituted.
- Also, it may be used as a bridge for patients with temporary cardiomyopathy from renal failure, myositis, or burns as well as a bridge to cardiac transplant.

ECMO Technique

- ECMO (Figure 46.3) may include venoarterial bypass or venovenous bypass.
- The venoarterial technique is most widely used.
- A cannula is placed into the right atrium via the right internal jugular vein.
- Blood is drained to a venous reservoir located 3 to 4 ft below the heart level.
- The blood is pumped by a roller pump through an oxygenator, where gas exchange occurs.
- The blood is warmed by the heat exchanger and returned to the patient via the cannula placed in the aortic arch via the right carotid artery.
- Systemic heparinization is administered via the circuit with activated clotting times of 180 to 240 seconds.
- This should be monitored frequently.
- Venoarterial ECMO achieves higher PaO_2 levels; lower perfusion rates are needed; and this technique bypasses the pulmonary circulation, decreases pulmonary artery pressures, and provides cardiac support to assist systemic circulation in comparison with venovenous.

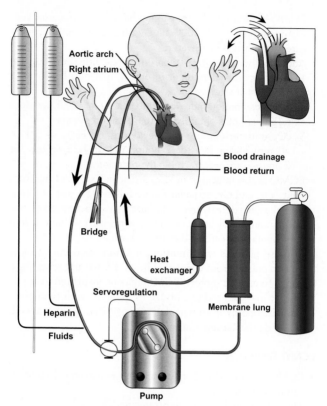

Figure 46.3 ECMO setup. (Reprinted with permission from Lippincott Nursing Advisor 2013. © Wolters Kluwer.)

- Venovenous bypass is performed using a double-lumen cannula placed into the right atrium via the right internal jugular vein.
- Desaturated blood is aspirated from the right atrium via the outer fenestrated venous catheter, and oxygenated blood is returned via the inner lumen of the catheter and is directed across the tricuspid valve.

MULTIORGAN SYSTEM MANAGEMENT DURING ECMO

- Cardiovascular management during ECMO includes maintaining systemic perfusion and monitoring intravascular volume by measuring urine output, central venous pressure, and mean arterial pressure as well as clinical examination findings.

- Echocardiography should be used to guide treatment and to exclude other congenital cardiac anomalies. Inotropic support may be required.
- Typical ventilatory settings with ECMO include an FiO_2 of 21% to 30%, peak inspiratory pressure of 15 to 25 cm water, a positive end-expiratory pressure of 3 to 5 cm water (higher PEEP values may avoid atelectasis and has been found to shorten bypass time), and intermittent mechanical ventilation of 10 to 20 breaths per minute.
- Oliguria and acute tubular necrosis associated with capillary leak and intravascular volume depletion within the first 24 to 48 hours of ECMO is common secondary to the acute inflammatory reaction from ECMO.
- After 48 hours, the patient should begin diuresing.
- If oliguria persists, consider giving diuretics.
- If renal failure ensues, hemodialysis may be added to the circuit.
- Hypoxia and acidosis may lead to central nervous system complications.
- Performing serial neurologic examinations, including the use of head ultrasonography, may be needed.
- Avoid paralytics, and if there is any suspicion of seizures, aggressive treatment is recommended.
- The patient's hemoglobin should be kept at 12 to 15 g/dL.
- Platelet transfusions may be required with the platelet consumption of ECMO.

COMPLICATIONS RELATED TO ECMO

- Care in placement of the cannulation devices is crucial.
- Venous damage with bleeding as well as arterial hemorrhage or dissection can occur in the carotid and/or aortic arch.
- Clots are the most common complication of ECMO.
- They can cause oxygenator failure, consumption coagulopathy, and systemic or pulmonary emboli.
- Systemic heparinization should be utilized while monitoring ACTs.
- Air in the circuit can dislodge the cannula devices, cause a small tear in the membrane, or cause high partial pressure of oxygen in the blood.
- A large air bolus can become fatal.
- If failure of the circuit occurs, clamp the venous line, open the bridge, and clamp the arterial line to remove the patient from the ECMO machine.

- Immediately bag the patient with 100% oxygen or place the patient on the pre-ECMO ventilatory settings.
- Other medical complications may include hemorrhagic complications (intrathoracic, GI/abdominal, pulmonary, or retroperitoneal) with decreased platelet counts, hemolysis, and consumption coagulopathy.
- Additionally, cardiac complications including hypertension, arrhythmias, tamponade, and myocardial stun may ensue.
- Pneumothorax, oliguria, and/or renal failure as well as neurologic complications may also occur.
- Monitoring for electrolyte abnormalities, metabolic derangements, and infectious complications is important.

WEANING ECMO

- The patient must be on reasonable ventilatory settings and demonstrate adequate gas exchange.
- The patient should be able to tolerate a pump flow of 10 to 20 mL/kg per minute with the minimum of 200 mL/min.

PEARLS AND PITFALLS

- ECMO is the most common form of pediatric mechanical circulatory support.
- Techniques include venovenous and venoarterial, the latter being the most common.
- The most common complication from ECMO cannulation is blood clots.

REFERENCES

1. Black MD, Coles JG, Williams WG, et al. Determinants of success in pediatric cardiac patients undergoing extracorporeal membrane oxygenation. *Ann Thorac Surg*. 1995;60:133-138.
2. del Nido PJ. Extracorporeal membrane oxygenation for cardiac support in children. *Ann Thorac Surg*. 1996;61:336-339; discussion 340-341.
3. Duncan BW. Pediatric mechanical circulatory support. *ASAIO J*. 2005;51:ix-xiv.
4. Duncan BW. Pediatric mechanical circulatory support in the United States: past, present, and future. *ASAIO J*. 2006;52:525-529.
5. Walters HL III, Hakimi M, Rice MD, et al. Pediatric cardiac surgical ECMO: multivariate analysis of risk factors for hospital death. *Ann Thorac Surg*. 1995;60:329-336; discussion 336-337.
6. Duncan BW. Matching the mechanical circulatory support device to the child with heart failure. *ASAIO J*. 2006;52:e15-e21.

7. Gibbon JH Jr. Application of a mechanical heart and lung apparatus to cardiac surgery. *Minn Med*. 1954;37(3):171-185.

8. Lillehei CW. A personalized history of extracorporeal circulation. *Trans Am Soc Artif Intern Organs*. 1982;28:5-16.

9. Kirklin JW, Donald DE, Harshbarger HG, Hetzel PS, Patrick RT, Swan HJ. Studies in extracorporeal circulation. I. Applicability of Gibbon-type pump-oxygenator to human intracardiac surgery: 40 cases. *Ann Surg*. 1956;144(1):2-8.

10. Rashkind WJ, Freeman A, Klein D, Toft RW. Evaluation of a disposable plastic, low volume, pumpless oxygenator as a lung substitute. *J Pediatr*. 1965;66:94-102.

11. Dorson W Jr, Baker E, Cohen ML, et al. A perfusion system for infants. *Trans Am Soc Artif Intern Organs*. 1969;15:155-160.

12. Baffes TG, Fridman JL, Bicoff JP, Whitehill JL. Extracorporeal circulation for support of palliative cardiac surgery in infants. *Ann Thorac Surg*. 1970;10(4):354-363.

13. Bartlett RH, Gazzaniga AB, Jefferies MR, Huxtable RF, Haiduc NJ, Fong SW. Extracorporeal membrane oxygenation (ECMO) cardiopulmonary support in infancy. *Trans Am Soc Artif Intern Organs*. 1976;22:80-93.

SECTION 4

Pediatric Surgical Oncology

Chapter 47

Wilms Tumor

Nawara Alawa

- The Wilms tumor, also known as a nephroblastoma, is a renal malignancy typically occurring in children that is thought to have been first described in 1814 by Thomas. F Rance (Figure 47.1).
- It was also subsequently described by Joseph Eberth's 1872 manuscript on a young child who presented with bilateral renal tumors.
- However, it is named after Dr Max Wilms, a German surgeon who formally described the tumor and its histology in 1899 through the addition of several cases of children's kidney tumors to the literature.[1]
- Before the 1920s, very few surgeons attempted to remove these tumors from the bodies of their young patients and those who did experienced mortality rates as high as 25%.[2]
- Two-year survival rates of children with this tumor have evolved from less than 10% in 1915 to 90% in 1985. There has been continuous improvement in survival rates owing to advances in management such as radiotherapy and modulated chemotherapy.[3]
- M. Wittenborg, a radiation oncologist, developed one of the innovative treatment techniques that are still used to supplement surgical resection.

RELEVANT ANATOMY

- Wilms tumor arises from primitive embryonic renal tissue and is typically an intrarenal solid tumor located in the retroperitoneum.

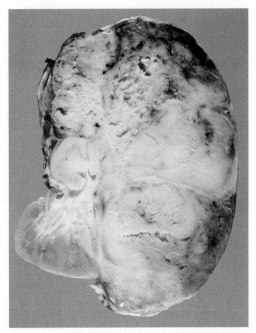

Figure 47.1 Wilms tumor. Typical gross appearance of Wilms tumor with large, bulging variegated mass showing areas of necrosis and hemorrhage. (Reprinted with permission from Jennette JC, Heptinstall RH, eds. *Heptinstall's Pathology of the Kidney.* 6th ed. Philadelphia, PA: Lippincott Williams & Wilkins; 2007.)

- The retroperitoneum, defined as the space between the posterior parietal peritoneum and the transversalis fascia, can be divided into 3 zones:
  - The central zone: aorta, inferior vena cava, pancreas, and duodenum
  - Two lateral zones: the kidneys, ureters, and ascending/descending colon
  - Pelvic zone: rectosigmoid, iliac vessels, and urogenital organs[4]
- Wilms tumors adhere to adjacent structures including but not limited to the diaphragm, liver, and the spleen.
- Careful attention to vessels including the aorta, renal vein, inferior vena cava, and superior mesenteric vessels is crucial to prevent iatrogenic injury.

EPIDEMIOLOGY AND ETIOLOGY

- Wilms tumor is the most common primary renal malignancy of childhood.

- It accounts for 95% of renal tumors in children <15 years of age and 6% of all pediatric malignancies.[5]

Incidence: The annual incidence of renal tumors is about 8.1 cases per million children, resulting in 600 to 700 new cases each year in North America.[6]

- Two-thirds of cases are diagnosed before the age of 5 years, 95% are diagnosed before the age of 10, and the mean age of diagnosis is 3 years of age.
- African-American children are at a greater risk of developing Wilms tumor, while Asian children have reduced risk.[7]
- Wilms tumor is associated with loss of function mutations of a number of tumor suppressors and transcription genes, including mutations of WT1, p53, FWT1, and FWT2 genes.

Etiology: There are a number of theories surrounding the etiology of Wilms tumors, but the exact etiology is still unknown.

CLINICAL PRESENTATION

Classic presentation: Children with Wilms tumor commonly present with a palpable abdominal mass. Other common symptoms include swelling, hematuria, fever, and hypertension.[8]

- A small subset of patients can present with subcapsular hemorrhage and can present with rapid abdominal enlargement, anemia, hypertension, and sometimes fever.
- The most common site of **metastasis** is the lung; however, children rarely present with respiratory symptoms.
- **Other common renal tumors** of childhood include clear cell sarcoma, rhabdoid tumors, renal cell carcinoma, and mesoblastic nephroma.
- These collectively account for about 5% of renal tumors in childhood.
- The **classic physical examination finding** is a firm, nontender, smooth mass that is eccentrically located and rarely crosses the midline.
- Between 5% and 10% of cases present with bilateral Wilms tumor, and this presentation is common in patients with a genetic predisposition to Wilms tumor, such as Beckwith-Wiedemann syndrome (Figure 47.2), WAGR syndrome, or Denys-Drash syndrome.
  - Additional associations include hemihypertrophy, Klippel-Trenaunay-Weber, Perlman syndrome, and genitourinary malformations such as horseshoe kidney.

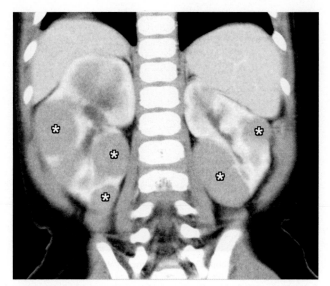

Figure 47.2 An 11-month-old girl with Beckwith-Wiedemann syndrome, bilateral nephroblastomatosis, and presumed bilateral Wilms tumor. Coronal contrast-enhanced CT image shows multiple bilateral low-attenuation renal masses (asterisks) due to nephrogenic rests and multifocal Wilms tumor. (Reprinted with permission from Lee EY. *Pediatric Radiology: Practical Imaging Evaluation of Infants and Children.* Philadelphia, PA: Wolters Kluwer; 2018.)

DIAGNOSIS

Imaging Findings

- With the classic presentation of an abdominal mass, imaging will narrow the differential diagnosis and provide important information for staging of the tumor.
- Abdominal ultrasound is the preferred initial imaging modality, as it is painless, is cost-effective, and does not subject the pediatric patient to ionizing radiation.
  - Doppler ultrasound imaging can be used to assess the renal vein and inferior vena cava for evidence of intravenous tumor extension and patency of vessels (Figure 47.3).
- Computed tomography (CT) scan of the abdomen will confirm renal origin of the mass and provide a better assessment of local extent of disease. CT is also effective in identifying patients with contralateral lesions (Figure 47.4).

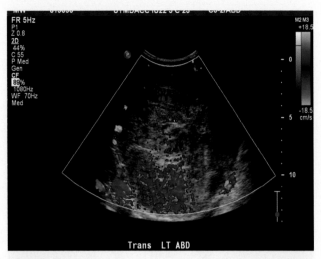

Figure 47.3 Color Doppler image of a large left Wilms tumor showing an area of increased flow. (Reprinted with permission from Dunnick R, Sandler C, Newhouse J. *Textbook of Uroradiology*. 5th ed. Philadelphia, PA: Lippincott Williams & Wilkins, a Wolters Kluwer Business; 2013.)

- It is important to image common sites of metastasis such as the liver and the lungs as well.
- In some cases CT is unable to differentiate Wilms tumor from hyperplastic or sclerotic nephrogenic rests, benign lesions that can undergo malignant degeneration.
- In these cases, MRI is useful to differentiate; however, it is not recommended in initial assessment of suspected nephroblastoma.
- Echocardiography is recommended to rule out intra-atrial extension of the tumor.

Laboratory Findings

- Laboratory studies including urinalysis, liver function, serum calcium, complete blood count, coagulation studies, and basic chemistries should be obtained to gauge baseline functioning and assess for organ dysfunction due to metastasis.

Staging

- Staging guidelines for Wilms tumor are presented in Table 47.1.

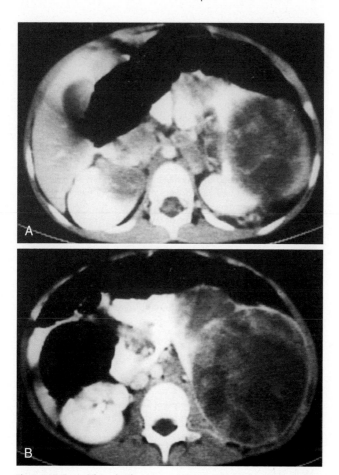

Figure 47.4 A, Bilateral Wilms tumor. A 5-year-old girl with left flank mass. Computed tomography (CT) sections of the upper abdomen with contrast medium enhancement show a necrotic mass arising from superior aspect of the left kidney. Note a small mass in the superior medial aspect of the right kidney. B, Bilateral Wilms tumor (same patient as in A). CT section of the abdomen with contrast medium enhancement shows extent of the large necrotic left Wilms tumor with periaortic adenopathy. (Reprinted with permission from Shaw KN, Bachur RG, eds. *Fleisher & Ludwig's Textbook of Pediatric Emergency Medicine.* 7th ed. Philadelphia, PA: Wolters Kluwer; 2016.)

MEDICAL AND SURGICAL MANAGEMENT

- Since it was first described, the mainstay of therapy for children diagnosed with Wilms tumor is a radical nephroureterectomy and retroperitoneal lymph node sampling.

TABLE 47.1

National Wilms Tumor Study Group/Children Oncology Group Tumor Staging

Stage I

Tumor is limited to the kidney and has been completely resected.

Tumor was not ruptured or biopsied before removal.

No penetration of the renal capsule or involvement of renal sinus vessels.

Stage II

Tumor extends beyond the capsule of the kidney but was completely resected with no evidence of tumor at or beyond the margins of resection.

Penetration of the renal capsule or invasion of the renal sinus vessels.

Stage III

Gross or microscopic residual tumor remains postoperatively including inoperable tumor, positive surgical margins, tumor spillage surfaces, regional lymph node metastases, positive peritoneal cytology, or transected tumor thrombus.

Tumor was ruptured or biopsied before removal.

Stage IV

Hematogenous metastases or lymph node metastases outside the abdomen (lung, liver, bone, brain).

Stage V

Bilateral renal involvement is present at diagnosis, and each side may be considered to have its own stage.

Reprinted by permission from Springer: Ehrlich PF. Wilms Tumor. In: Mattei P, Nichol PF, Rollins MD, et al. eds. *Fundamentals of Pediatric Surgery*. 2nd ed. New York, NY: Springer; 2010. Copyright © 2011 Springer Science+Business Media, LLC.

- Prognostic factors associated with increased risk of recurrence or death include the following:
  - Tumor histology: favorable histology (no anaplasia) versus unfavorable (focal or diffuse anaplasia) (Figure 47.5)
  - Tumor stage
  - Molecular genetic markers
  - Age >2 years
- The presence of these factors leads to a more aggressive treatment strategy, often requiring neoadjuvant or adjuvant chemotherapy and radiation therapy (Figure 47.6).

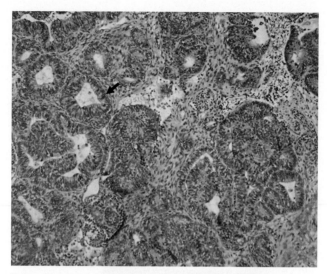

Figure 47.5 Favorable histology triphasic Wilms tumor with predominantly epithelial (tubular) differentiation (arrow). (Reprinted with permission from Constine LS, Tarbell NJ, Halperin EC. *Pediatric Radiation Oncology.* 6th ed. Philadelphia: Wolters Kluwer; 2016.)

Operative Intervention

- Transabdominal transperitoneal incision is standard; however, if the tumor is very large, a thoracoabdominal incision that extends through the eighth or ninth intercostal space provides adequate exposure (Figure 47.7).
- Examination of the abdomen is an important first step to assess for metastases or evidence of peritoneal seeding.
- Current guidelines do not mandate surgical exploration of the contralateral kidney in patients whose initial imaging studies suggest a unilateral process.
- Once the abdomen has been adequately explored, mobilization of the colon to the midline and the bowel is reflected to expose the kidney.
- Gerota fascia is opened, and it is important to palpate the anterior and posterior surfaces of the kidney and inspect hilar and regional lymph nodes.
- Dissection of the kidney is delicate, as these tumors have a tendency to rupture easily leading to the undesired complication of tumor spillage, which requires postoperative radiation.

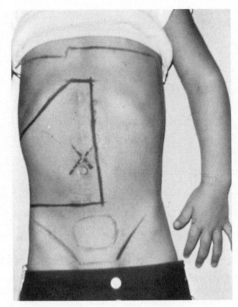

Figure 47.6 Anteroposterior portal for whole abdomen and flank portals used in irradiation of patients with stage III Wilms tumors. The upper margin of the abdominal field must include the diaphragm. The acetabulum and the femoral head should be excluded from the irradiated volume to decrease the probability of slipped femoral epiphysis. (Reprinted with permission from Thomas PRM. Wilms' tumor. In: Perez CA, Brady LW, eds. *Principles and Practice of Radiation Oncology*. 3rd ed. Philadelphia, PA: Lippincott–Raven; 1998:2107-2116.)

- Presently, there is no role for laparoscopic management of Wilms tumors due to the increased risk of rupture and spillage.
- It is rare for contiguous organs to be frankly invaded by Wilms tumor; however, *en bloc* resection is sometimes warranted.
- Ultimately however, extensive resection is not recommended and comes with significant risk and morbidity.
- In cases that may require a more extensive operation, biopsy and chemotherapy followed by a subsequent operation at a later date are advised.
- Two important factors affecting relapse include the failure to biopsy lymph nodes and tumor spillage.

POSTOPERATIVE CARE

- Postoperatively, observation of the surgical incision for erythema, drainage, or separation is important.

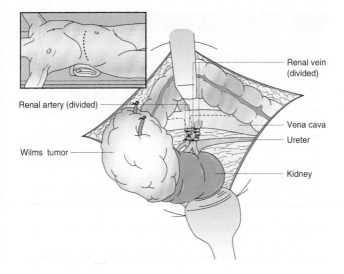

Figure 47.7 Anatomy and operative approach to resection of a Wilms tumor. Reprinted with permission from Mulholland MW, Lillemoe KD, Doherty GM, Upchurch GR, Alam HB, Pawlik TM. *Greenfield's Surgery: Scientific Principles and Practice.* 6th ed. Philadelphia, PA: Wolters Kluwer; 2017.)

- Monitor for signs of infection.
- Monitor IV fluid therapy and intake and output carefully.
- Diet should be advanced slowly to minimize risk of obstructive symptoms.
- Follow-up care should include screening for tumor recurrence with the patient's primary care physician.
- Pain control using multimodal analgesics is advised in kids, as there are no current guidelines about the safe and effective management of postoperative pain control in pediatrics.[9]

COMPLICATIONS

- Major complications include tumor rupture, tumor spillage, thrombus dislodgement, postoperative intussusception, intestinal obstruction, bleeding, and surgical site infections.[10]
- Recurrence occurs in about 10% to 15% of cases after surgical resection.[11]

PEARLS AND PITFALLS

- Wilms tumor or nephroblastoma is the most common renal malignancy of childhood.
- Overall survival of children with Wilms tumor is 85%.
- The initial assessment of an abdominal mass and suspected Wilms tumor should be with ultrasound and CT scan.
- Preoperative and intraoperative biopsies before removing the kidney are not recommended.
- Key prognostic factors include stage, histology, presence of loss of heterozygosity, age of child, and size of tumor.
- The presence of anaplasia on histologic evaluation is the most important predictor of adverse outcomes.
- Factors associated with a worse prognosis include recurrence, failure to sample lymph nodes, and intraoperative tumor spillage.
- Patients should be followed up for tumor recurrence by their primary care physician.

REFERENCES

1. Coppes-Zantinga AR, Coppes MJ. Max Wilms and "Die Mischgeschwülste der Niere" *CMAJ.* 1999;160:1196.
2. D'Angio GJ. Oncology seen through the prism of Wilms tumor. *Med Pediatr Oncol.* 1985;13:53-58.
3. de Camargo B, de Andrea ML, Franco EL. Catching up with history: treatment of Wilms' tumour in a developing country. *Med Pediatr Oncol.* 1987;15:270-276.
4. Tröbs RB. Anatomical basis for Wilms tumor surgery. *J Indian Assoc Pediatr Surg.* 2009;14(2):50-54. doi:10.4103/0971-9261.55151.
5. Bernstein L, Linet M, Smith MA, et al. *Cancer Incidence and Survival Among Children and Adolescents: United States SEER Program 1975-1995, SEER Program.* Bethesda, MD: National Cancer Institute; 1999:79.
6. Howlader N, Noone AM, Krapcho M, et al, eds. SEER Cancer Statistics Review, 1975-2012, National Cancer Institute. Bethesda, MD, based on November 2014 SEER data submission, posted to the SEER web site, April 2015.
7. Breslow N, Olshan A, Beckwith JB, Green DM. Epidemiology of Wilms tumor. *Med Pediatr Oncol.* 1993;21:172.
8. Fernandez C, Geller JI, Ehrlich PF, et al. Renal tumors. In: Pizzo P, Poplack D, eds. *Principles and Practice of Pediatric Oncology.* 6th ed. St. Louis: Lippincott Williams & Wilkins; 2011:861.
9. Lee JY, Jo YY. Attention to postoperative pain control in children. *Korean J Anesthesiol.* 2014;66(3):183-188. doi:10.4097/kjae.2014.66.3.183.
10. Erginel B. Chapter 4: Wilms tumor and its management in a surgical aspect. In: van den Heuvel-Eibrink MM, ed. *Wilms Tumor [Internet].* Brisbane, AU: Codon Publications; 2016.
11. Shamberger RC, Guthrie KA, Ritchey ML, et al. Surgery-related factors and local recurrence of Wilms' tumor in National Wilms Tumor Study 4. *Ann Surg.* 1999;229(2):292-297.

Chapter 48

Neuroblastoma

Reagan Lindsay Ross

- Neuroblastoma is the third most common childhood cancer, after leukemia and brain tumors, and is the most common solid extracranial tumor in children.

EPIDEMIOLOGY AND ETIOLOGY

- More than 600 cases are diagnosed in the United States each year, and neuroblastoma accounts for approximately 15% of all pediatric cancer fatalities.[1]
- The median age at diagnosis is 17.3 months, and 40% of patients are diagnosed before 1 year of age.[1,2]
- Neuroblastomas are the most common cancer among infants younger than 12 months, in whom the incidence rate is almost twice that of leukemia.[3]
- The incidence of neuroblastoma is greater among white than black infants (ratio of 1.7:1 and 1.9:1 for males and females, respectively), but less if any racial difference is apparent among older children.[1]
- Neuroblastoma is slightly more common among boys compared with girls.[1]

EMBRYOLOGY

- Neuroblastoma is commonly used to refer to a spectrum of neuroblastic tumors (including neuroblastomas, ganglioneuroblastomas, and ganglioneuromas) that arise from primitive sympathetic ganglion cells.
- The neuroectodermal cells that comprise neuroblastic tumors originate from the neural crest during fetal development and migrate to the adrenal medulla and sympathetic nervous system.

PATHOLOGY

- The International Neuroblastoma Pathology Classification classifies tumors of neuroblastic origin according to the balance between neural-type cells and Schwann-type cells into neuroblastoma, ganglioneuroblastoma, or ganglioneuroma.

- Neuroblastomas are the most undifferentiated and aggressive of this family of tumors.[4]
- The degree of differentiation and stromal component of neuroblastoma tumors can be predictive of outcome and are used for treatment considerations.
- Neuroblastomas are composed almost entirely of neuroblasts, with very few Schwannian (or stromal) cells (Figure 48.1).
- These are called "stroma-poor" tumors.[5]
- Ganglioneuroblastomas are "intermixed stroma-rich" tumors because of the increased proportion of Schwannian cells.
- These tumors generally have intermediate malignant potential, between that of neuroblastomas and ganglioneuromas.
- Ganglioneuromas are predominantly composed of Schwannian cells studded with maturing or fully mature ganglion cells.[4,6-7]
- These tumors tend to occur in older children aged 5 to 7 years rather than the more aggressive neuroblastomas.
- They are considered to be benign but can metastasize.[8-10]
- The prognosis is excellent, even when complete tumor removal is not possible.[11]

RISK FACTORS

- Risk factors can include maternal, fetal, and genetic factors.

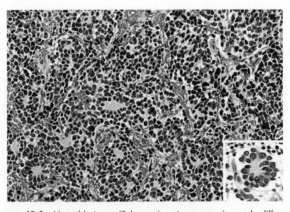

Figure 48.1 Neuroblastoma (Schwannian stroma-poor), poorly differentiated subtype is the most common form of tumor in the neuroblastoma group. Neuroblastoma cells produce neurites and can show rosette formations. Inset: Typical Homer-Wright rosette. (Reprinted with permission from Stocker JT, Dehner LP, Husain AN. *Stocker and Dehner's Pediatric Pathology.* 3rd ed. Philadelphia, PA: Lippincott Williams & Wilkins; 2010.)

- Folate deficiency, other congenital abnormalities, maternal opiate consumption, small- or large-for-gestational-age babies, and maternal gestational diabetes mellitus have all shown a correlation with and may play a role in development of neuroblastoma.
- A higher incidence of neuroblastoma has been suggested in girls with Turner syndrome.[12]
- Hirschsprung disease, central hypoventilation, and neurofibromatosis type 1 have also been described in association with neuroblastoma.[13-16]
- There is a family history of neuroblastoma in 1% to 2% of cases, but most are sporadic.[17-19]
- The inheritance pattern appears to be autosomal dominant with incomplete penetrance and a broad spectrum of clinical behavior.[20]
- Inherited cases usually present at an earlier age than sporadic cases (mean age 9 vs 17 mo), and a large proportion have bilateral adrenal or multifocal disease.

CLINICAL PRESENTATION

- Neuroblastomas can arise anywhere throughout the sympathetic nervous system (Figure 48.2).
- 40% of neuroblastomas arise from the adrenal gland followed by 25% from the abdominal cavity, 15% from the thoracic region, 5% from the cervical region, and 5% in the pelvic sympathetic ganglia.[21]
- Less commonly, tumors arise within the central or autonomic nervous systems.[22] Neuroblastoma has been shown to metastasize to lymph nodes, bone marrow, cortical bone, dura, orbits, liver, and skin, and less frequently to pulmonary and intracranial sites.[23]
- Some of patients presenting symptoms may include abdominal pain or constipation with or without a palpable abdominal mass.
- Palpable, asymptomatic nodules can also appear.
- Localized back pain or weakness from spinal cord compression may be present.
- Scoliosis, bladder dysfunction, bone pain, or anemia may also be present.
- Additionally, patients may present with Horner syndrome, periorbital ecchymoses, or proptosis.
- Opsoclonus-myoclonus syndrome has been described, as well as heterochromia iridis.

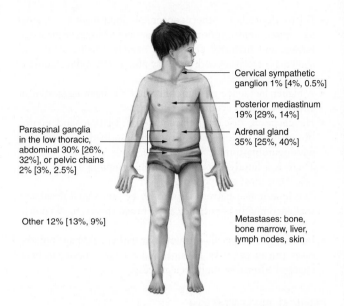

Cervical sympathetic
ganglion 1% [4%, 0.5%]

Posterior mediastinum
19% [29%, 14%]

Paraspinal ganglia
in the low thoracic,
abdominal 30% [26%,
32%], or pelvic chains
2% [3%, 2.5%]

Adrenal gland
35% [25%, 40%]

Other 12% [13%, 9%]

Metastases: bone,
bone marrow, liver,
lymph nodes, skin

Figure 48.2 Common locations of primary tumors in neuroblastoma. The percentage is derived from data on 8369 tumors from the International Neuroblastoma Risk Group project. Tumors arising in the neck and thorax were significantly more common in children <18 months of age. (Reprinted with permission from Constine LS, Tarbell NJ, Halperin EC. *Pediatric Radiation Oncology.* 6th ed. Philadelphia, PA: Wolters Kluwer; 2016. Data from Vo KT, Matthay KK, Neuhaus J, et al. Clinical, biologic, and prognostic differences on the basis of primary tumor site in neuroblastoma: a report from the international neuroblastoma risk group project. *J Clin Oncol.* 2014;32:3169–3176.)

- Some patients have presented with unexplained secretory diarrhea and systemic systems, hypertension, or unilateral nasal obstruction.
- Opsoclonus-myoclonus and secretion of vasoactive intestinal polypeptide are 2 unique paraneoplastic syndromes that can be associated with both localized and disseminated neuroblastomas.

DIAGNOSIS AND STAGING

- All patients should undergo a complete history and physical examination as well as laboratory evaluation including blood counts, serum chemistries, and liver function tests.
- Evaluation of urine or serum catecholamine metabolite levels, vanillylmandelic acid (VMA), and homovanillic acid (HVA) should be obtained to assist in diagnosis and monitoring of

disease response, as levels are elevated in greater than 90% of patients with neuroblastoma.

- In addition, it is recommended to test for ferritin and lactate dehydrogenase (LDH) concentrations, as they may be elevated and can be expected to return to normal during adequate treatment.
- Histologic confirmation is required for definitive diagnosis.
- Tissue is usually obtained by incisional biopsy of the primary tumor or bone marrow biopsy/aspirate in patients who are suspected to have metastatic disease in the marrow.
- For tumors that appear to be localized and resectable without substantial morbidity, the initial diagnostic procedure may include a complete or near-complete resection of the primary tumor and sampling of nonadherent ipsilateral and contralateral lymph nodes.
- The initial procedure should not include resection of vital structures or major motor or sensory nerves.
- As most children will undergo an abdominal ultrasound as initial imaging studies during workup for an abdominal mass, a CT or MRI for further evaluation of the primary tumor site and nodal sites of metastatic disease is recommended in suspected cases of neuroblastoma (Figure 48.3).
- These more advanced imaging studies may reveal a heterogeneous mass, possibly containing calcifications.

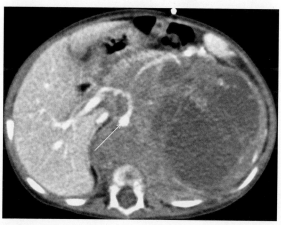

Figure 48.3 Neuroblastoma. Axial postcontrast CT image of the abdomen shows large heterogeneously enhancing mass in the retroperitoneum on left side crossing the midline and causing encasement and displacement of aorta and celiac axis (arrow) compatible with neuroblastoma. (Reprinted with permission from White, AJ. *The Washington Manual of Pediatrics.* 2nd ed. Philadelphia, PA: Lippincott Williams & Wilkins; 2016.)

- If the mass is near the spine, an MRI is recommended to evaluate for spinal canal involvement.
- Those patients who are diagnosed with neuroblastoma must be evaluated for metastatic bone disease with an I123-MIBG scan, which has a sensitivity of approximately 90%.[24]

TREATMENT

- Surgery is the primary treatment for children, with 3 exceptions, with low-risk disease when complete resection is feasible (Figure 48.4).
- Those exceptions include patients with low-risk tumors that cannot be completely resected or that have life-threatening complications.
- Consideration of chemotherapy and/or radiation therapy may be required.
- In patients with asymptomatic 4S disease, observation may be an option, as there is a high rate of spontaneous regression.
- For infants younger than 6 months of age with small, localized adrenal masses, expectant observation with serial ultrasound and urine catecholamines is recommended.

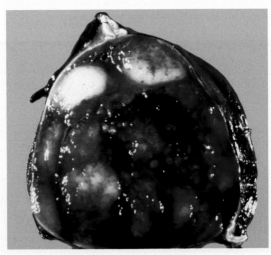

Figure 48.4 Neuroblastoma. Adrenal neuroblastoma (Schwannian stroma-poor), poorly differentiated subtype, measuring 5 × 4.5 cm in the greatest dimension, shows a friable and hemorrhagic appearance. (Reprinted with permission from Stocker JT, Dehner LP, Husain AN. *Stocker and Dehner's Pediatric Pathology.* 3rd ed. Philadelphia, PA: Lippincott Williams & Wilkins; 2010.)

- In children with intermediate-risk disease, a combined modality approach that includes chemotherapy and surgical resection is standard.

PEARLS AND PITFALLS

- Neuroblastoma is the most common extracranial tumor in children.
- 40% of neuroblastomas arise from the adrenal gland.
- This tumor more commonly crosses the midline (than Wilms tumor).

- The degree of surgical resection and duration of chemotherapy required are still uncertain.
- The role of radiation therapy is less clear, except in the context of disease progression despite chemotherapy plus surgery or for complications such as spinal cord compression.
- For those with high-risk neuroblastoma, aggressive combined modality approaches are recommended.
- These generally include chemotherapy, surgical resection, high-dose chemotherapy with stem cell rescue, radiation therapy, and biologic/immunologic therapy.
- These approaches have improved event-free survival, but the majority of patients eventually relapse and die of their disease.

REFERENCES

1. Goodman MT, Gurney JG, Smith MA, Olshan AF. Sympathetic nervous system tumors. In: Ries LA, Smith MA, Gurney JG, et al, eds. *Cancer Incidence and Survival among Children and Adolescents: United States SEER Program, 1975-1995*. Bethesda, MD: National Cancer Institute; 1999:35.
2. Brodeur GM, Hogarty MD, Mosse YP, Maris JM. Neuroblastoma. In: Pizzo PA, Poplack DG, eds. *Principles and Practice of Pediatric Oncology*. Philadelphia: Lippincott Williams & Wilkins; 2011:886.
3. Gurney JG, Ross JA, Wall DA, et al. Infant cancer in the U.S.: histology-specific incidence and trends, 1973 to 1992. *J Pediatr Hematol Oncol*. 1997;19:428.
4. Shimada H, Ambros IM, Dehner LP, et al. The International Neuroblastoma Pathology Classification (the Shimada system). *Cancer*. 1999;86:364.
5. Schwab M, Shimada H, Joshi V, Brodeur GM. Neuroblastic tumours of adrenal gland and sympathetic nervous system. In: Kleihues P, Cavenee WK, eds. *Pathology and Genetics of Tumours of the Nervous System*. Lyon; 2000:153.

6. Origone P, Defferrari R, Mazzocco K, et al. Homozygous inactivation of NF1 gene in a patient with familial NF1 and disseminated neuroblastoma. *Am J Med Genet.* 2003;118A:309.

7. Shimada H, Chatten J, Newton WA Jr, et al. Histopathologic prognostic factors in neuroblastic tumors: definition of subtypes of ganglioneuroblastoma and an age-linked classification of neuroblastomas. *J Natl Cancer Inst.* 1984;73:405.

8. Koch CA, Brouwers FM, Rosenblatt K, et al. Adrenal ganglioneuroma in a patient presenting with severe hypertension and diarrhea. *Endocr Relat Cancer.* 2003;10:99.

9. Meyer S, Reinhard H, Ziegler K, et al. Ganglianeuroma: radiological and metabolic features in 4 children. *Pediatr Hematol Oncol.* 2002;19:501.

10. Geoerger B, Hero B, Harms D, et al. Metabolic activity and clinical features of primary ganglioneuromas. *Cancer.* 2001;91:1905.

11. De Bernardi B, Gambini C, Haupt R, et al. Retrospective study of childhood ganglioneuroma. *J Clin Oncol.* 2008;26:1710.

12. Blatt J, Olshan AF, Lee PA, Ross JL. Neuroblastoma and related tumors in Turner's syndrome. *J Pediatr.* 1997;131:666.

13. Shahar E, Shinawi M. Neurocristopathies presenting with neurologic abnormalities associated with Hirschsprung's disease. *Pediatr Neurol.* 2003;28:385.

14. Nemecek ER, Sawin RW, Park J. Treatment of neuroblastoma in patients with neurocristopathy syndromes. *J Pediatr Hematol Oncol.* 2003;25:159.

15. Stovroff M, Dykes F, Teague WG. The complete spectrum of neurocristopathy in an infant with congenital hypoventilation, Hirschsprung's disease, and neuroblastoma. *J Pediatr Surg.* 1995;30:1218.

16. Kushner BH, Hajdu SI, Helson L. Synchronous neuroblastoma and von Recklinghausen's disease: a review of the literature. *J Clin Oncol.* 1985;3:117.

17. Arenson EB Jr, Hutter JJ Jr, Restuccia RD, Holton CP. Neuroblastoma in father and son. *J Am Med Assoc.* 1976;235:727.

18. Maris JM, Chatten J, Meadows AT, et al. Familial neuroblastoma: a three-generation pedigree and a further association with Hirschsprung disease. *Med Pediatr Oncol.* 1997;28:1.

19. Kushner BH, Gilbert F, Helson L. Familial neuroblastoma. Case reports, literature review, and etiologic considerations. *Cancer.* 1986;57:1887.

20. Perri P, Longo L, McConville C, et al. Linkage analysis in families with recurrent neuroblastoma. *Ann N Y Acad Sci.* 2002;963:74.

21. Neuroblastic tumours of adrenal gland and sympathetic nervous system. In: *Pathology and Genetics of Tumours of the Nervous System.* Lyon: World Health Organization, IARC; 2000:153.

22. Goodman MT, Gurney JG, Smith MA, Olshan AF. Sympathetic nervous system tumors. In: Ries LA, Smith MA, Gurney JG, et al, eds. *Cancer Incidence and Survival among Children and Adolescents: United States SEER Program, 1975-1995.* Bethesda, MD: National Cancer Institute; 1999:35.

23. DuBois SG, Kalika Y, Lukens JN, et al. Metastatic sites in stage IV and IVS neuroblastoma correlate with age, tumor biology, and survival. *J Pediatr Hematol Oncol.* 1999;21:181.

24. Vik TA, Pfluger T, Kadota R, et al. (123)I-mIBG scintigraphy in patients with known or suspected neuroblastoma: results from a prospective multicenter trial. *Pediatr Blood Cancer.* 2009;52:784.

Chapter 49

Pancreatic Tumors in Children

Isolina R. Rossi

- An extremely rare entity, and until 2004, studies relied on case reports and series for their data.
- Most recently, the National Cancer Institute Surveillance, Epidemiology, and End Results (SEER) published data from 1973 to 2004.[1]
- The first successful laparoscopic distal pancreatectomy in a child was documented in 2003.[2]

RELEVANT ANATOMY

- Normal pancreas anatomy is demonstrated in Figure 49.1.
- Lying in an oblique orientation, the pancreas is a retroperitoneal organ.
- There are 4 regions to the pancreas: head, neck, body, and tail.
- Its head rests in the C-shaped duodenum, anterior to the vena cava, right renal artery, and both renal veins. The common bile duct is in the deep posterior groove behind the head.
- The splenic artery and vein run along the posterosuperior aspect of the body (Figure 49.2).
- The lesser sac lies in the space between the pancreas and the stomach, which are lined by peritoneum.
- A plane can usually be developed between the neck of the pancreas and the portal and superior mesenteric vein during a pancreatic resection.
- The vascular supply to the pancreas originates from the celiac trunk and is shared with the duodenum.
- The exception to this rule is the inferior pancreatic head and uncinate process, which is supplied by the superior mesenteric artery.[3]

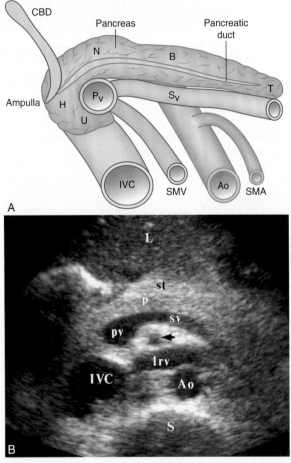

Figure 49.1 Normal pancreas anatomy. A diagram (A) and an ultrasound in transverse plane (B) demonstrate the normal anatomy of the pancreas. The majority of the pancreas (p) lies anterior to the splenic vein (sv) and its junction with the superior mesenteric vein (SMV) forming the portal vein (pv). The head (H) and uncinate process (U) of the pancreas cradle the origin of the portal vein. The pancreatic neck (N) is anterior to the SV-SMV confluence, and the uncinate process and inferior vena cava (IVC) are posterior to the confluence. The superior mesenteric artery (SMA, arrow) arises from the aorta (Ao) dorsal to the splenic vein. The left renal vein (lrv) passes between the SMA and aorta to the inferior vena cava. The left lobe of the liver (L) offers a good sonographic window to the pancreas. The stomach (st) and lesser sac (collapsed) are anterior to the pancreas. CBD, common bile duct; S, spine; B, body of the pancreas; T, tail of the pancreas; p, pancreas. (Reprinted with permission from Brant WE, Helms C. *Fundamentals of Diagnostic Radiology*. 4th ed. Philadelphia, PA: Wolters Kluwer/Lippincott Williams & Wilkins Health; 2012.)

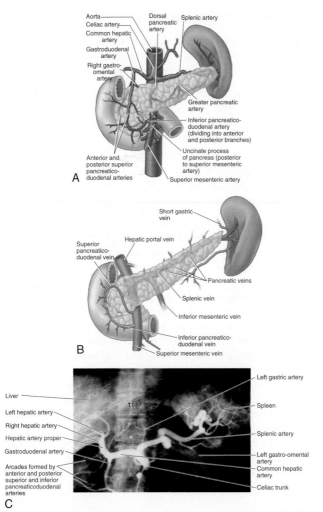

Figure 49.2 Arterial supply and venous drainage of pancreas. Because of the close relationship of the pancreas and duodenum, their blood vessels are the same in whole or in part. A, Arteries (anterior view). Except for the inferior part of the pancreatic head (including uncinate process), the spleen and pancreas receive blood from the celiac artery. B, Venous drainage (anterior view). C, Celiac (anteroposterior view). (Reprinted with permission from Moore KL, Dalley AF, Agur AMR. *Clinically Oriented Anatomy.* 7th ed. Philadelphia, PA: Lippincott Williams & Wilkins; 2014.)

EPIDEMIOLOGY AND ETIOLOGY

Incidence: A review of all documented cases in the United States from 1973 to 2004 suggests an incidence of 1.8 cases of pediatric pancreatic tumors per million children.

- Has a female to male ratio of 1.9:1 and is more common in Asian ethnicities.
- The strongest independent risk factors are stage, histology, and surgical intervention.[1]

Classification: The 3 most common pediatric pancreatic neoplasms are *pancreatoblastoma, solid pseudopapillary neoplasms,* and *pancreatic endocrine tumors.*

- Tumors can arise from either exocrine or endocrine cells.
- *Pancreatoblastoma* (ie, Frantz tumor) is the most common malignant pediatric pancreatic tumor, with both recurrence and metastasis.
- Can be associated with Beckwith-Wiedemann and familial adenomatous polyposis; has a predicted 5-year survival of 66%.[1]
- *Solid pseudopapillary neoplasm* is most common in 20-year-old women but less gender predominant in the pediatric groups.[1]
- Has a 5-year predicted survival of 95% after complete resection, recurrence rate of 10%, and metastatic potential of 19.5% metastatic rate.[2]
- *Pancreatic endocrine tumor* is most common in genetic syndromes such as multiple endocrine neoplasia 1/2 (MEN1/2), von Hippel-Lindau, neurofibromatosis 1, and tuberous sclerosis.[1]
- Insulinomas have a 5-year predicted survival of 85% after surgical resection and 6% incidence of malignancy.
- Higher rates of recurrence have been associated with syndromic tumors.[2]

Etiology

- *Pancreatoblastomas* make up 30% to 50% of all pediatric pancreatic tumors.[4]
- They are embryogenic in origin, considered to be the analogous tumor of hepatoblastoma to the liver and nephroblastoma to the kidney.
- It has both epithelial and mesenchymal cellular makeup.[5]
- *Solid pseudopapillary neoplasms* make up 1% to 3% of all pancreatic tumors.
- They are not generally associated with genetic syndromes or tumor markers.

- They are often thought to originate from embryonic stem cells or ovarian-related cells that migrate during embryogenesis.[6]
- *Pancreatic endocrine tumors:* One-third of gastroenteropancreatic neuroendocrine tumors are located in the pancreas.
- They can be associated with genetic syndromes such as MEN1/2, von Hippel-Lindau, and tuberous sclerosis.[2]

CLINICAL PRESENTATION

- An otherwise healthy child presenting with incidental mass on imaging, palpable mass with abdominal pain, or hypoglycemia.
- *Pancreatoblastoma:* incidental abdominal mass noticed in the first decade of life with a mean of 2.4 years.
- Equal occurrence in tail and head of pancreas.
- Recurrence and metastasis are more common than in other pancreatic tumors.[2]
- Rarely occurs in children over the age of 10 years.
- Congenital forms are almost always associated with Beckwith-Wiedemann syndrome.
- They account for 30% to 50% of pediatric pancreatic neoplasms.[2]
- *Solid pseudopapillary neoplasm:* most common in 20-year-old women, but less gender predominant in the pediatric group.
- Generally a low-grade neoplasm. unlike adults, children are usually symptomatic with abdominal discomfort and pain.[2]
- *Pancreatic endocrine tumor:* most commonly an insulinoma.
- Generally, they are benign lesion with equal occurrence in head and tail of pancreas.
- Children often present with severe postprandial hypoglycemia and may often be initially worked up for seizures.
- Whipple triad is classic: fasting hypoglycemia, symptoms of hypoglycemia, relief of symptoms with glucose administration.[2]
- *Insulinomas (pancreatic endocrine tumor)* must be differentiated from congenital hyperinsulinism.
- On histopathology, insulinomas do NOT preserve the lobular architecture.[7]

DIAGNOSIS

Laboratory Findings

- *Pancreatoblastoma:* Although numerous cases of elevated alpha-fetoprotein have been documented, it is not considered a sensitive marker.
- Initial measurement of this marker may allow for surveillance of recurrence after treatment.[5]

- *Solid pseudopapillary neoplasm*: Elevated alpha-1-antitrypsin, alpha-1-antichymotrypsin, neuron-specific enolase (NSE), vimentin, and progesterone receptor have been documented, but these are not considered sensitive markers.[4]
- *Pancreatic endocrine tumor:* This may or may not be symptomatic.
- Insulinomas may present with Whipple triad of fasting hypoglycemia, symptoms of hypoglycemia, and resolution of symptoms with glucose administration.
- When hypoglycemia occurs in children, imaging and workup are indicated to rule out insulinoma.
- Gastrinomas can cause Zollinger-Ellison syndrome, reflux, and secretory diarrhea.[2]

Imaging Findings

- Imaging modality of choice for pancreatic mass in a child is ultrasonography, particularly in children with vague abdominal pain.[8]
- The pancreas and retroperitoneal fat can be difficult to differentiate owing to similar echogenicity; thus cross-sectional imaging is indicated if a mass is identified.
- Computed tomography (CT) and magnetic resonance imaging (MRI) are both acceptable modalities that also allow for staging.[8]
- Aggressive attempt at preoperative tissue diagnosis (ie, biopsy, fine needle aspiration) is most important if alternative diagnoses are being considered.
- Biopsy is discouraged if a *solid pseudopapillary neoplasm* is suspected.[2]
- *Pancreatic endocrine tumor:* Arterial stimulus with venous sampling (ASVS) and transhepatic portal venous sampling (THVS) can be used to diagnose *insulinoma* when all other imaging has failed.[2]

TNM Staging

- Tumor-node-metastasis (TNM) staging is used for pancreatic neoplasms.

SURGICAL MANAGEMENT

- *Pancreatoblastoma:* High-stage tumors are recommended for neoadjuvant chemotherapy for improved resection rates (EXPeRT trial).[9]

- Surgical resection is the standard for both primary and metastatic tumors.
- Irradiation is recommended for surgical intervention that does not successfully remove all tumor.
- Unresectable disease is often invasive of porta hepatis, invasive of major vasculature (aorta, inferior vena cava), or metastatic.
- Such invasion should be screened for on imaging.[8]
- *Solid pseudopapillary neoplasm*: Complete resection with negative margins is often curative.
- Enucleation has been linked to higher recurrence rates.
- Owing to high risk of recurrence, biopsy is also discouraged.[2]
- *Pancreatic endocrine tumor:* Complete resection of primary and metastatic disease is curative (Figure 49.3).
- If the tumor is in the head, neck, or proximal body, then enucleation should be performed.
- It is common that the tumor cannot be localized before surgery.
- Intraoperative ultrasound is ideal in this situation.
- A thorough search for the tumor focus includes medially mobilizing the pancreatic tail and spleen for bimanual palpation.

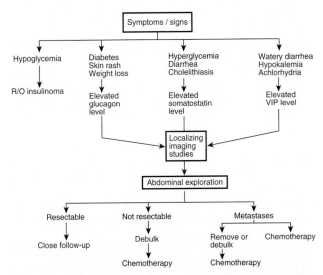

Figure 49.3 Treatment algorithm for common endocrine tumors of the pancreas. (Reprinted from Schwartz MZ. Unusual peptide-secreting tumors in adolescents and children. *Semin Pediatr Surg.* 1997;6:141-146; Copyright 1997, with permission from Elsevier.)

- If serum hormone levels are elevated before surgery, repeat levels 20 minutes after removal of the specimen can determine the efficacy of resection and need for further dissection.[10]

OPERATIVE INTERVENTION

- Distal pancreatectomy: necessary for removal of masses in the pancreatic tail.
- The spleen should be preserved as often as possible in benign or low-grade tumors to avoid postsplenectomy infections.
- Total pancreatectomy: avoided if possible by partial or subtotal pancreatectomies and enucleation.
- Pancreaticoduodenectomy: necessary for removal of malignancy of pancreatic head or common bile duct, which is rarely seen in children.
- En bloc removal of pancreatic head, distal common bile duct, duodenum, jejunum, and gastric antrum.
- Pylorus preserving techniques have been considered in the absence of abnormal lymph nodes along the hepatic artery and when a free margin of at least 3 cm exists between the pylorus and the mass, but does not reduce morbidity or mortality.[11]
- Extended lymphadenectomy of nodes from the celiac axis, iliac bifurcation, portal vein, and SMA increases morbidity with no change in mortality.[12]
- Open procedures are generally performed for multiple reasons: there is no proven advantage of laparoscopy in pediatric pancreatic tumors, the need for smaller instruments for the pediatric population, and lack of formal training due to low case volume.[13]
- At the time of this publication, there is no existing randomized control trial that compares open versus laparoscopic distal pancreatectomy for pancreatic cancer in children.
- Many case series have reported noninferior results with laparoscopic versus open distal pancreatectomy, particularly for *solid pseudopapillary neoplasms*.[14]
- Neoadjuvant chemotherapy is indicated for high-stage *pancreatoblastomas* for improved resection rates.[9]
- Management of vasculature with electrocautery (monopolar or bipolar) has become the preferred method of hemostasis.

- It is important to take down the venous pancreatic branches that drain into the splenic vein and the splenic arterial branches.
- During pancreatic head resections, the vessels supplying the third and fourth sections of the duodenum must remain intact to prevent duodenal ischemia.
- These vessels arise from the celiac trunk proximally and the SMA distally.[7]

Open Approach

- Pancreatic exposure can be achieved by transecting the gastrocolic ligament to enter the lesser sac and by mobilizing the splenic flexure.
- Splenic vessels can then be identified on the superior aspect of the pancreas.
- Management of these vessels depends on whether the spleen will be preserved or removed.
- Liver, visceral, and parietal peritoneal surfaces should be surveyed to ensure proper resection.
- For a distal pancreatectomy, the tail of the pancreas is transected with suture ligation of the pancreatic duct.
- The spleen should be conserved if possible.
- A drainage tube is left in place, to be removed 3 weeks postoperatively.
- For a pancreaticoduodenectomy, gastrohepatic omentum is opened and celiac axis should be assessed for abnormal nodes.
- Ascending colon and hepatic flexure should be medially freed from duodenum and head of the pancreas.
- Kocher maneuver allows for dissection posterior to the pancreatic head (Figure 49.4).
- The gastroepiploic artery and vein are ligated to avoid injury (Figure 49.4).
- Mesenteric vascular involvement should be determined preoperatively with imaging and not by intraoperative palpation.
- An aberrant right hepatic artery exists in 20% of the population.
- It branches from the SMA posterior to the pancreas and is also best assessed on imaging preoperatively.
- The gastroduodenal artery is ligated, and the pancreatic neck should be easily dissected from the anterior portal vein in the absence of tumor invasion.
- A cholecystectomy follows, and the duodenum is divided (location depends on pylorus preservation).

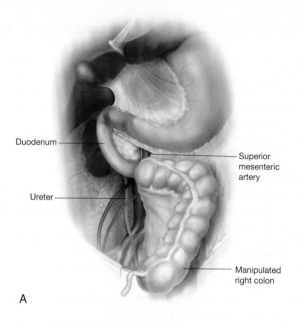

Duodenum

Superior
mesenteric
artery

Ureter

Manipulated
right colon

A

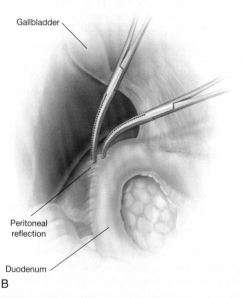

Gallbladder

Peritoneal
reflection

Duodenum

B

Figure 49.4 Kocher maneuver. An extended Kocher maneuver allows lifting of the pancreatic head out of the retroperitoneum for palpation (C) after mobilization of the right colon (A) and incision of the peritoneal reflection along the duodenum (B). Separation from the transverse mesocolon allows for complete mobilization of the pancreas and palpation of the pancreatic body and tail (D). (Reprinted with permission from Mulholland MW, Albo D, Dalman R, Hawn M, Hughes S, Sabel M, eds. *Operative Techniques in Surgery.* Philadelphia, PA: Wolters Kluwer Health; 2015.)

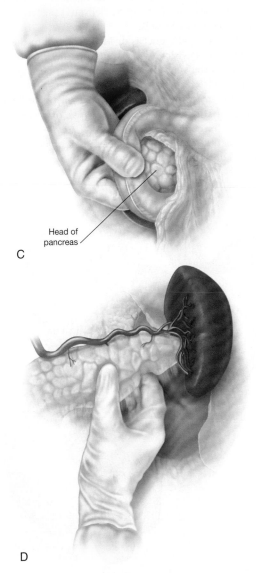

C

Head of
pancreas

D

Figure 49.4—cont'd

- The jejunum is divided distal to the ligament of Treitz and mesentery ligated until it can be delivered posterior to the superior mesenteric vessels.
- The common hepatic duct is divided proximal to the cystic duct entrance. Division of the pancreatic neck occurs anterior to the portal vein with dissection of the head and uncinate process from the surrounding structures.
- It is important to meticulously remove all tissue from the surrounding structures to reduce the risk of recurrence or incomplete resection.
- Reconstruction ensues with anastomoses of pancreas, bile duct, and duodenum/stomach[3] (Figure 49.5).

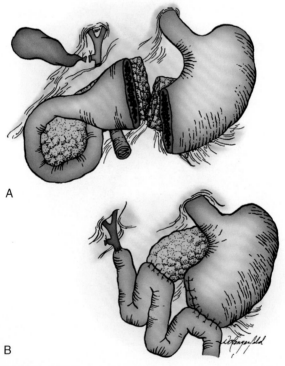

Figure 49.5 Whipple procedure. A, The head of the pancreas, distal common bile duct, gastric antrum, and duodenum are removed. B, The GI tract, pancreatic duct, and bile duct are reconstructed. (Reprinted with permission from Jarrell BE, Kavick SM. *NMS Surgery*. 6th ed. Philadelphia, PA: Wolters Kluwer; 2016.)

Laparoscopic Approach (Distal Pancreatectomy)

- Patients are supine with legs open.
- Trocar positioning varies with surgeon preference.
- Port size will also vary depending on the size of the patient and the size of laparoscopic tools available.
- Two working ports are placed in left lateral epigastric and right lateral umbilical.
- Another larger working port is placed right lateral to the previous port.
- The optic port is placed periumbilical (Figure 49.6).
- Upon entry, the lesser sac can be accessed.
- The posterior wall of the stomach close to the greater curvature is then sutured to the abdominal wall to provide visualization of the pancreatic tail.
- The pneumoperitoneum will aid in suspending the stomach to maintain your operative view.
- At this point, intraoperative ultrasound can be used to identify the lesion if necessary.
- Dissection of the pancreas can be performed sharply, with staples or with ultrasonic shears.
- The inferior border is mobilized and rotated forward so that the posterior surface is exposed.

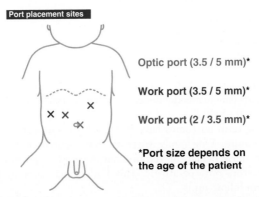

Figure 49.6 Laparoscopic pancreatectomy access points. Location of port sites for pediatric laparoscopic pancreatectomy. (Reprinted with permission from Wulkan ML. Pancreatectomy. In: Saxena AK, Höllwarth ME, eds. *Essentials of Pediatric Endoscopic Surgery*. Berlin, Heidelberg: Springer Berlin Heidelberg; 2009:349-354. Copyright © 2009 Springer-Verlag Berlin Heidelberg.)

- The pancreas can be maneuvered atraumatically with either nylon tape or a penrose drain.
- The pancreatic duct is suture ligated, and the specimen is removed with a specimen bag.[11]
- Laparoscopic approach is rapidly becoming an acceptable route of intervention, particularly for solid pseudopapillary tumors due to low malignancy potential.
- Laparoscopic distal pancreatectomies have been shown to have quicker recovery times, fewer occurrences of adhesive ileus, and aesthetic benefits.[11]
- Current case series have been limited by selection of smaller size and less malignant tumors for the laparoscopic cases.
- At the time of this publication, a randomized control trial is being developed in the Netherlands (LEOPARD).[15]

POSTOPERATIVE CARE

- Postoperative care is similar after both open and laparoscopic approaches.
- Partial pancreatectomies may require continuous IV glucose infusion and sometimes require temporary IV insulin infusion.[7]
- Drains are often left in place but have not had proven benefit.[16]
- Irradiation treatment may be indicated if incomplete negative margins were not obtained.

Complications

- The major complications include delayed gastric emptying, postoperative ileus, splenic infarction, chylous drainage, and pancreatic fistula.
- Leaks and morbidity are higher in distal pancreatectomy versus pancreaticoduodenectomy, but mortality remains the same for both.[16]
- Long-term outcomes have been rarely documented in the literature. One study suggests that recurrence for even the most benign of tumors can develop at greater than 10 years postoperatively. This finding may support long-term follow-up.[11]

PEARLS AND PITFALLS

■ There are 1.8 cases of pediatric pancreatic tumors per million children.

■ Most common tumors are pancreatoblastoma, solid pseudo-papillary neoplasm, and pancreatic endocrine tumors.

■ These may be an incidental finding and symptomatic and may have palpable mass, pain, diarrhea, or Whipple triad.

■ Ultrasound is the best initial imaging modality for diagnosis, with follow-up cross-sectional imaging.

■ Although majority of cases are still performed open, laparoscopic distal pancreatectomies are becoming common for solid pseudopapillary neoplasms in children.

REFERENCES

1. Brecht IB, Schneider DT, Klopperl G. Malignant pancreatic tumors in children and young adults: evaluation of 228 patients identified through the surveillance, epidemiology, and end result database (SEER). *Klin Pediatr.* 2011;223:341-345.

2. Hsieh L, Burjonrappa S. Pediatric pancreatic tumors: a review of current concepts. *JP (Online).* 2016;17(3):257-262.

3. Brunicardi FC, Andersen DK, Billiar TR, et al. *Chapter 33: Pancreas.* In: *Schwartz's Principles of Surgery.* 10th ed. New York: McGraw-Hill; 2015:1168-1169, 1217-1225.

4. Hamilton SR, Aaltonen LA, eds. World Health Organization Classification of Tumours. *Pathology and Genetics of Tumours of the Digestive System.* Lyon: IARC Press; 2000.

5. Defachelles AS, Rocourt N, Branchereau S, et al. Pancreatoblastoma in children: diagnosis and therapeutic management. *Bull Cancer.* 2012;99(7-8):793-799.

6. Mao C, Guvendi M, Domenico DR, et al. Papillary cystic and solid tumors of the pancreas: a pancreatic embryonic tumor? Studies of three cases and cumulative review of the world's literature. *Surgery.* 1995;118:821-828.

7. Mattei P, ed. Chapter 79: Congenital hyperinsulinism. In: *Fundamentals of Pediatric Surgery.* New York: Springer; 2011:610-615.

8. Shet NS, Cole BL, Iyer RS. Imaging of pediatric pancreatic neoplasms with radiologic-histopathologic correlation. *Am J Roentgenol.* 2014;202:1337-1348. doi:10.2214/AJR.13.11513.

9. Bien E, Godzinski J, Dall'igna P, et al. Pancreatoblastoma: a report from the European cooperative study group for paediatric rare tumours (EXPeRT). *Eur J Cancer.* 2011;47(15):2347-2352.

10. Mattei P, ed. Chapter 80: Disorders of the pancreas. In: *Fundamentals of Pediatric Surgery.* New York: Springer; 2011:620-621.

11. Huttner FJ, Fitzmaurice C, Schwarzer G, et al. Pylorus-preserving pancreaticoduodenectomy (pp Whipple) versus pancreaticoduodenectomy (classic Whipple) for surgical treatment of periampullary and pancreatic carcinoma. *Cochrane Database Syst Rev.* 2016;2:CD006053.

12. Kennedy EP, Yeo CJ. Pancreaticoduodenectomy with extended retro-peritoneal lymphadenectomy for periampullary adenocarcinoma. *Surg Oncol Clin N Am*. 2007;16(1):157-176.

13. Namgoong JM, Kim DY, Kim SC, et al. Laparoscopic distal pancreatectomy to treat Solid Pseudopapillary Neoplasms in children: transition from open to laparoscopic approaches in suitable cases. *Pediatr Surg Int*. 2014;30:259-266.

14. Riviere D, Gurusamy KS, Kooby DA, et al. Laparoscopic versus open distal pancreatectomy for pancreatic cancer. *Cochrane Database Syst Rev*. 2016;4:CD011391.

15. De Rooij T, van Hilst J, Vogel JA, et al. Minimally invasive versus open distal pancreatectomy (LEOPARD): study protocol for a randomized controlled trial. *Trials*. 2017;18:166.

16. Klingensmith ME, Aziz A, Bharat A, et al. *Chapter 13: pancreas*. In: *The Washington Manual of Surgery*. 6th ed. Philadelphia: Lippincott Williams & Wilkins; 2012:338-339.

Chapter 50

Hepatic Neoplasms in Children

Ann M. Polcari

- The liver is an intraperitoneal organ located below the diaphragm in the right upper quadrant (RUQ) of the abdomen, extending from the fourth to fifth rib to just below the costal margin (Figure 50.1).
- It is covered almost entirely by Glisson capsule, a tough, fibrous sheath. The posterior surface has a "bare area" where the inferior vena cava (IVC) and gallbladder lie.
- The liver has dual blood supply:
  - Hepatic system (25%) includes the hepatic artery, which originates from the celiac trunk.
  - Portal system (75%) includes the portal vein, which carries nutrient filled blood from the gastrointestinal system to the liver, as well as venous blood from the spleen.
- Venous drainage from the liver is via the IVC.
- The gallbladder is located on the posteroinferior surface of the liver. It holds bile, which is removed from the liver via the hepatic duct.
- The "porta hepatis," or the hepatoduodenal ligament, contains the portal vein posteriorly, hepatic artery medially, and common bile duct laterally.

EPIDEMIOLOGY AND ETIOLOGY

Prevalence

- Hepatic neoplasms in children are rare, comprising only 1% to 2% of all childhood cancers.[1]
- Metastatic tumors (eg, Wilms tumor, lymphoma, neuroblastoma) to the liver are more common than primary hepatic tumors.[2]

Etiology

- Etiology varies by tumor type. Some are associated with genetic syndromes; many arise from de novo mutations.
- Primary hepatic neoplasms in children can be identified as benign or malignant.

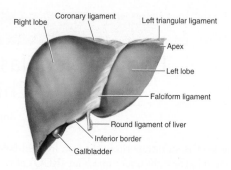

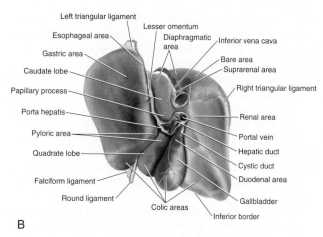

Figure 50.1 Peritoneal and visceral relationships of liver. A, The liver is divided into right and left lobes by the falciform and coronary ligaments (anterior view, diaphragmatic surface). B, The posteroinferior aspect of the liver (visceral surface). (Reprinted with permission from Moore KL, Dalley AF, Agur AMR. *Clinically Oriented Anatomy.* 7th ed. Philadelphia, PA: Lippincott Williams & Wilkins; 2014.)

- The benign tumors include (Table 50.1) the following:
  - Infantile hemangioendothelioma
  - Mesenchymal hamartoma
  - Focal nodular hyperplasia
  - Hepatocellular adenoma
- The malignant lesions include (Table 50.2) the following:
  - Hepatoblastoma
  - Hepatocellular carcinoma
  - Undifferentiated embryonal carcinoma
  - Rhabdomyosarcoma of the biliary tree

Clinical Presentation

Classic presentation: Clinical presentation also varies by the type of tumor (Tables 50.1 and 50.2), but symptoms are most often nonspecific and one must have a high level of suspicion.

- Most pediatric hepatic neoplasms are almost always found incidentally on imaging.
- Some tumors grow so rapidly that they present with a palpable mass in the RUQ, with nausea or vomiting due to local compressive symptoms.
- RUQ pain and jaundice are also common.

DIAGNOSIS

Laboratory Findings

- Significant laboratory findings differ by tumor type (Tables 50.1 and 50.2).
- Alpha-fetal protein (AFP) is elevated in many hepatic tumors and is typically followed after treatment to determine response.

Imaging Findings

- The initial modality of choice is ultrasound, particularly when a patient presents with RUQ pain or palpable mass. However, additional imaging and even biopsy are typically required to make the diagnosis.
- Some hepatic tumors can be diagnosed by CT with contrast alone; others are better visualized by MRI with contrast. See Tables 50.1 and 50.2 for information about key findings in particular liver neoplasms.

SURGICAL MANAGEMENT

- **Conservative management with serial ultrasound or CT imaging is appropriate for most benign, asymptomatic lesions.**
- Chemotherapy is appropriate for known-responsive lesions, which are neoadjuvant or adjuvant depending on the type of tumor.

Operative Intervention

Liver Resection

- The Pretreatment Extent of Disease (PRETEXT) system was developed by the International Society of Pediatric Oncology on Childhood Liver Tumors (SIOPEL) group to identify suitable candidates for primary resection (Figure 50.2).[3]

TABLE 50.1				
Benign Pediatric Liver Tumors				
	Infantile Hepatic Hemangioma (Also Termed "Infantile Hemangioendothelioma")	Mesenchymal Hamartoma	Focal Nodular Hyperplasia	Hepatocellular Adenoma
Epidemiology	Most common benign solid liver tumor in children **Age:** <6 mo; almost all <2 mo **Gender:** slight female predominance	Second most common benign pediatric tumor **Age:** <2 y **Gender:** male predominance	4%-10% of benign pediatric tumors **Age:** 2-5 y **Gender:** female predominance	Very rare—4% of all tumors in children **Age:** >10 y **Gender:** female predominance, especially those using oral contraceptives (OCPs)
Etiology and associations	**Syndromes:** Osler-Weber-Rendu, Klippel-Trenaunay-Weber, Ehlers-Danlos, Beckwith-Wiedemann	Heterogeneous genetic causes	Liver trauma, hemochromatosis, Klinefelter syndrome, possibly OCP use	**Infants and young children:** >50% associated with glycogen storage disease, Fanconi anemia, or tyrosinemia **Older children:** OCP use, anabolic steroid use

(continued)

Clinical presentation	• May be asymptomatic • Classic complex: hepatomegaly, congestive heart failure (CHF), and anemia • Often with cutaneous hemangiomas	• **Neonates:** High-output CHF with pulmonary hypertension • **Older children:** abdominal distension, ascites, with or without a palpable mass (ascites) • Nausea or vomiting due to compression	• **Typically asymptomatic** • If symptomatic: abdominal pain, hepatomegaly, decreased appetite with weight loss and fatigue	• **Typically asymptomatic** • May have intermittent abdominal pain • 10% present with acute abdominal pain due to hemorrhage into tumor
Laboratory findings	Anemia (50%), AFP may be elevated	AFP may be elevated	LFTs may be elevated	–

TABLE 50.1 (CONTINUED)

Benign Pediatric Liver Tumors

	Infantile Hepatic Hemangioma (Also Termed "Infantile Hemangioendothelioma")	Mesenchymal Hamartoma	Focal Nodular Hyperplasia	Hepatocellular Adenoma
Imaging	Best modality: MRI with contrast Note: Biopsies are avoided owing to vascularity	• Multiseptated, multicystic (fluid-filled) mass • R-sided predilection	CT with contrast will show early enhancement with central scar	• CT with contrast shows multiple feeding vessels (differentiates from FNH) • May show areas of calcification or hemorrhage

(continued)

Pathology			
Gross: • May be solitary, multifocal (up to 25 lesions), or diffuse • Range from 1 to 13 cm **Microscopic:** • Layers of flat endothelial cells on a supporting fibrous stroma • GLUT-1 positive	**Gross:** • Large, well-circumscribed, solitary lesion • 8-10 cm diameter **Microscopic:** • Mixture of bile ducts, liver cells, mesenchyme with dilated bile and lymphatic ducts	**Gross:** • Well circumscribed, lobulated, unencapsulated • Single feeding artery with central stellate scar **Microscopic:** • Disorganized hepatocyte hyperplasia in nodules • Overexpression of ANGPT1 and 2	**Gross:** • Solitary, unencapsulated **Microscopic:** • Large sheets of cells resembling normal hepatocytes separated by dilated vessels • No portal vessels or bile ducts

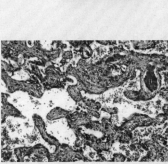
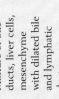
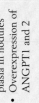
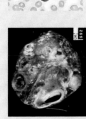
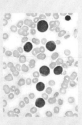
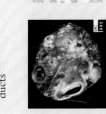

TABLE 50.1 (CONTINUED)				
Benign Pediatric Liver Tumors				
	Infantile Hepatic Hemangioma (Also Termed "Infantile Hemangioendothelioma")	**Mesenchymal Hamartoma**	**Focal Nodular Hyperplasia**	**Hepatocellular Adenoma**
Treatment	• Some regress spontaneously after 1 y of age • **Asymptomatic:** Serial ultrasounds to monitor growth. Propranolol recently proposed • **Symptomatic:** Consider surgical resection or embolization • Transplant is last resort • **Note: Monitor for resolution, malignant transformation has been reported**	• Spontaneous resolution is rare • **Recommended therapy is excision and can be curative** • Risk of development into undifferentiated embryonal sarcoma	• **Asymptomatic:** Observation with serial ultrasound • **Symptomatic, >5 cm, progression:** biopsy followed by resection • No malignant potential	• Remove offending agent (OCPs, anabolic steroids). • If stable, observe • **Resection is definitive treatment**

Data from Zheng H, Finn LS, Murray KF. Neoplasms of the liver. In: Wyllie R, Hyams JS, Kay M, eds. *Pediatric Gastrointestinal and Liver Disease*. 5th ed. Philadelphia: Elsevier; 2016:582-589.e4; Andrews WS. Lesions of the liver. In: Holcomb GW, Murphy JP, eds. *Ashcraft's Pediatric Surgery*. 5th ed. Philadelphia: Saunders Elsevier; 2010:895-914; and Sebire NJ, Ashworth M, Malone M, Jacques TS, Rogers BB, eds. *Diagnostic Pediatric Surgical Pathology*. 1st ed. Philadelphia: Elsevier; 2010. Images reprinted with permission from Pizzo PA, Poplack DG. *Principles and Practice of Pediatric Oncology*. 7th ed. Philadelphia: Wolters Kluwer Health; 2016; Sanders RC. *Clinical Sonography: A Practical Guide*. 5th ed. Philadelphia: Wolters Kluwer Health; 2016; Fiser S. *The ABSITE Review*. 5th ed. Philadelphia: Wolters Kluwer Health; 2017; Brant WE, Helms C. *Fundamentals of Diagnostic Radiology*. 4th ed. Philadelphia: Wolters Kluwer Health; 2013; Husain AN, Stocker JT, Dehner LP. *Stocker and Dehner's Pediatric Pathology*. 6th ed. Philadelphia: Wolters Kluwer Health; 2016; Stocker JT, Dehner LP, Husain AN. *Stocker and Dehner's Pediatric Pathology*. 3rd ed. Philadelphia: Wolters Kluwer Health; 2011; and Rubin R, Strayer DS, Rubin R. *Rubin's Pathology*. Philadelphia: Wolters Kluwer Health; 2012.

TABLE 50.2

Malignant Pediatric Liver Tumors

	Hepatoblastoma	Hepatocellular Carcinoma	Undifferentiated Embryonal Carcinoma	Rhabdomyosarcoma of the Biliary Tree
Epidemiology	Most common pediatric liver malignancy; incidence 0.5-1.5 cases per million children <15 y in developed countries **Age:** <5 y, mostly <2 y **Gender:** male predominance	Second most common pediatric liver malignancy **Age:** >10 y; fibrolamellar variant in adolescents **Gender:** no gender distinction	9%-13% of all solid liver tumors in children; incidence 0.5-1 per million in Western countries **Age:** 5-10 y **Gender:** male predominance	Most common sarcoma in children **Age:** <5 y **Gender:** no gender distinction
Etiology and associations	• Most result from sporadic mutations • Beckwith-Wiedemann, trisomies • Familial adenomatous polyposis (FAP) • Extreme prematurity and low birth weight	Most commonly de novo mutations in children	Heterogeneous genetic causes	Heterogeneous genetic causes

(continued)

TABLE 50.2 (CONTINUED)

Malignant Pediatric Liver Tumors

	Hepatoblastoma	Hepatocellular Carcinoma	Undifferentiated Embryonal Carcinoma	Rhabdomyosarcoma of the Biliary Tree
Clinical presentation	• Typically asymptomatic • 80% with palpable RUQ mass • Precocious puberty if secreting HCG • Hemorrhage with hypovolemia if ruptured • Jaundice is uncommon	• Abdominal mass or RUQ pain • Nonspecific symptoms: nausea and vomiting, anorexia, malaise, weight loss • 10% present with rupture and hemoperitoneum	• RUQ or epigastric pain, with or without palpable mass • Nonspecific symptoms: vomiting, anorexia, lethargy	• Jaundice (80%) with palpable abdominal mass/distention • Nonspecific symptoms: fever, nausea, vomiting
Laboratory findings	• 70% anemia • 50% thrombocytosis (>500 000) • >90% have significantly elevated AFP that can exceed 1 million	• 70%-85% with elevated AFP • Mild elevations in LFTs and LDH	• Typically within normal limits	• Biliary ductal obstruction: elevated direct bilirubin, alkaline phosphatase, and LFTs

(continued)

Imaging	• CT may show calcifications within mass (50%) • 20% have metastasis, often to lungs, at diagnosis • Note: Confirmation requires biopsy	• Hallmark: hepatic blood supply dependent • CT/MRI with contrast to determine local involvement • Note: Biopsy to differentiate from hepatoblastoma	**Dichotomy between modalities:** • Ultrasound: solid lesion • CT/MRI: cystic lesion • Note: Confirmation requires FNA or biopsy	• Ultrasound will show biliary dilation and possibly a mass • Consider MRCP or percutaneous cholangiogram

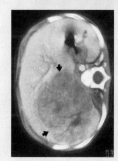

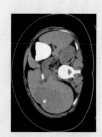

TABLE 50.2 (CONTINUED)

Malignant Pediatric Liver Tumors

	Hepatoblastoma	Hepatocellular Carcinoma	Undifferentiated Embryonal Carcinoma	Rhabdomyosarcoma of the Biliary Tree
Pathology	Gross: • Solitary • Can be 15 cm, extending into pelvis and chest • R lobe predominant Microscopic: • 6 histologic types, highly variable • Appearance of immature hepatocytes: embryonal cells at 6- to 8-wk gestation	Gross: • May be solitary or multi-focal (33%) Microscopic: • 60% have surrounding cirrhosis • Adolescents and young adults have fibrolamellar type (20%): coarse granular eosinophilic cytoplasm	Gross: • Encapsulated **R lobe predominant** • Average size 14-21 cm Microscopic: • Spindle and stellate cells with many mitoses	Gross: • Average size: 8 cm Microscopic: • Similar to other rhabdomyosarcomas: stellate and spindle cells surrounded by myxoid stroma

	Resection		Radical excision is the only chance for cure	Resection with adjuvant chemotherapy, and possibly radiation
Treatment	• **Resection**	• Size of tumor and degree of surrounding cirrhosis determines **resection or transplant**	• **Radical excision is the only chance for cure**	Resection with adjuvant chemotherapy, and possibly radiation
	• 85% are resectable after neoadjuvant chemotherapy (cisplatin-based regimen)	• If rupture and hemodynamically stable, conservative management	• Usually fatal owing to involvement of nearby structures	
	• Consider adjuvant chemotherapy or transplant for those with vascular invasion	• If rupture and unstable, embolize tumor	• Transplant is last effort	
Prognosis	75% 5-year survival (note: Children's Oncology Group [COG] and Pretreatment Extent of Disease [PRETEXT] are 2 prognosis estimators)	Poor survival rates overall: 10%-30%	37.5% 5-year survival	66% 5-year survival

Data from Zheng H, Finn LS, Murray KF. Neoplasms of the liver. In: Wyllie R, Hyams JS, Kay M, eds. *Pediatric Gastrointestinal and Liver Disease.* 5th ed. Philadelphia: Elsevier; 2016:582–589.e4; Andrews WS. Lesions of the liver. In: Holcomb GW, Murphy JP, eds. *Ashcraft's Pediatric Surgery.* 5th ed. Philadelphia: Saunders Elsevier; 2010:895-914; and Sebire NJ, Ashworth M, Malone M, Jacques TS, Rogers BB, eds. *Diagnostic Pediatric Surgical Pathology.* 1st ed. Philadelphia: Elsevier; 2010. Images reprinted with permission from Mulholland MW, Lillemoe KD, Doherty GM, Maier RV, Upchurch GR. *Greenfield's Surgery.* 4th ed. Philadelphia: Wolters Kluwer Health; 2006; Pizzo PA, Poplack DG. *Principles and Practice of Pediatric Oncology.* 7th ed. Philadelphia: Wolters Kluwer Health; 2016; Mills SE. *Histology for Pathologists.* 4th ed. Philadelphia: Wolters Kluwer Health; 2013; and Husain AN, Stocker JT, Dehner LP. *Stocker and Dehner's Pediatric Pathology.* 4th ed. Philadelphia: Wolters Kluwer Health; 2016.

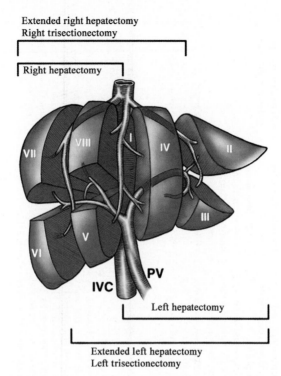

Figure 50.2   Diagrammatic representation of liver segments with standard liver resections demonstrated. IVC, inferior vena cava; PV, pulmonary vein. (Reprinted with permission from Gabrielli A, Layon AJ, Yu M. *Civetta, Taylor, & Kirby's Critical Care.* 4th ed. Philadelphia, PA: Lippincott Williams & Wilkins; 2008.)

- Invasion of local vasculature or centrally located lesions are more often deemed unresectable.
- The area of resection is typically based on Couinaud system of segmentation.

Open Approach[4]

- Begins with bilateral subcostal incisions, followed by an intraoperative ultrasound of the liver to determine accurate tumor margins and locate nearby vasculature. After marking the liver itself, electrocautery and often a LigaSure device are used to resect the tumor. In addition, argon beam coagulation is used for hemostasis.

- Right hepatectomy is performed more often than left hepatectomy. Both involve dividing the hilar plate of the liver before ligating either the right hepatic artery and right branch of the portal vein or left hepatic artery and left branch of the portal vein. Next, the appropriate hepatic vein is ligated.

Laparoscopic Approach

- This approach is termed "Minimally Invasive Liver Resection" (MILR).
- Aside from case reports, published data is lacking.
- A 2016 retrospective study of outcomes in 36 pediatric patients undergoing MILR for both benign and malignant conditions found the technique to have good oncologic results with minimal morbidities (eg, seroma, wound infection). There were no reoperations, tumor recurrences, or mortalities at 1-year follow-up.[5]

Complications

- Intraoperative complications include hemorrhage, tumor or air embolism, and iatrogenic bile duct injury.
- Postoperative complications include bleeding, infection with possible abscess formation, bile leak, and wound infection.

Orthotopic Transplant

- It is primarily used for unresectable tumors.
- Also, a last resort treatment when previous management fails.
- 3% of all liver transplants in children are for hepatoblastoma. A 70% 5-year survival rate has been reported.[4]

Complications

- The worst complication is rejection of the transplanted organ.
- Other complications include hepatic artery or portal vein thrombosis, bile leak or stricture, and infection due to immunosuppression from posttransplant therapy.

POSTOPERATIVE CARE

- Adequate fluid replacement.
- Albumin, vitamin K, and clotting factor supplementation are typically required for the first 3 to 4 days.
- LFTs normalize around 2 weeks.
- **AFP should be monitored at 3- to 6-month intervals as appropriate for tumor type.**[4]

PEARLS AND PITFALLS

- Metastatic hepatic tumors are more common than primary hepatic neoplasms in children.
- The majority of pediatric liver tumors are found incidentally on imaging.
- AFP is the most commonly elevated laboratory value.
- Biopsy may be required for diagnosis.
- Liver resection is the mainstay of treatment.

REFERENCES

1. Zheng H, Finn LS, Murray KF. Neoplasms of the liver. In: Wyllie R, Hyams JS, Kay M, eds. *Pediatric Gastrointestinal and Liver Disease*. 5th ed. Philadelphia: Elsevier; 2016:582-589.e4.
2. Andrews WS. Lesions of the liver. In: Holcomb GW, Murphy JP, eds. *Ashcraft's Pediatric Surgery*. 5th ed. Philadelphia: Saunders Elsevier; 2010:895-914.
3. Rapkin LB, Olson TA. Hepatic tumors. In: Lanzkowsky P, Lipton JM, Fish JD, eds. *Lanzkowsky's Manual of Pediatric Hematology and Oncology*. 6th ed. Dan Diego: Elsevier; 2016:569-576.
4. Gow KW. *Pediatric Liver Tumors. Medscape [Internet]*; September 15, 2016. [cited 2017 July 1]. Available from: http://emedicine.medscape.com/article/940516-overview?pa=FW2pbsoaXUmuNlcft5915z8m3X-eIGC%2BtBBzQi1Q5AYnl8dRKUC4tWlo8hJtxurI6NFsYx-Duz%2Fz2hge3aAwEFsw%3D%3D#a4.
5. Veenstra MA, Koffron AJ. Minimally-invasive liver resection in pediatric patients: initial experience and outcomes. *HPB*. 2016:18(6):518-522.

Chapter 51

Adrenal Tumors in Children

Scott J. Revell, Carly M. Conway, and Jessica L. Buicko

- The first successful adrenalectomy was performed by John Knowsley Thornton who removed a 20-lb en bloc adrenal tumor with left kidney from a 36-year-old woman in 1889.
- Since that time anterior, posterior, thoracoabdominal, and laparoscopic approaches have been developed for both the benign and malignant pathologies.
- The adrenalectomy has become the treatment mainstay for adrenal hyperplasia, large nonfunction adrenal tumors, benign endocrinologically active or enlarging adenomas, adrenal cancers, and adrenal metastasis.

RELEVANT ANATOMY

- The adrenal glands are triangular dark yellow structures located superior and medial to the kidneys in the retroperitoneum at the level of the 11th thoracic vertebrae.
- The adrenal gland is composed of 2 independent exocrine organs made up of tissue from different embryological origins, the outer cortex, and the inner medulla.
- The adrenal cortex is divided into 3 layers, each dedicated to its synthetic function.
- The outermost layer that is composed of steroid-producing cells of the zona glomerulosa is devoted to synthesis of mineralocorticoids and makes up 15% of the adrenal gland.
- The zona fasciculata devoted to glucocorticoid production makes up 75% of the gland.
- The zona reticularis synthesizes and secretes androgens.
- The medulla arises from neuroectoderm and contains the Chromaffin cells, which produce the catecholamines: norepinephrine and epinephrine.
- The adrenals are highly vascular and receive arterial supply from 3 sources.
- Superiorly they receive multiple branches from the phrenic arteries.
- The medial aspect is supplied by the direct aortic perforator, and inferiorly small branches originate off the renal arteries.

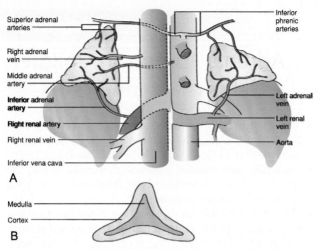

Figure 51.1 Adrenal gland anatomy. A, Arterial (dark shaded) and venous (light shaded) anatomy of the adrenal glands. B, Schematic showing outer adrenal cortex (light shaded) and inner adrenal medulla (dark shaded). (Reprinted with permission from Fiser S. *The ABSITE Review*. 5th ed. Philadelphia, PA: Wolters Kluwer Health; 2017.)

- Care must be taken to identify and cauterize these small branches to prevent bleeding.
- The venous outflow from the adrenals occurs via a single dominate vein.
- On the left, it drains into the left renal vein.
- On the right, the adrenal vein drains directly into the IVC several centimeters cephalad to the right renal vein[1] (Figure 51.1).

EPIDEMIOLOGY AND ETIOLOGY

- Adrenal tumors other than the neuroblastoma occur rarely in childhood.
- Neuroblastoma, covered in chapter 48, is the most common adrenal tumor and may occur anywhere along the sympathetic nervous system, with 40% originating in the adrenals.
- Neuroblastoma is the most common extracranial solid tumor diagnosed in the pediatric population accounting for 8% to 10% of all childhood malignancies and 15% of pediatric cancer deaths.

- With an incidence of 1/100 000 persons-years, they account for more than 90% of adrenal tumors.[2]
- Tumors derived for the adrenal cortex are uncommon and account for only 0.2% of malignancies in the US pediatric population.[3,4]
- There is an increased incidence associated with several genetic syndromes including Beckwith-Wiedemann, Li-Fraumeni, multiple endocrine neoplasia-type 1, and familial adenomatous polyposis coli, which has led to investigations examining oncogenes and tumor suppressor genes, yet the exact etiology remains elusive.[5,6]
- The other neoplasm discussed in this chapter is the pheochromocytoma (PCC), which originate from adrenal chromaffin cells of the medulla.
- Within the pediatric population, the estimated incidence of PCC and paragangliomas (extra-adrenal PCC) is 0.8 to 1.6 per million.[7-10]
- Roughly 80% of these tumors will produce catecholamines, and PCC may account for up to 90% of the pediatric population with sustained hypertension.[8]

CLINICAL PRESENTATION

Adrenal Cortical Tumors

- Adrenal carcinomas are extremely aggressive tumors, and a good prognosis largely depends on early detection.
- Approximately 90% of adrenal cortical tumors (ACTs) in children are functional, producing androgens, cortisol, aldosterone, estrogen, or a combination of steroids.
- About 80% of these tumors produce androgens making the sequalae virilization the most common presenting signs.
- Presenting signs and symptoms depend on age and sex.
- Female infants are likely to present with ambiguous genitalia such as fusion of the labioscrotal folds, clitoromegaly, or external male genitalia with bilateral cryptorchidism.
- The signs in male infants will be more subtle, likely presenting as penile enlargement and accelerated growth as the child ages.
- In older children, hirsutism, accelerated growth, short stature due to premature closure of growth plates, early acne, amenorrhea (primary and secondary), clitoromegaly, and precocious puberty should prompt investigation.[11]
- It is important to note that congenital adrenal hyperplasia (CAH) is the most common cause of virilization and ambiguous genitalia in newborns.

- Roughly 90% of cases are caused by defects in 21-hydroxylase, leading to improper synthesis of cortisol and aldosterone and shunting of steroid precursor molecules to the androgenic intermediaries.
- CAH can be differentiated from virilizing tumors by administering dexamethasone 0.5 mg po q 6 hours for 48 hours, which will suppress urinary and plasma excess androgens in cases of CAH.
- Additionally, CAH exhibits concomitant glucocorticoid and mineralocorticoid deficiencies.
- Cushingoid features secondary hypercortisolism is another common presentation.
- In the pediatric population, impaired linear growth is an important sign of hypercortisolism.
- Signs common in adults are common in children as well.
- The redistribution of fat to the upper back and face is pathognomonic, but central obesity, hypertension, easy bruising, osteoporosis, striae, acne, and menstrual irregularity should all prompt investigation.
- Adrenal cortical carcinoma is a very aggressive tumor, which metastasizes to the lungs, liver, and lymph nodes.
- Prognosis is based on size and resectability.

Pheochromocytoma

- PCC typically presents in children ages 8 to 14 years as sustained hypertension associated with acute onset of headaches, palpitations, blurry vision, sweating, nausea, weight loss, and polydipsia or polyuria
- Failure to recognize early symptoms can lead to heart failure, encephalopathy, and hypertensive retinitis.
- On examination, patients are normally hypertensive, tachycardic, and diaphoretic.

DIAGNOSIS

Laboratory Findings and Imaging Findings

Virilization

- The initial step in the workup for virilization is biochemical testing in the form of elevated urine and plasma androgens.
- The commonly elevated urine in androgens in patients with virilization are dehydroepiandrosterone (DHEA), its sulfate form (DHEA-S), 17-ketosteroids, and pregnanetriol.

- Elevated plasma levels of DHEA and DHEA-S, 17-hydroxy-progesterone, testosterone, and androstenedione should also prompt further investigation.[12,13]
- The next step is to differentiate adrenal tumors for CAH, which is done with the dexamethasone suppression test mentioned earlier.
- If androgen production is not suppressed, computed tomography (CT), magnetic resonance imaging (MRI), or ultrasound should be used to attempt to localize the tumor.

Cushingoid Features

- Patients with signs and symptoms of Cushing syndrome should first undergo biochemical testing to determine if there is overproduction of adrenocorticotropic hormone (ACTH) or cortisol and whether feedback inhibition is present.
- Before 6 years of age, cortisol excess is likely to be a result of an adrenal tumor.
- Whereas in older children, oversecretion of ACTH by the pituitary is more likely to be the culprit.
- The first-line screening tests include a late night salivary cortisol or plasma cortisol, which has a sensitivity of 93% and specificity of 96% and testing for the lack of the normal diurnal variation in cortisol secretion by checking fasting serum cortisol at 8 AM and 6 PM.[14]
- This test has an 80% sensitivity for Cushing syndrome.
- The most sensitive test is the 24-hour urine cortisol of free cortisol or 17-hydroxycorticosteroid.
- If cortisol excess is demonstrated, the next step is to distinguish between pituitary and nonpituitary causes.
- Plasma ACTH levels or a high-dose dexamethasone suppression test can be utilized at this point.
- Plasma ACT levels are usually elevated with ectopic ACTH-producing tumors, moderately elevated with pituitary neoplasms and low with adrenal sources of cortisol excess.
- In the high-dose dexamethasone test, 24-hour urine free cortisol or 17-hydroxycorticosteroid levels are collected after administering 2 mg dexamethasone q 6 hours for 48 hours.
- If the hypercortisolism is caused by adrenal hyperplasia secondary to pituitary oversecretion of ACTH, then steroid secretion will be suppressed. Steroid secretion is not suppressed with ACTs.

- An additional test that may be utilized is the corticotropin-releasing hormone (CRH) stimulation test, where 1 μg per kg of CRH is given IV and serial plasma levels of ACTH and cortisol are monitored for 3 hours.
- When hypercortisolism is a result of adrenal tumors or ectopic ACTH production, there will be no response due to chronic suppression of the pituitary.
- Patients with Cushing disease will typically have a marked elevation in ACTH and cortisol.
- If biochemical tests are suggestive of Cushing disease, an MRI of the pituitary should be performed.
- In the case of results suggestive of adrenal tumor, MRI or CT should be used to attempt to localize the tumor.

PCC

- Diagnosis is based on the detection of elevated urine or plasma levels of fractionated metanephrines.
- Previously the 24-hour urine collection was considered the gold standard, but this can be problematic in children.
- Both urine and plasma levels are considered to be nearly 100% sensitive, with a specificity of 97%.
- Positive biochemical tests should lead to imaging studies for localization.
- The modern imaging modalities have made several past tests obsolete.
- Venous sampling, adrenal arteriography, and histamine/phentolamine provocation tests have largely been replaced by ultrasound, MRI, CT, and metaiodobenzylguanidine (MIBG) scintigraphy owing to their increased sensitivity, speed, and safety (Figure 51.2).
- MRI provides better assessment of locoregional invasion but may require sedation.
- With CT, radiation dose must be considered, and while it detects up to 95% of tumors, it is likely to miss very small tumors <1.5 cm.
- MIBG scintigraphy has nearly a 100% specificity and is useful when clinical suspicion remains high after negative MRI or CT scan.
- It is important to remember that between 19% and 38% of PCC will be bilateral on imaging.

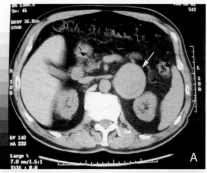

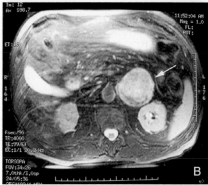

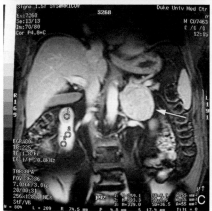
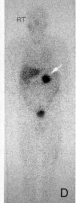

Figure 51.2 Imaging of pheochromocytoma (arrows). A, Computed tomography scan shows well-circumscribed left adrenal mass. B, T2-weighted magnetic resonance imaging (MRI) shows the mass to be heterogeneously bright, consistent with pheochromocytoma. C and D, Coronal contrast-enhanced MRI and near-simultaneous 131I-metaiodobenzylguanidine (131I-MIBG; RT, radioactive tracer) scanning show location of the pheochromocytoma and relationship to surrounding structures. (Reprinted with permission from Mulholland MW. *Greenfield's Surgery*. 5th ed. Philadelphia, PA: Wolters Kluwer Health; 2017.)

SURGICAL MANAGEMENT

- While the treatment for ACT and PCC is primarily surgical, perioperative management is exceedingly important owing to the widespread physiological consequences of endocrine surgery.
- Surgery for functional adrenal tumors inherently involves dramatic physiological changes postoperatively that affect multiple organs systems.

ACT

- Patients with Cushing syndrome from cortisol secreting tumors have chronically suppressed normal adrenal tissue and are typically started on IV hydrocortisone in the immediate preoperative period and transitioned to oral hydrocortisone postoperatively to prevent adrenal crisis.

PCC

- Patients with PCC are at risk for intraoperative hemodynamic lability. Intraoperative complications can be greatly decreased by preoperative alpha-blockade with phenoxybenzamine or doxazosin to achieve normotension for 1 to 2 weeks preoperatively.[15]
- Preoperative intravascular volume expansion with hydration from high-salt and high-fluid diets have also been recommended to prevent intraoperative hypotension.
- Beta-blockade can be added in cases for cardiac arrhythmias, persistent tachycardia, or pure epinephrine-producing tumors.
- Alpha-blockade must be achieved first to prevent the catecholamine-induced myopathy from direct effects on the myocardium and ischemia from vasoconstriction.
- In the case of bilateral PCC, the tumors should be cored out if possible, leaving viable adrenal tissue to avoid the long-term steroid supplementation.

OPERATIVE INTERVENTION

- The classic surgical procedure for all adrenal tumors is the adrenalectomy.
- This can be performed either laparoscopically or open, with open adrenalectomy typically being performed for malignancies, large masses (Figure 51.3).

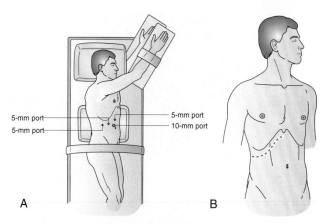

5-mm port
5-mm port

5-mm port
10-mm port

A

B

Figure 51.3 Incisions for right adrenalectomy. Shown are typical incisions for (A) laparoscopic approach and (B) open, anterior approach. (Reprinted with permission from Mulholland MW. *Greenfield's Surgery*. 5th ed. Philadelphia, PA: Wolters Kluwer Health; 2017.)

Open Approach

- For open adrenalectomy, several approaches have been described, but most commonly in children, a transabdominal approach is utilized.
- For this approach typically either a transverse abdominal or partial chevron incision is used.

Left Adrenalectomy

- The left adrenalectomy is simpler owing to the left adrenal being longer, draining into the left renal vein, and the gland being more anteriorly located (Figure 51.4).
- To expose the left adrenal, the splenocolic ligament is taken down and the colon is reflected medially.
- The splenorenal ligament can then be divided and plane bluntly developed between the tail of the pancreas and the kidney.
- The spleen and pancreas are retracted medially.
- The adrenal can be difficult to identify when nestled in surrounding perinephric fat.
- The medial, inferior, and lateral borders of the adrenal are dissected out.
- The adrenal vein should then be identified at the superior aspect of the renal vein where it is ligated and divided.
- The superior and posterior attachments are the taken down to free the gland.

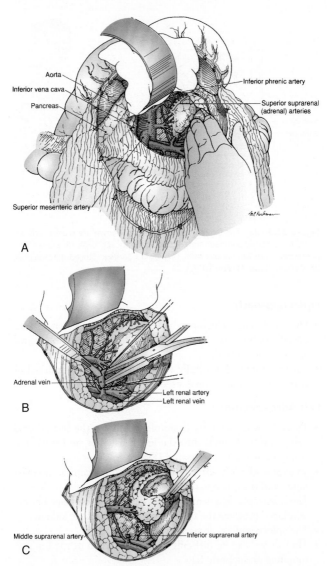

Figure 51.4 Left adrenalectomy. A, Exposure by creating a large window into the lesser sac. B, Division of adrenal vein. C, Division of remaining attachments may be completed with ties or harmonic scalpel. (Reprinted with permission from Scott-Conner CE. *Scott-Conner and Dawson: Essential Operative Techniques and Anatomy.* 4th ed. Philadelphia, PA: Wolters Kluwer Health; 2013.)

Right Adrenalectomy

- To expose the right adrenal, the triangular ligament must be divided from the inferior border of the liver cephalad to the diaphragm.
- The liver can then be retracted medially and the adrenal identified.
- The plane between the vena cava and the adrenal is dissected by opening to the posterior peritoneum.
- The adrenal is dissected from medial border and continued superiorly and inferiorly.
- The arterial branches are taken with cautery or clipped.
- The adrenal vein most often emerges from the middle of the adrenal and enters the IVC posterior and lateral.
- The vein should be ligated doubly with clips or a vascular stapler because it can be easily avulsed from the IVC.
- Care should also be taken to avoid accessory hepatic veins.
- The adrenal is then retracted away from the IVC.
- The diaphragm should be visible posteriorly and the dissection should continue along the inferomedial aspect of the adrenal and until the posterior and lateral attachments can be freed.

Laparoscopic Approach

- For transabdominal laparoscopic adrenalectomy, the patient is positioned in a modified 45° lateral decubitus position with the table flexed.
- This allows for gravity to partially retract the liver or spleen.

Left Adrenalectomy

- Using open technique, a 5-mm umbilical port is placed and the abdominal cavity is insufflated.
- This port becomes the left-hand working port.
- Under direct visualization, a second 5-mm port is then placed in the midline 2 fingerbreadths below the xiphoid, which is primarily utilized as the camera port.
- Next a 10-mm port is placed in the midclavicular line halfway between the umbilicus and iliac crest and will become the right-hand working port.
- After port placement, the procedure can proceed as described in the left open adrenalectomy section.

Right Adrenalectomy

- For the right adrenalectomy, the 5-mm umbilical and subxiphoid ports are placed as above.
- A 10-mm subumbilical port is then placed in the right midclavicular line.

- Lastly, for liver retraction, an additional 5-mm port is placed in the midaxillary line.
- At this point, the procedure may proceed as described in the right open adrenalectomy section.

Retroperitoneal Approach

- The retroperitoneal approach in children is typically reserved for those that are suspected to have intra-abdominal adhesions from previous surgery.
- The working space is tight and must be carefully developed.
- With the patient in the lateral position, the tip of the 12th rib is located and a 1-cm incision is made.
- The tissues are then bluntly dissected, and the retroperitoneum is entered by penetrating the lumbodorsal fascia.
- The retroperitoneal space is then developed, and a 10-mm port is placed and the space is insufflated.
- A 5-mm port is then placed at the same level on the anterior axillary line.
- The final port is placed at the same level but on the posterior axillary line.
- The procedure can then proceed in a similar fashion, as the transperitoneal approaches mentioned earlier.

POSTOPERATIVE CARE

ACT

- Cushingoid
  - In patients with hypercortisolism ACT, the contralateral adrenal will be suppressed.
  - To avoid postoperative adrenal crisis, cortisone should be given in the immediate preoperative period and continued postoperatively tapering the dose incrementally until maintenance levels are reached.
    - Depending on the length of suppression in the tapering period, it may last up to a year.

PCC

- Patients should be monitored carefully for signs of hypotension and hypoglycemia.
- After tumor excision, circulating catecholamine levels may drop precipitously, resulting in hypotension from decrease systemic resistance.

- Additionally, hypoglycemia can result from the loss of the catecholamine stimulation of glycogenolysis.
- In the case that blood pressures do not return to normal within 2 weeks postoperatively, a workup for additional tumors or metastasis should begin.

PEARLS AND PITFALLS

- Adrenalectomy is indicated for functional tumors.
- Adrenal adenomas and carcinomas are indistinguishable on imaging.
- Virilization is the most common presenting sign in adrenocortical cancer.
- In patients with PCC, preoperative alpha-blockade is crucial to optimize blood pressure in 1 to 2 weeks preceding surgery.
- Alpha-blockade should be initiated before beta-blockade to avoid cardiomyopathy.

REFERENCES

1. Standring S. *Gray's Anatomy: The Anatomical Basis of Clinical Practice.* London: Elsevier; 2005.
2. Hsieh MH, Meng MV, Walsh TJ, et al. Increasing incidence of neuroblastoma and potentially higher associated mortality of children from nonmetropolitan areas: analysis of the surveillance, epidemiology, and end results database. *J Pediatr Hematol Oncol.* 2009;31:942-946.
3. Young Jr JL, Miller RW. Incidence of malignant tumors in U.S. children. *J Pediatr.* 1975;86:254-258.
4. Lack EE, Mulvihill JJ, Travis WD, et al. Adrenal cortical neoplasms in the pediatric and adolescent age group: clinicopathologic study of 30 cases with emphasis on epidemiological and prognostic factors. *Pathol Annu.* 1992;27:1-53.
5. Libe R, Fratticci A, Bertherat J. Adrenocortical cancer: pathophysiology and clinical management. *Endocr Relat Cancer.* 2007;14:13-28.
6. Latronico AC, Chrousos GP. Adrenocortical tumors. *J Clin Endocr Metab.* 1997;82:1317-1324.
7. Ludwig AD, Feig DI, Brandt ML, et al. Recent advances in the diagnosis and treatment of pheochromocytoma in children. *Am J Surg.* 2007;194:792-797.
8. Havekes B, Romijn JA, Eisenhofer G, et al. Update on pediatric pheochromocytoma. *Pediatr Nephrol.* 2009;24:943-950.
9. Ciftci AO, Tanyel FC, Senocak ME, et al. Pheochromocytoma in children. *J Pediatr Surg.* 2001;36:447-452.
10. Bissada NK, Safwat AS, Seyam RM, et al. Pheochromocytoma in children and adolescents: a clinical spectrum. *J Pediatr Surg.* 2008;43:540-543.

11. Michalkiewicz E, Sandrini R, Figuereido B, et al. Clinical and outcome characteristics of children with adrenocortical tumors: a report from the international pediatric adrenocortical tumor registry. *J Clin Oncol.* 2004;22:838-845.

12. Forest MG. Recent advances in the diagnosis and management of congenital adrenal hyperplasia due to 21-hydroxylase deficiency. *Hum Reprod Update.* 2004;10(6):469-485.

13. Jaier JH, Louchart J, Cahill GF. Adrenal virilism. II. Metabolic studies. *J Clin Invest.* 1952;31(10):880-884.

14. Carroll T, Raff H, Findling J. Late-night salivary cortisol for the diagnosis of cushing syndrome: a meta-analysis. *Endocr Pract.* 2009;15(4):335-342.

15. Goldstein RE, O'Neill Jr JA, Holcomb III GW, et al. Clinical experience over 48 years with pheochromocytoma. *Ann Surg.* 1999;229:755-764.

Chapter 52

Mediastinal Tumors

Marcus E. Eby

- **The mediastinum** is the central compartment of the thoracic cavity, which is surrounded by loose connective tissue and enclosed laterally by the left and right pleurae.
- The mediastinum is the **most common** location of chest masses in children where a wide variety of both benign and malignant tumors may occur.[1]
- Mediastinal tumors are classified based on 1 of 3 mediastinal compartments (anterior, middle, or posterior) in which they originate (Figure 52.1).

ANTERIOR MEDIASTINUM

Normal Contents

- Thymus gland, internal mammary artery and vein, lymph nodes, and adipose tissue

Boundaries

- Anterior: sternum
- Posterior: the anterior pericardium
- Lateral: parietal pleurae
- Superior: imaginary line extending from sternal angle to T4 vertebrae
- Inferior: surface of diaphragm

Most Common Anterior Mediastinal Neoplasms

- Mnemonic: 4Ts = **T**eratoma (and other germ cell tumors), **T**errible lymphoma, **T**hymoma, and **T**hyroid neoplasms (from ectopic thyroid tissue)

MIDDLE MEDIASTINUM

Normal Contents

- Pericardium and its contents, ascending aorta, superior and inferior vena cava, brachiocephalic artery and vein, central portion of pulmonary arteries and veins, phrenic and upper vagus nerves, trachea, the main bronchi, and lymph nodes

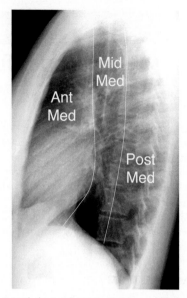

Figure 52.1 Lateral chest radiograph showing mediastinal divisions. The anterior mediastinum (Ant Med) lies posterior to the sternum and anterior to a line drawn along the anterior tracheal wall in the upper mediastinum and the posterior border of the heart in the lower mediastinum. The posterior mediastinum (Post Med) lies posterior to a line 1 cm behind the anterior margin of the vertebral column and anterior to the chest wall. The middle mediastinum (Mid Med) lies between these. (Reprinted with permission from Webb WR, Higgins CB. *Thoracic Imaging.* 2nd ed. Philadelphia, PA: Wolters Kluwer/Lippincott Williams & Wilkins Health; 2010.)

Boundaries

- Anterior and posterior: the pericardium
- Lateral: parietal pleurae
- Superior: imaginary line extending from sternal angle to T4 vertebrae
- Inferior: surface of diaphragm

Most Common Middle Mediastinal Neoplasms Bronchogenic Cyst

- Lymphoma, cardiac tumor, cystic hygroma, pericardial cyst

POSTERIOR MEDIASTINUM

Normal Contents

- Descending aorta, esophagus, thoracic duct, azygos and hemiazygos veins, and lymph nodes

Boundaries

- Anterior: the posterior pericardium
- Posterior: T5-T12 vertebrae
- Lateral: parietal pleurae
- Superior: imaginary line extending from sternal angle to T4 vertebrae
- Inferior: surface of diaphragm

MOST COMMON NEOPLASMS

- Neurogenic tumors, meningomyelocele, neuroenteric abnormalities
  - **Note: the most common pediatric mediastinal mass = neurogenic tumor** (~20% of all mediastinal tumors), usually found in the **posterior mediastinum.**[2]
  - As mediastinal masses can be either benign or malignant, definitive tumor diagnosis via biopsy (obtained via CT guided, bronchoscopy, or surgical) is desired before definitive intervention to determine the nature of the tumor and whether chemotherapy might reduce the size of the tumor for easier resection if indicated.[2]

Neurofibroma

OVERVIEW

- Neurofibromas are nerve-sheath tumors that can arise from peripheral nerves, sympathetic ganglia, or mediastinal chemoreceptors of the paraganglion system[3,4]
- **Most common benign tumor** of the mediastinum in children
- **Most frequently** located in the **posterior mediastinum**
  - **Note:** neurofibromas can present in isolation or as one of multiple tumors seen in neurofibromatosis type 1

PRESENTATION

- Often presents with tracheal compression as tumor grows in size, resulting in upper respiratory symptoms or with the development of scoliosis; usually first suspected on plain radiographs and confirmed with MRI (Figure 52.2)

SURGICAL INTERVENTION

- Surgical resection is the standard treatment option. A thoracoscopic approach is increasingly used to access neurogenic tumors of the posterior mediastinum.[5]

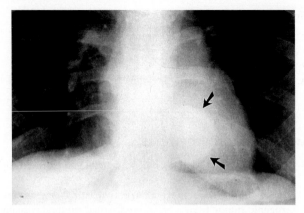

Figure 52.2 Neurofibroma presenting as a posterior mediastinal mass in a PA chest radiograph. Observe the dense radiopaque nodular lesion seen through the left ventricle of the heart (arrows). This lesion is in the posterior mediastinum and represents a neurofibroma. (Reprinted with permission from Yochum TR, Rowe LJ. *Yochum and Rowe's Essentials of Skeletal Radiology.* 3rd ed. Philadelphia, PA: Lippincott Williams & Wilkins; 2004.)

- **Note:** Complete resection can be difficult, as neurofibromas can be large in size with a tendency for local invasiveness and involvement of critical nerves; thus, this may require an open approach for best chance of reducing recurrence rates.[6]

Germ Cell Tumors

OVERVIEW

- Germ cell tumors originate from primordial germ cells, which may contain components of fetal endoderm, mesoderm, and ectoderm. As such, germ cell tumors may present as cystic, solid, or mixed lesions capable of containing hair, sebaceous glands, teeth, bone, and muscle, as well as well-differentiated thyroid, adrenal, or pancreatic tissue.[7]
- These are the third **most common** mediastinal tumor **in children**.
- Teratomas are the **most common mediastinal germ cells tumors**.
  - Almost always located in the anterior mediastinum and almost always benign

PRESENTATION

- Germ cell tumors may be detected on prenatal ultrasonography and be associated with fetal hydrops and polyhydramnios.
- Benign teratomas are commonly asymptomatic and are discovered as anterior mediastinal calcifications on routine chest radiograph in older children.
- Large teratomas present with respiratory distress caused by compression of the trachea and/or adjoining parenchyma.

SURGICAL INTERVENTION

- Surgery is indicated to relieve symptoms and to rule out malignant elements. Resection is generally achieved via median sternotomy or thoracotomy.
  - **Note:** Even if the tumor is benign, any recurrence has a high risk of being malignant, so long-term follow-up is required.[8]

Lymphoma

OVERVIEW

- Lymphoma is the **most common** cause of **anterior** and **middle** mediastinal masses in children.
- Most non-Hodgkin tumors found in the mediastinum are of a lymphoblastic T-cell origin because these cells arise from T-cell precursors. The thymus has a major role in producing these cells.
- Approximately 70% of children with lymphoblastic lymphoma will have an anterior mediastinal mass.[9]

PRESENTATION

- A mediastinal lymphoma may present as an incidental finding on a chest radiograph.
- Respiratory distress, cough, chest pain, neck swelling, or superior vena cava syndrome may be presenting symptoms if there is compression of the trachea or the upper central venous system.[9–11]
  - **Non-Hodgkin lymphomas** grow quickly and frequently cause notable, if not severe, respiratory compromise. Pleural effusions are present in 50% to 70% of these cases.[10]
  - **Hodgkin lymphomas** may present with fever or systemic symptoms in addition to cervical or mediastinal adenopathy.

Thymoma

OVERVIEW

- Neoplasms of epithelial or lymphocytic origin arising from within the parenchyma of the thymus
  - **Note: rare in children** (but **most common neoplasms of the anterior mediastinum in adults** and commonly associated with myasthenia gravis)[11]

PRESENTATION

- Typically present on imaging as a soft tissue mass within the anterior mediastinum and may have cystic components with calcifications (Figure 52.3)
- Biopsy recommended to confirm tissue diagnosis
- Malignant potential is determined by the presence and extent of microscopic or macroscopic invasion beyond the capsule of the gland[12]

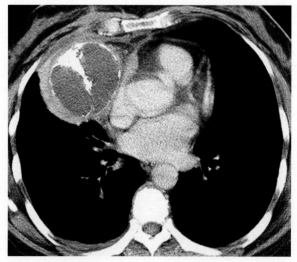

Figure 52.3 Cystic thymoma, noninvasive. CT shows a cystic mass in the right cardiophrenic angle. The mass shows dense calcification, including calcification of its capsule. A noninvasive cystic thymoma was found at surgery. (Reprinted with permission from Webb WR, Higgins CB. *Thoracic Imaging.* 2nd ed. Philadelphia, PA: Wolters Kluwer/Lippincott Williams & Wilkins Health; 2010.)

SURGICAL INTERVENTION

- Total surgical excision is recommended.
- Radiation and chemotherapy may be required for advanced stages of malignancy or partially resected or unresectable disease.[12,13]

Osteochondroma

OVERVIEW

- **Most common** of all **benign bone tumors**
- 3:1 male predominance
- Usually present in the first to third decade of life

PRESENTATION

- Originate from the rib cortex; can present as a painless mass or with complications of hemothorax, pneumothorax, rib fracture, or nerve/vascular impingement[14,15]
- Chest radiograph often reveals a pedunculated mass with a cartilaginous cap

SURGICAL INTERVENTION

- Surgical resection is indicated, as only 10% of all rib tumors are benign and malignant transformation of osteochondromas can occur.
  - **Note:** Surgery should be delayed until after puberty except in cases of increasing size or symptoms.[14]

PEARLS AND PITFALLS

- Mediastinal tumors are classified based on **one of three mediastinal compartments** (anterior, middle, or posterior) in which they originate.
- Neurofibromas are the **most common** benign tumor of the mediastinum in children and **most commonly** found in the posterior mediastinum.
- Lymphomas are the **most common** tumor of the anterior and middle mediastinum in children.
- Thymomas are rare in children but are the **most common** anterior mediastinal tumor in adults.

REFERENCES

1. Shochat SJ. Tumors of the lung. In: Grosfeld JL, O'Neill JA, Fonkalsrud EW, et al. eds. *Pediatric Surgery*. 6th ed. Philadelphia: Mosby; 2006:640-648.

2. Petroze R, McGahren ED. Pediatric chest II. *Surg Clin North Am*. 2012;92(3):645-658.

3. Azarow KS, Pearl RH, Zurcher R, et al. Primary mediastinal masses. A comparison of adult and pediatric populations. *J Thorac Cardiovasc Surg*. 1993;106(1):67-72.

4. Grosfeld JL, Weinberger M, Kilman JW, et al. Primary mediastinal neoplasms in infants and children. *Ann Thorac Surg*. 1971;12(2):179-190.

5. Lacreuse I, Valla JS, de Lagausie P, et al. Thoracoscopic resection of neurogenic tumors in children. *J Pediatr Surg*. 2007;42(10):1725-1728.

6. Fraga JC, Aydogdu B, Aufieri R, et al. Surgical treatment for pediatric mediastinal neurogenic tumors. *Ann Thorac Surg*. 2010;90(2):413-418.

7. Azizkhan RG. Teratomas and other germ cell tumors. In: Grosfeld JL, O'Neill JA, Fonkalsrud EW, et al, eds. *Pediatric Surgery*. 6th ed. Philadelphia: Mosby; 2006:554-574.

8. Lakhoo K, Boyle M, Drake DP. Mediastinal teratomas: review of 15 pediatric cases. *J Pediatr Surg*. 1993;28(9):1161-1164.

9. Garey CL, Laituri CA, Valusek PA, et al. Management of anterior mediastinal masses in children. *Eur J Pediatr Surg*. 2011;21:310-313.

10. Mauch PM, Kalish LA, Kadin M, et al. Patterns of presentation of Hodgkin disease: implication for etiology and pathogenesis. *Cancer*. 1993;71:2062-2071.

11. Ingram L, Rivera GK, Shapiro DN. Superior vena cava syndrome associated with childhood malignancy: analysis of 24 cases. *Med Pediatr Oncol*. 1990;18: 476-481.

12. Rothstein DH, Voss SD, Isakoff M, et al. Thymoma in a child: case report and review of the literature. *Pediatr Surg Int*. 2005;21:548-551.

13. Pollack A, Komaki R, Cox JD, et al. Thymoma: treatment and prognosis. *Int J Radiat Oncol Biol Phys*. 1992;23:1037-1043.

14. Smith SE, Keshavjee S. Primary chest wall tumors. *Thorac Surg Clin*. 2010;20(4):495-507.

15. Marino-Nieto J, Lugo-Vicente H. Rib osteochondroma in a child: case report and review of literature. *Bol Asoc Med P R*. 2011;103(1):47-50.

Chapter 53

Tumors of the GI Tract in Children

Nicholas Cortolillo

- There are many different tumors that affect the gastrointestinal (GI) tract in the pediatric population.
- This chapter will serve to highlight the major features of the most relevant tumors and syndromes including familial adenomatous polyposis (FAP), hereditary nonpolyposis colorectal cancer (HNPCC), juvenile polyposis syndrome (JPS), Peutz-Jeghers syndrome (PJS), Cowden syndrome (CS), Burkitt lymphoma (BL), and appendiceal carcinoid.

Familial Adenomatous Polyposis

EPIDEMIOLOGY AND ETIOLOGY

- FAP is the most common adenomatous polyposis syndrome in children.
- It is characterized by early onset of hundreds, possibly thousands, of adenomatous polyps in the colon beginning in early adolescence.
- Most patients with FAP will develop colorectal adenocarcinoma by age 40 years without intervention.
- The disease is inherited in an autosomal dominant fashion.
- The genetic defect is due to a germ line mutation in the APC gene (adenomatous polyposis coli), which is a tumor suppressor gene located on chromosome 5q21-22.[1]
- Patients with FAP are also at increased risk of periampullary cancers and mesenteric fibromatosis (desmoid tumors), which are the second and third most lethal complications of this syndrome, respectively.

Associated Syndromes (Gardner, Turcotte, and APCC)

- Closely related polyposis syndromes that are associated with the APC mutation include Gardner syndrome and Turcotte syndrome.

- Gardner syndrome is characterized by the aforementioned colorectal adenomatous polyps plus dental abnormalities, osteomas, epidermoid cysts, and desmoid tumors. Turcotte syndrome is associated with medulloblastomas.
- A milder variant of the FAP syndrome is attenuated familial adenomatous polyposis (AFAP), which is notable for fewer polyps, more right-sided than left-sided polyps, and a later age of polyposis onset in the fourth decade of life.

CLINICAL PRESENTATION

- Most patients with FAP are asymptomatic until the development of cancer, occurring at a mean age of 39 years.[2]
- Early diagnosis allows rigorous screening and affords colectomy before the onset of adenocarcinoma.
- Nonspecific symptoms include unexplained hematochezia, abdominal pain, or diarrhea in adolescent patients.
- A slit lamp examination may reveal congenital hypertrophy of the retinal pigment epithelium, which are discrete flat and pigmented lesions of the retina and are highly specific for FAP.
- Nearly 80% of patients will report a family history of early-onset colorectal cancer (CRC), but 20% with spontaneous APC mutations will have no remarkable family history.[3]

DIAGNOSIS

Screening

- Recommendations are largely based on expert opinion and observational data.
- Screening for cancers associated with FAP should occur in patients with known APC mutations as well as in patients at risk for FAP, including first-degree relatives of those with FAP who either have not yet undergone genetic evaluation or who have indeterminate genetic testing results.
- For patients with classic FAP, CRC screening begins annually at age 10 to 12 years[4] (Figure 53.1).
- Flexible sigmoidoscopy is recommended, and if adenomas are found, then complete colonoscopy is indicated.
- Several biopsies should be obtained to sample for dysplasia.
- Notes should be made of size, number, and distribution of polyps to guide surgical planning.
- Endoscopic control is unrealistic except in cases of AFAP where the number of polyps is multiple orders less in scale, and polypectomy can obviate the need for colectomy.

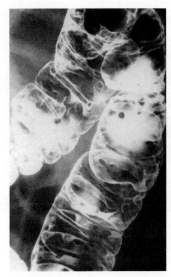

Figure 53.1 Familial polyposis. Small uniform polyps virtually carpet the colon. This patient had familial adenomatous polyposis. (Reprinted with permission from Swischik LE. *Imaging of the Newborn, Infant and Young Child.* 4th ed. Philadelphia, PA: Lippincott Williams & Wilkins; 1997.)

- Screening for AFAP is recommended to begin at the age of 25 years and every 1 to 2 years thereafter.
- Screening of the upper GI tract is recommended for both classic FAP and AFAP, given the high prevalence of gastric and duodenal polyps and risk of cancer.
- Screening with upper endoscopy should begin at the onset of polyposis or at the age of 25 years whichever comes first.[5,6]
- If no polyps are detected, screening is repeated every three years if the patient remains asymptomatic.
- Unlike lower endoscopy, screening for the upper GI tract has not been consistently shown to decrease mortality.

MEDICAL AND SURGICAL MANAGEMENT

- Colectomy is indicated for documented or suspected cancer, any biopsy of high-grade dysplasia, recurrent bleeding, multiple adenomas larger than 6 mm, marked increase in polyp number on consecutive endoscopies, inability to adequately survey the colon due to diminutive polyps (Figure 53.2).

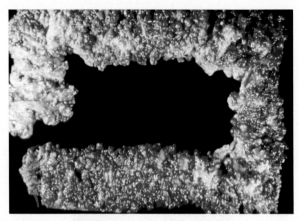

Figure 53.2 Familial adenomatous polyposis surgical specimen. (Reprinted with permission from Schaaf CP, Zschocke J, Potocki L. *Human Genetics.* Philadelphia, PA: Wolters Kluwer Health; 2012.)

- Surgical options include total proctocolectomy with end ileostomy, proctocolectomy with ileal pouch-anal anastomosis, or subtotal colectomy with ileorectal anastomosis.
- For patients with few rectal polyps (<10) and low risk of desmoid tumors, subtotal colectomy with ileo-rectal anastomosis may offer better quality of life.[7]

POSTOPERATIVE CARE

- Postoperatively, routine screening continues annually to survey the remaining rectal mucosa.
- Up to 20% of patients will develop desmoid tumor after colectomy, and this is the second most lethal complication of FAP, as it encases bowel, arteries, veins, and ureters.
- Life expectancy is greatly expanded in patients who undergo colectomy.
- Desmoid tumors and upper GI cancers are the next most common causes of death postcolectomy.[8]
- The cumulative probability of developing any non-CRC, mostly periampullary cancer, is 11% at 50 years and 52% at 75 years.[9]
- Screening for non-CRCs must be continued throughout life in FAP patients, including annual thyroid ultrasound to screen for thyroid nodules and abdominal CT scan to screen for desmoid tumor in the patient with bowel obstruction or a palpable abdominal mass.

Lynch Syndrome—Hereditary Nonpolyposis Colorectal Cancer

EPIDEMIOLOGY AND ETIOLOGY

- The most common form of hereditary CRC is known as Lynch syndrome and accounts for up to 5% of all colorectal carcinomas.[10]
- The disease is inherited in an autosomal dominant fashion as a result of defective DNA mismatch repair genes.
- HNPCC is divided into 2 groups, Lynch I and Lynch II (Figure 53.3).
- Patients with HNPCC Lynch I and Lynch II are at higher risk for CRC at much earlier ages.
- However, those with Lynch II are at increased risk of many other cancers including endometrial carcinoma and cancers of other sites such as small bowel, ureter, renal pelvis, ovary, and stomach.
- Despite the name of the disease containing the term "nonpolyposis," HNPCC patients do have polyps with the average age of polyp onset in the late second or early third decade of life.[11]

CLINICAL PRESENTATION

- Making the diagnosis of HNPCC requires family history, tumor testing, and genetic evaluation.
- Patients often are asymptomatic in early stages.
- May have nonspecific symptoms such as fatigue, anemia, or change in bowel habits.

DIAGNOSIS

- A pedigree should be drawn of each patient considered for HNPCC or any familial cancer syndrome, for that matter.
- Lynch syndrome is a diagnosis given to patients AND their families who fulfill the Amsterdam criteria, best memorized and applied in the 3-2-1 rule.[12]
- Three or more family members with HNPCC-related cancers, one of whom is a first-degree relative of the other two.
- Two successive affected generations (one of the patients is a first-degree family member of the other patients).
- One or more of the HNPCC-related cancers diagnosed younger than 50 years.
- FAP has been excluded.

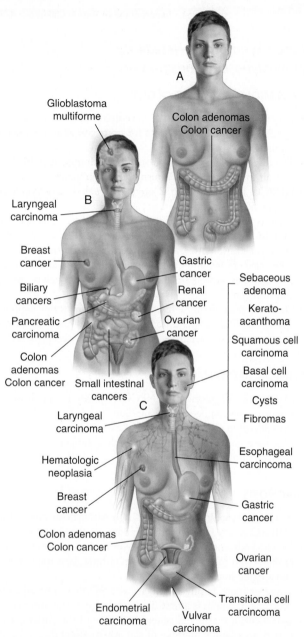

Figure 53.3 Neoplasms arising in patients with hereditary cancer syndromes. A, Lynch I syndrome. B, Lynch II syndrome. C, Muir-Torre syndrome. (Adapted from Noffsinger AE. *Fenoglio-Prieser's Gastrointestinal Pathology.* Philadelphia, PA: Wolters Kluwer Health; 2018.)

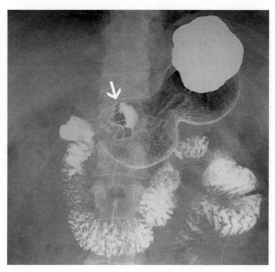

Figure 53.4 This is an example of a Lynch syndrome family with a classical phenotype but in which evaluations by several different highly competent laboratories have failed to identify mismatch repair mutations. Stars indicate individuals who have been tested. (Reprinted with permission from Tan D, Lauwers G. *Advances in Surgical Pathology: Gastric Cancer*. Philadelphia, PA: Wolters Kluwer Health; 2012.)

- Additionally, Lynch syndrome refers to any patients and their families who have a documented germ line mutation in one of the DNA mismatch repair genes.

Screening

- Patients with Lynch syndrome should undergo CRC screening with colonoscopy every 1 to 2 years beginning at age 20 to 25 years, or 5 years earlier before the age of the first diagnosed cancer in the family, whichever comes first[13] (Figure 53.4).

MEDICAL AND SURGICAL MANAGEMENT

- The diagnosis of CRC or the presence of an endoscopically unresectable polyp is an indication for total abdominal colectomy with ileorectal anastomosis, followed by annual surveillance of the rectal stump.[14]
- In addition, women with Lynch syndrome who do not plan to have future children should be offered prophylactic hysterectomy and bilateral salpingo-oophorectomy at the time of colectomy.

- A screening program should also be established for the other cancer types in the family. Women with Lynch syndrome are recommended to receive annual pelvic examinations and endometrial biopsies, plus transvaginal ultrasound for ovarian cancer starting at 30 to 35 years of age, or 3 to 5 years earlier than the earliest age of cancer diagnosis in the family.[11,13]
- Screening for gastric cancer is recommended to begin at age 30 to 35 years and repeated every 2 to 3 years for those with gastric cancer risk factors.
- Treatment of *Helicobacter pylori* has been shown to significantly reduce the risk of gastric cancer in Lynch syndrome.[15]
- For urinary tract cancers, annual random urinalysis is recommended to begin at age 30 to 35 years.[16]
- Microscopic analysis of the urine is controversial.
- Note that these recommendations are based largely on expert opinion and observational studies, and any screening program should be individualized to the patient and family history.

Juvenile Polyposis Syndrome

EPIDEMIOLOGY AND ETIOLOGY

- JPS is an autosomal dominant condition characterized by multiple hamartomatous polyps in the GI tract and confers an increased risk for colon and gastric cancer.[5]
- This is differentiated from sporadic juvenile polyps, which can occur in up to 2% of children younger than 10 years and confer no increased risk of malignancy.
- JPS is a rare disorder affecting 1 out of every 100 000 individuals.
- The disease occurs as a result of germ line mutations in the SMAD4 or BMPR1A, genes that are involved in the TGF-B signaling pathway.[17]

CLINICAL PRESENTATION

- Polyps begin to appear in the first decade of life, and patients can experience up to 100 polyps in their lifetime.
- JPS is a clinical diagnosis based on the presence of either
  - More than 5 juvenile polyps in the colorectum
  - Multiple juvenile polyps in other parts of the GI tract OR
  - Any number of juvenile polyps in a patient with a known history of JPS
  - PLUS the absence of clinical findings of other hamartomatous polyposis syndromes such as PJS and PTEN syndrome[14]

- JPS due to SMAD4 mutations may also be associated with hereditary hemorrhagic telangiectasia (HHT), which presents with telangiectasias of the skin and buccal mucosa, epistaxis, and iron deficiency anemia from bleeding.[18]
- Over 90% of polyps are located in the colon, but 14% of polyps are seen in the stomach, 10% in the duodenum and jejunum, and 7% in the ileum.[19]
- The most common presenting symptom is blood per rectum.
- Most patients are symptomatic by 20 years.
- Disease onset in infancy is associated with a poorer prognosis and is characterized by diarrhea, bleeding, and intussusception.

MEDICAL AND SURGICAL MANAGEMENT

- The cumulative risk of CRC in patients with JPS is 20% by age 35 years and 68% by age 60 years.
- JPS also predisposes to gastric cancer, with a lifetime risk of 20% to 30% and a mean age at diagnosis of 58 years.[20]
- Screening for CRC and upper GI cancers with esophagogastroduodenoscopy (EGD) and colonoscopy should be performed every 1 to 3 years beginning at age 12 years or at the onset of symptoms.[14,21]
- If polyps are found, then screening should continue annually.
- The small bowel is typically monitored with balloon enteroscopy or capsule endoscopy; however, the timing and intervals for these screenings are controversial.
- Laboratory analysis assessing for iron-deficiency anemia and protein-losing enteropathy should be included as adjuncts.
- Most polyps in this syndrome can be managed endoscopically.
- Surgical management is reserved for intractable symptoms (ie, bleeding), biopsy-proven cancer, or when polyps cannot be managed endoscopically.
- The decision for proctocolectomy with ileal pouch–anal anastomosis versus subtotal colectomy with ileorectal anastomosis is both patient and disease specific.

Peutz-Jeghers Syndrome

EPIDEMIOLOGY AND ETIOLOGY

- PJS is an autosomal dominant inherited disorder characterized by hamartomatous polyps in the GI tract, mucocutaneous pigmentation, and 10- to 20-fold increased risk of GI cancers and non-GI cancers.[22]

- The disease occurs due to germ line mutations in the LKB1 gene encoding a serine threonine kinase on chromosome 19, a designated tumor suppressor gene.[23]
- Approximately 10% to 20% of cases are due to spontaneous mutations.[24]
- Extraintestinal tumors include ovarian sex cord tumors, cervical adenoma malignum, testis Sertoli cell tumors, and breast carcinoma.

CLINICAL PRESENTATION

- Pigmented mucocutaneous macules are seen in over 95% of PJS patients and are seen as flat, blue-gray to brown spots 1 to 5 mm in size (Figure 53.5).
- Locations include the lips and perioral region in 94%, palms of the hands in 74%, buccal mucosa in 66%, and soles of the feet in 62%.[25]
- These spots will appear in the first one to two years of life.
- Malignant transformation is rare.
- Most fade after puberty.
- The median time of first presentation with polyps is age 11 to 13 years; approximately 50% of individuals have experienced symptoms by age 20 years.

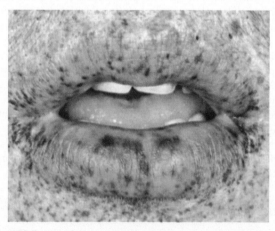

Figure 53.5 Peutz-Jeghers syndrome. When pigmented spots on the lips are more prominent than freckling of the surrounding skin, suspect this syndrome. Pigment in the buccal mucosa helps to confirm the diagnosis. Pigmented spots may also be found on the face and hands. Multiple intestinal polyps are often associated. (Reprinted with permission from Bickley LS. *Bates' Guide to Physical Examination and History Taking*. Philadelphia, PA: Wolters Kluwer Health; 2003.)

- Rectal bleeding, iron-deficiency anemia, abdominal pain, and obstruction are the most common complications.[26]
- Nearly 50% of patients will experience intussusception during their lifetime.
- The small bowel is the most commonly affected location 60% to 90%, followed by the colon 50% to 64%, and stomach 15% to 30%.[25]
- On histology, PJ polyps are hamartomas and contain a proliferation of smooth muscle extending into the lamina propria, but the overlying epithelium is normal.[27]

MEDICAL AND SURGICAL MANAGEMENT

- Individuals who meet clinical criteria for PJS should have confirmatory genetic testing for the LKB1 gene.
- About 48% of patients with PJS develop and die from cancer by age 57 years.
- Others may have a normal life span.
- The mean age at first diagnosis of cancer is 42.9 years, ±10.2 years.[28]
- The most common sites for malignancy are the colon in 40%, stomach in 29%, small bowel in 13%, and pancreas in 11% to 36%.
- Non-GI cancers account for over half of the malignancies seen in PJS.[29]
- Women with PJS have increased lifetime risk of breast cancer in 36% to 54%, ovary in 21%, and cervix in 10%.[30]
- In particular, the variant of cervical adenoma malignum is known to be highly aggressive.
- Surveillance should be offered to patients with PJS in the form of annual physical examinations with pelvic examinations, testicular examinations, and complete blood count.
- Baseline endoscopy with colonoscopy, capsule endoscopy, and EGD should be obtained before age 10 years and repeated annually if polyps are found.
- Annual GI screening may occur at age 18 years if no polyps are found at baseline screening.
- For females, annual Pap smear and transvaginal ultrasound is recommended starting at age 21 years.
- Annual mammography or breast MRI should commence at age 25 years.
- Pancreatic screening is controversial, but some centers advocate rigorous screening in the form of annual magnetic resonance cholangiopancreatography or endoscopic ultrasound beginning at age 30 years.[11]

Cowden Syndrome (PTEN Hamartoma Tumor Syndrome)

EPIDEMIOLOGY AND ETIOLOGY

- Germ line mutations in the phosphatase and tensin homolog (PTEN) gene have been described in a variety of rare phenotypic patterns.
- The defining feature of these disorders is hamartomas.
- CS is the most studied PTEN hamartoma tumor syndrome (PHTS), and it carries autosomal dominant heritance.[31]
- In addition to hamartomas, patients with CS have dermatology disorders including oral fibromas, trichilemmomas, oral fibromas, macrocephaly, and penile lentigines.
- In addition, CS confers increased risk of breast, thyroid, endometrial, kidney, and CRCs.
- It affects 1 in 200 000 people. Spontaneous mutations are responsible for 10% to 30% of diagnoses.[32]

CLINICAL PRESENTATION

- What is known about clinical manifestations of CS come from small case series; thus the true frequencies of the clinical features are unknown (Figure 53.6).
- Breast cancer is the most common malignancy in CS, afflicting around 25% to 50% of women, usually in the fourth or fifth decade of life.[33]
- Thyroid disease is also common in this population; it is estimated two-thirds of patients experience will have benign thyroid abnormalities, including multinodular goiter, adenomas, and lymphocytic thyroiditis.[34]
- CS confers increased risk of thyroid cancer as well, up to 24% in one series of 2723 patients.[35]
- Papillary carcinomas predominate in most series.
- Colorectal adenocarcinoma affects 9% to 18% of patients with CS.[36]

MEDICAL AND SURGICAL MANAGEMENT

- Children or adults presenting with suspected CS may qualify for PTEN testing if they meet strict clinical criteria.
- Cancer surveillance is the main focus of management and is National Comprehensive Cancer Network-supported for CS.

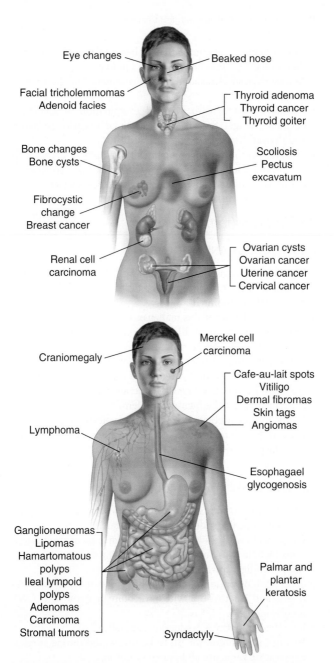

Figure 53.6 Diagrammatic representation of many of the intestinal and extraintestinal lesions found in patients with Cowden syndrome. (Adapted from Noffsinger AE. *Fenoglio-Prieser's Gastrointestinal Pathology.* Philadelphia: Wolters Kluwer Health; 2018.)

- Colonoscopy is recommended to begin at age 35 years and then every 5 years if no polyps are found.
- Annual thyroid ultrasound should commence at the time of diagnosis.
- Annual comprehensive physical examination is advocated beginning at age 18 years, with particular attention to breast and thyroid tissues.
- With regard to women, annual mammography or breast MRI is recommended starting at age 30 to 35 years or 5 to 10 years before the earliest known relative with breast cancer.

Burkitt Lymphoma

EPIDEMIOLOGY AND ETIOLOGY

- BL is a highly aggressive B cell non-Hodgkin lymphoma characterized by the translocation and deregulation of the c-MYC gene on chromosome 8.
- There are 3 forms of this malignancy.
- The endemic form of BL is caused by Epstein-Barr virus (EBV) infection and presents as a jaw for facial bone tumor in 60%, and the GI tract is usually not the primary site.[37]
- The sporadic form most often arises from the distal ileum or stomach; however, unlike the endemic form, EBV infection is frequently not the inciting problem.[38]
- Lastly, immunodeficiency-related BL typically involves bone marrow, lymph nodes, and the CNS while sparing the abdomen, face, or jaw.[39]

CLINICAL PRESENTATION

- The sporadic form of BL comprises 30% of pediatric lymphomas with a peak incidence of age 11 years.
- For patients with the sporadic form of BL, presenting symptoms include those related to GI bleeding or bowel obstruction, including intussusception.
- Over 25% of patients will also have jaw or facial involvement, and up to 30% will have bone marrow and CNS involvement.
- Lymphadenopathy is frequently generalized.
- It is not uncommon for BL to be discovered during surgical exploration for acute abdominal symptoms.
- If the tumor can be resected safely and easily in such settings, then it is recommended to do so.

- Otherwise, the main role of surgery in BL is for obtaining a tissue biopsy.
- Histology will reveal diffuse infiltrate of neoplastic cells in a starry sky pattern.
- High mitotic counts and >95% staining for Ki67 are common.[28]

MEDICAL AND SURGICAL MANAGEMENT

- Children with biopsy proven BL should be enrolled in a trial, whenever possible.
- Multiagent combination chemotherapy (ifosfamide, carboplatin, etoposide) with or without immunotherapy (rituximab) is preferred at most centers.
- Depending on the stage of disease, chemotherapy may last 6 weeks up to 8 months. BL is highly sensitive to chemotherapy.
- Stage I and II disease has an event-free survival of 98% at 4 years.[40]
- Relapses are considered more aggressive than the initial disease and typically occur within the first 2 years.

Appendiceal Carcinoid

EPIDEMIOLOGY AND ETIOLOGY

- The term "carcinoid" pertains to well-differentiated neuroendocrine tumors originating in the GI tract (50%), lungs (30%), or rarely the kidneys or ovaries.[41]
- The "carcinoid syndrome" is applied to patients with metastatic neuroendocrine tumors to liver who present with a constellation of symptoms, primarily flushing and diarrhea.
- This is caused by systemic effects of GI peptides and hormones, which bypass the usual hepatic metabolism, including serotonin, 5-hydroxytryptophan, histamine, prostaglandins, catecholamines, and bradykinins.
- Despite carcinoid tumors having median age of 63 years at diagnosis with an age-adjusted incidence of 5 per 100 000, it remains well-documented diagnosis in the pediatric population.

CLINICAL PRESENTATION

- Similar to adults, the appendix is the most common site of a carcinoid tumor in children.
- Children with carcinoid of the proximal appendix usually present with acute appendicitis.[42]

- Presentation of the tumor in the context of carcinoid syndrome is exceedingly rare in children. Ileal and colonic carcinoids are more likely to present as a palpable mass due to their larger sizes, as virtually all tumors are over 2 cm at the time of discovery.[43]
- For the rare carcinoid that is not discovered surgically, 5-HIAA levels may be elevated in 24-hour urine specimen.
- On pathology, carcinoid tumors have multiple well-demarcated islands of closely packed cells with peripheral palisading that are separated by fibrotic stroma.
- The tumor cells have round nuclei with "salt and pepper" chromatin that are surrounded by a moderate amount of lightly eosinophilic granular cytoplasm.

MEDICAL AND SURGICAL MANAGEMENT

- When the tumor is less than 2 cm in diameter, appendectomy alone is adequate therapy.
- Lesions over 2 cm with invasion of the mesoappendix or the appendiceal base require right hemicolectomy.[44]
- Survival is excellent for localized disease that undergoes resection.
- The disease-free 5-year survival for carcinoid of the appendix is 89% with only 4% having liver metastasis.[45]
- Carcinoid tumors arising from elsewhere in the GI tract have higher rates of local and distant metastases.
- Patients with metastatic disease to the liver may be palliated medically with octreotide for secretory diarrhea, albuterol inhalers as needed for bronchospasm, and alpha-receptor blockade for flushing.
- Aggressive chemotherapy and surgical debulking offer no benefit in these circumstances.
- Transcatheter arterial chemoembolization of liver metastases has been shown to have palliative benefit.[46]

Other Intestinal Polyps

- A variety of nonhereditary nonmalignant neoplasms may also be found in the GI tract of children.
- Inflammatory polyps, also known as pseudopolyps, may be found in children with inflammatory bowel disease or may also occur as a result of necrotizing enterocolitis.
- Histologically, these may be different to distinguish from benign juvenile polyps.

- Benign lymphoid polyps are a frequent cause of intussusception in children.
- These lesions usually occur in the ileum or rectum and may be numerous; however, they are typically small <5 mm, sessile, and umbilicated.
- They are regarded as a self-limiting reactive process to other benign GI tract pathology.

PEARLS AND PITFALLS

- FAP is the most common adenomatous polyposis syndrome in children characterized by hundreds of polyps throughout the colon. A germ line mutation in the APC gene is the signature genetic defect in APC.
- Lynch syndrome (HNPCC) is inherited in an autosomal dominant fashion as a result of defective DNA mismatch repair genes. The diagnosis is given to patients AND their families who fulfill the Amsterdam criteria, best memorized and applied in the 3-2-1 rule (see above).
- JPS is an autosomal dominant condition characterized by multiple hamartomatous polyps in the GI tract.
- PJS is an autosomal dominant inherited disorder characterized by hamartomatous polyps in the GI tract, mucocutaneous pigmentation, and 10- to 20-fold increased risk of GI cancers and non-GI cancers.
- The sporadic form of BL comprises 30% of pediatric lymphomas with a peak incidence of age 11 years.

REFERENCES

1. Nieuwenhuis MH, De Vos Tot Nederveen Cappel W, Botma A, et al. Desmoid tumors in a Dutch cohort of patients with familial adenomatous polyposis. *Clin Gastroenterol Hepatol.* 2008;6:215-219.
2. Nieuwenhuis MH, Mathus-Vliegen LM, Slors FH, et al. Genotype-phenotype correlations as a guide in the management of familial adenomatous polyposis. *Clin Gastroenterol Hepatol.* 2007;5:374-378.
3. Heiskanen I, Kellokumpu I, Järvinen H. Management of duodenal adenomas in 98 patients with familial adenomatous polyposis. *Endoscopy.* 1999;31:412-416.
4. Vasen HF, Moslein G, Alonso A, et al. Guidelines for the clinical management of familial adenomatous polyposis (FAP). *Gut.* 2008;57:704-713.
5. Syngal S, Brand RE, Church JM, Giardiello FM, Hampel HL, Burt RW. ACG clinical guideline: genetic testing and management of hereditary gastrointestinal cancer syndromes. *Am J Gastroenterol.* 2015;110:223-262; quiz 263.
6. Bisgaard ML, Fenger K, Bülow S, Niebuhr E, Mohr J. Familial adenomatous polyposis (FAP): frequency, penetrance, and mutation rate. *Hum Mutat.* 1994;3:121-125.

7. Petersen GM, Slack J, Nakamura Y. Screening guidelines and premorbid diagnosis of familial adenomatous polyposis using linkage. *Gastroenterology*. 1991;100:1658-1664.

8. Burt RW, DiSario JA, Cannon-Albright L. Genetics of colon cancer: impact of inheritance on colon cancer risk. *Annu Rev Med*. 1995;46:371-379.

9. Leoz ML, Carballal S, Moreira L, Ocaña T, Balaguer F. The genetic basis of familial adenomatous polyposis and its implications for clinical practice and risk management. *Appl Clin Genet*. 2015;8:95-107.

10. Moreira L, Balaguer F, Lindor N, et al. Identification of Lynch syndrome among patients with colorectal cancer. *JAMA*. 2012;308:1555-1565.

11. American Gastroenterological Association. American Gastroenterological Association medical position statement: hereditary colorectal cancer and genetic testing. *Gastroenterology*. 2001;121:195-197.

12. Win AK, Buchanan AD, Rosty C, et al. Role of tumour molecular and pathology features to estimate colorectal cancer risk for first-degree relatives. *Gut*. 2015;64:101-110.

13. Giardiello FM, Allen JI, Axilbund JE, et al. Guidelines on genetic evaluation and management of Lynch syndrome: a consensus statement by the US multi-society task force on colorectal cancer. *Dis Colon Rectum*. 2014;57:1025-1048.

14. Kalady MF, McGannon E, Manlich E, Fazio VW, Church JM. Risk of colorectal adenoma and carcinoma after colectomy for colorectal cancer in patients meeting Amsterdam criteria. *Ann Surg*. 2010;252:507-511; discussion 511–3.

15. Vasen HFA, Blanco I, Aktan-Collan K, et al. Revised guidelines for the clinical management of Lynch syndrome (HNPCC): recommendations by a group of European experts. *Gut*. 2013;62:812-823.

16. Myrhøj T, Andersen M-B, Bernstein I. Screening for urinary tract cancer with urine cytology in Lynch syndrome and familial colorectal cancer. *Fam Cancer*. 2008;7:303-307.

17. Latchford AR, Neale K, Phillips RKS, Clark SK. Juvenile polyposis syndrome: a study of genotype, phenotype, and long-term outcome. *Dis Colon Rectum*. 2012;55:1038-1043.

18. Howe JR, Roth S, Ringold JC, et al. Mutations in the SMAD4/DPC4 gene in juvenile polyposis. *Science*. 1998;280:1086-1088.

19. O'Malley M, LaGuardia L, Kalady MF, et al. The prevalence of hereditary hemorrhagic telangiectasia in juvenile polyposis syndrome. *Dis Colon Rectum*. 2012;55:886-892.

20. Grotsky HW, Rickert RR, Smith WD, Newsome JF. Familial juvenile polyposis coli. A clinical and pathologic study of a large kindred. *Gastroenterology*. 1982;82:494-501.

21. Brosens LAA, van Hattern A, Hylind LM, et al. Risk of colorectal cancer in juvenile polyposis. *Gut*. 2007;56:965-967.

22. Howe JR, Bair JL, Sayed MG, et al. Germline mutations of the gene encoding bone morphogenetic protein receptor 1A in juvenile polyposis. *Nat Genet*. 2001;28:184-187.

23. Jeghers H, McKUSICK VA, Katz KH. Generalized intestinal polyposis and melanin spots of the oral mucosa, lips and digits; a syndrome of diagnostic significance. *N Engl J Med*. 1949;241:993, illust; passim.

24. Jenne DE, Reomann H, Nezu J, et al. Peutz-Jeghers syndrome is caused by mutations in a novel serine threonine kinase. *Nat Genet*. 1998;18:38-43.

25. Hernan I, Roid I, Martin B, Gamundi MJ, Martinez-Gimeno M, Carballo M. De novo germline mutation in the serine-threonine kinase STK11/LKB1 gene associated with Peutz-Jeghers syndrome. *Clin Genet.* 2004;66:58-62.

26. Utsunomiya J, Gocho H, Miyanaga T, Hamaguchi E, Kashimure A. Peutz-Jeghers syndrome: its natural course and management. *Johns Hopkins Med J.* 1975;136:71-82.

27. Hinds R, Philp C, Hyer W, Fell JM. Complications of childhood Peutz-Jeghers syndrome: implications for pediatric screening. *J Pediatr Gastroenterol Nutr.* 2004;39:219-220.

28. ClinicalKey. Available from: https://www.clinicalkey.com/#!/content/book/3-s2.0-B9780443068089000142?scrollTo=%23hl0010188. Accessed: January 22, 2018.

29. van Lier MGF, Wagner A, Mathus-Vliegen EMH, Kuipers EJ, Steyerberg EW, van Leerdam ME. High cancer risk in Peutz-Jeghers syndrome: a systematic review and surveillance recommendations. *Am J Gastroenterol.* 2010;105:1258-1264; author reply 1265.

30. Rebsdorf Pedersen I, Hartvigsen A, Fischer Hansen B, Toftgaard C, Konstantin-Hansen K, Bullow S. Management of Peutz-Jeghers syndrome. Experience with patients from the Danish polyposis register. *Int J Colorectal Dis.* 1994;9:177-179.

31. Marsh DJ, Kum JB, Lunetta KL, et al. PTEN mutation spectrum and genotype-phenotype correlations in Bannayan-Riley-Ruvalcaba syndrome suggest a single entity with Cowden syndrome. *Hum Mol Genet.* 1999;8:1461-1472.

32. Mester J, Eng C, Estimate of de novo mutation frequency in probands with PTEN hamartoma tumor syndrome. *Genet Med.* 2012;14:819-822.

33. Pilarski R. Cowden syndrome: a critical review of the clinical literature. *J Genet Couns.* 2009;18:13-27.

34. Hall JE, Abdollahian DJ, Sinard RJ. Thyroid disease associated with Cowden syndrome: a meta-analysis. *Head Neck.* 2013;35:1189-1194.

35. Ngeow J, Mester J, Rybicki LA, Ni Y, Milas M, Eng C. Incidence and clinical characteristics of thyroid cancer in prospective series of individuals with Cowden and Cowden-like syndrome characterized by germline PTEN, SDH, or KLLN alterations. *J Clin Endocrinol Metab.* 2011;96:E2063-E2071.

36. Heald B, Mester J, Rybicki L, Orloff MS, Burke CA, Eng C. Frequent gastrointestinal polyps and colorectal adenocarcinomas in a prospective series of PTEN mutation carriers. *Gastroenterology.* 2010;139:1927-1933.

37. Ogwang MD, Bhatia K, Biggar RJ, Mbulaiteye SM. Incidence and geographic distribution of endemic Burkitt lymphoma in northern Uganda revisited. *Int J Cancer.* 2008;123:2658-2663.

38. Morton LM, Wang SS, Devesa SS, Hartge P, Weisenburger DF, Linet MS. Lymphoma incidence patterns by WHO subtype in the United States, 1992-2001. *Blood.* 2006;107:265-276.

39. Guech-Ongey M, Simard EP, Anderson WF, et al. AIDS-related Burkitt lymphoma in the United States: what do age and CD4 lymphocyte patterns tell us about etiology and/or biology? *Blood.* 2010;116:5600-5604.

40. Gerrard M, Cairo MS, Weston C, et al. Excellent survival following two courses of COPAD chemotherapy in children and adolescents with resected localized B-cell non-Hodgkin's lymphoma: results of the FAB/LMB 96 international study. *Br J Haematol.* 2008;141:840-847.

41. Maggard MA, O'Connell JB, Ko CY. Updated population-based review of carcinoid tumors. *Ann Surg*. 2004;240:117-122.
42. Andersson A, Bergdahl L. Carcinoid tumors of the appendix in children. A report of 25 cases. *Acta Chir Scand*. 1977;143:173-175.
43. Soga J. Carcinoids of the colon and ileocecal region: a statistical evaluation of 363 cases collected from the literature. *J Exp Clin Cancer Res*. 1998;17:139-148.
44. Moertel CG, Weiland LH, Nagorney DM, Dockerty MB. Carcinoid tumor of the appendix: treatment and prognosis. *N Engl J Med*. 1987;317:1699-1701.
45. Shebani KO, Souba WW, Finkelstein DM, et al. Prognosis and survival in patients with gastrointestinal tract carcinoid tumors. *Ann Surg*. 1999;229:815.
46. Roche A, Girish BV, de Baere T, et al. Trans-catheter arterial chemoembolization as first-line treatment for hepatic metastases from endocrine tumors. *Eur Radiol*. 2003;13:136-140.

Chapter 54

Testicular Tumors in Children

Kenan Ashouri, and Fawaz M. Ashouri

- Pediatric testicular tumors are rare in the prepubescent male (Figure 54.1).
- Germ cell tumors (GCTs) comprise the majority of testicular tumors in the pediatric population.

EPIDEMIOLOGY AND ETIOLOGY

- The most common type of GCT in the pediatric population is **yolk sac tumors,** followed by **teratomas.**[1]
  - Yolk sac tumors are malignant and express alpha fetoprotein (AFP).
  - In contrast to adults, teratomas in children are often benign and lack immature components.[2,3]
- **Epidermoid cysts** are another common benign testicular tumor in children.
- The next most common category is gonadal stromal tumors, including sertoli cell tumors, leydig cell tumors, and juvenile granulosa cell tumors, in respective order of approximate incidence.
- Seminomatous GCTs are rare in children.
- Paratesticular rhabdomyosarcomas are the most common malignant tumor of the paratesticular structures.
  - Often arise from the spermatic cord, tunicae, or epididymis.
  - Highly aggressive and warrant retroperitoneal lymph node dissection (RPLND) and metastatic workup.[4]
- Secondary tumors are most commonly leukemia or lymphoma.
- Cryptorchidism is classically associated with an increased relative risk of GCT (RR~3-8) in the undescended testicle, which is only reduced but not eliminated (RR~2-3) after prepubertal orchiopexy.[5]

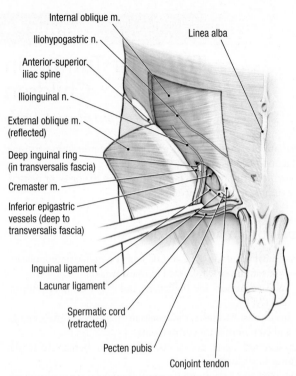

Internal oblique m.

Iliohypogastric n.

Anterior-superior
iliac spine

Ilioinguinal n.

External oblique m.
(reflected)

Deep inguinal ring
(in transversalis fascia)

Cremaster m.

Inferior epigastric
vessels (deep to
transversalis fascia)

Inguinal ligament

Lacunar ligament

Spermatic cord
(retracted)

Pecten pubis

Linea alba

Conjoint tendon

Figure 54.1 Inguinal anatomy. Note: Scarpa fascia (not depicted) is more predominant both near the pelvis and in children. (Reprinted with permission from Detton AJ. *Grant's Dissector*. 16th ed. Philadelphia, PA: Wolters Kluwer; 2017.)

CLINICAL PRESENTATION

- Testicular tumors typically present as a painless testicular mass incidentally found by the patient or parent or on clinical examination.
- There is often an associated hydrocele occurring in ~1 in 5 patients.[6]

DIAGNOSIS

- **AFP is elevated in yolk sac tumors (YSTs)** and is critical in diagnosing, staging, and monitoring recurrence of YSTs; however, it can be physiologically elevated in infants for up to 1 year.[7]
- If AFP is elevated, chest X-ray and CT abdomen/pelvis are needed for staging.[1]

- Ultrasonography is useful in differentiating a testicular tumor from other testicular pathology, such as torsion or paratesticular tumor (Figure 54.2).
- Although ultrasound can be used to characterize tumors by common appearance, it is difficult to truly differentiate malignant versus benign testicular tumors ultrasonographically.[8]
  - Yolk sac tumor will appear as a well-circumscribed, heterogenous mass with central hemorrhage or necrosis.
  - Teratomas will have a complex, heterogenous appearance with mixed composition representative of 3 germ cell layers such as acoustic-shadowing from calcification.
  - Epidermoid cysts are keratin-lined with "onion-skinning" or alternating hyper- and hypoechoic layered appearance surrounding a cystic center.
- Leydig cell tumors are implicated in testicular masses with associated precocious puberty.[9]

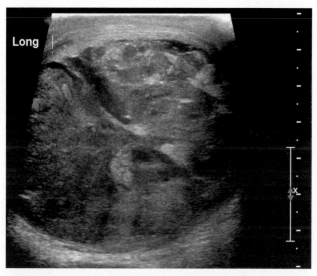

Figure 54.2 Gray-scale image of the right scrotum in an adolescent shows complete replacement of the right testicle by a large heterogeneous mass. Heterogeneity of mass favors germ cell tumor as likely histopathology, and this was confirmed after radical orchiectomy. Tumor was predominantly mature teratoma with components of yolk sac tumor and embryonal carcinoma. (Reprinted with permission from Iyer R, Chapman T. *Pediatric Imaging: The Essentials*. Philadelphia, PA: Wolters Kluwer Health; 2016.)

MEDICAL AND SURGICAL MANAGEMENT

- **Most yolk sac tumors present as clinical stage I**, confined to the testis, and **can be managed with radical inguinal orchiectomy** with high ligation of the cord.
  - Clinical stage II or higher warrants the addition of a platinum-based chemotherapy regimen.
  - Recurrence can be managed with salvage chemotherapy with favorable outcome.
  - Recurrence after chemotherapy or clinical stage III or IV disease warrants RPLND.[10]
- In children teratomas rarely harbor immature elements and thus are rarely malignant in the prepubertal population.
- **Both teratomas and epidermoid cysts should be managed with testis-sparing surgery.**[2,3]

SURGICAL MANAGEMENT

Radical Orchiectomy

- A 5-cm transverse incision in the abdominal crease should be made overlying the deep inguinal ring.
- After dissecting through the subcutaneous fat and Scarpa fascia, identify and defat the external oblique aponeurosis to the superficial inguinal ring.
- Using the metzenbaum scissors with specific care not to injure the underlying tissue, enter the aponeurosis at the level of the deep inguinal ring and divide it toward the superficial inguinal ring.
- Dissect the elements of the spermatic cord and displace the ilioinguinal nerve laterally.
- Free the spermatic cord to its origin at the deep inguinal ring until the peritoneal reflection is visualized.
- Place a penrose drain or vessel loop around the cord, occluding the vascular supply.
- Deliver the cord and testicle with its tunica vaginalis from the scrotum and transect the gubernaculum, at which point 2 suture ligatures should be placed across the proximal spermatic cord above the level of the penrose or vessel loop and 1 suture distally, below the penrose or vessel loop with approximately 1 cm in-between the proximal and distal suture ligatures.
- At our center, we prefer a nonabsorbable polyester 2-0 suture.

- Specific care should be taken not to incorporate any bowel or hernia contents within the ligation.
- At this point, the spermatic cord can be divided to remove the testicle and spermatic cord en bloc.
- Irrigate the tissue space.
- Scrotal exploration is not necessary.
- Reapproximate the superficial inguinal ring and external oblique aponeurosis using either interrupted vicryl or silk.
- Reapproximate the subcutaneous tissue and close skin.

Testis-Sparing Surgery—Partial Orchiectomy

- Inguinal incision should be made in similar fashion as above; however, in this case we will not enter the external oblique aponeurosis.
- Place a vessel loop or penrose drain over spermatic cord.
- Deliver testicle and tunica vaginalis through inguinal incision.
- After making an incision in the tunica vaginalis, excise the lesion in elliptical fashion with negative gross margins (use ultrasound guidance if necessary).
- Frozen section is recommended.
- Approximate tunica albuginea with running 5-0 PDS.
- Benign lesions should be managed with testis-sparing surgery if possible.

POSTOPERATIVE CARE

- Yolk sac tumors should be monitored postradical orchiectomy with monthly AFP for 2 years, chest X-rays every 2 months for 2 years, and CT every 3 months for 1 year then every 6 months the second year.[11]
  - RPLND should be performed in children with rise in AFP despite orchiectomy and chemotherapy.[1,11]

PEARLS AND PITFALLS

- Inguinal incision is used in both radical orchiectomy and testis-sparing approach.
- A scrotal approach or biopsy in the context of a yolk sac tumor will upstage disease to stage II.
- During radical inguinal orchiectomy, take specific care not to incorporate peritoneal contents in the ligation of the cord.
- Yolk sac tumors will stain for PAS and AFP and classically have Schiller-Duval bodies on pathologic analysis.
- Teratomas are typically benign in children.
- In prepubertal children, RPLND is reserved or patients with persistent retroperitoneal mass or elevated AFP after definitive management of orchiectomy and chemotherapy.
- Disorders of sexual development increase the risk of testicular cancer in situations with hypovirilization and cryptorchidism.
- Orchiopexy reduces the risk of GCT in the involved testis but does not return the risk to baseline.

REFERENCES

1. Agarwal PK, Palmer JS. Testicular and paratesticular neoplasms in prepubertal males. *J Urol*. 2006;176(3):875-881.
2. De Backer A, Madern GC, Pieters R, et al. Influence of tumor site and histology on long-term survival in 193 children with extracranial germ cell tumors. *Eur J Pediatr Surg*. 2008;18(1):1-6.
3. Grady RW, Ross JH, Kay R. Epidemiological features of testicular teratoma in a prepubertal population. *J Urol*. 1997;158(3 pt 2):1191-1192.
4. Raney RB, Anderson JR, Barr FG, et al. Rhabdomyosarcoma and undifferentiated sarcoma in the first two decades of life: a selective review of intergroup rhabdomyosarcoma study group experience and rationale for Intergroup Rhabdomyosarcoma Study V. *J Pediatr Hematol Oncol*. 2001;23(4):215-220.
5. Wood HM, Elder JS. Cryptorchidism and testicular cancer: separating fact from fiction. *J Urol*. 2009;181(2):452-461.
6. Metcalfe PD, Farivar-Mohseni H, Farhat W, McLorie G, Khoury A, Bagli DJ. Pediatric testicular tumors: contemporary incidence and efficacy of testicular preserving surgery. *J Urol*. 2003;170(6 pt 1):2412-2415; discussion 5-6.
7. Ross JH. Prepubertal testicular tumors. *Urology*. 2009;74(1):94-99.
8. Shah RU, Lawrence C, Fickenscher KA, Shao L, Lowe LH. Imaging of pediatric pelvic neoplasms. *Radiol Clin North Am*. 2011;49(4):729-748, vi.
9. Cortez JC, Kaplan GW. Gonadal stromal tumors, gonadoblastomas, epidermoid cysts, and secondary tumors of the testis in children. *Urol Clin North Am*. 1993;20(1):15-26.
10. Ahmed HU, Arya M, Muneer A, Mushtaq I, Sebire NJ. Testicular and paratesticular tumours in the prepubertal population. *Lancet Oncol*. 2010;11(5):476-483.
11. Wu HY, Snyder III HM. Pediatric urologic oncology: bladder, prostate, testis. *Urol Clin North Am*. 2004;31(3):619-627, xi.

Chapter 55

Ovarian Tumors in Children

Ann M. Polcari

RELEVANT ANATOMY

- The ovary is a female reproductive organ suspended within the pelvis.
- It is kept in close proximity to the uterus and fallopian tubes by several ligaments (Figure 55.1A):
  - Directly connected to the uterus via the ovarian ligament.
  - Directly connected to the pelvic wall via the suspensory, or infundibulopelvic, ligament.
  - Covered by the broad ligament, a wide, fibrous tissue connecting and covering the uterus, fallopian tubes, and ovaries. It is divided into 3 continuous parts: the mesometrium, mesosalpinx, and mesovarium.
- The ovary has dual blood supply: from the uterine arteries, found within the broad ligament, and from the ovarian artery, found in the suspensory ligament (Figure 55.1B).
  - The uterine artery branches off of the internal iliac, whereas the ovarian artery branches directly off the descending aorta.
- Venous drainage parallels the arterial supply.
- The ureters pass just posterior to the uterine artery to reach the bladder. This is a potential site of ureteral damage during pelvic surgery.

EPIDEMIOLOGY AND ETIOLOGY

- Ovarian masses are the most common genital neoplasm in children.[1]

Etiology

- Most ovarian tumors in children and adolescents are germ cell tumors (GCTs), meaning they arise from the precursor cells of the ovum (Figure 55.2).[2]
  - Other, rarer tumors, are derived from the epithelial lining, stromal tissue (ie, hormone-producing cells), or a mixture of these tissue types (Figure 55.3).

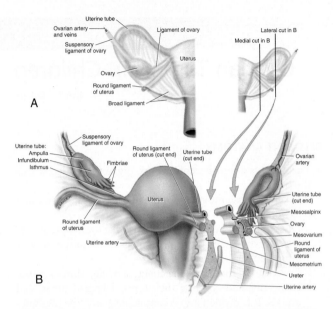

Figure 55.1 Uterus, uterine tubes, and broad ligament. Relationship of the broad ligament to the ovary and its ligaments (A, anterior view). Sagittal sections showing the mesentery of the uterus (mesometrium), ovary (mesovarium), and uterine tube (mesosalpinx) (B, anterolateral view). (Reprinted with permission from Moore KL, Agur AMR, Dalley AF. *Essential Clinical Anatomy.* 5th ed. Philadelphia, PA: Wolters Kluwer Health; 2015.)

- Some are associated with syndromes, such as Peutz-Jeghers syndrome, Ollier disease, and Maffucci syndrome.[3]
  - Gonadoblastoma, a mixed germ cell-stromal tumor, is found in girls with Turner syndrome and those with gonadal dysgenesis.[2]

Incidence

- Benign and malignant ovarian lesions occur in 2.6 per 100 000 girls less than 15 years of age.[3]

Prevalence

- 1.2% of ovarian cancers are found in woman less than 19 years of age.
  - 15% of ovarian tumors in children are epithelial-derived. These are more common in adults.[3]

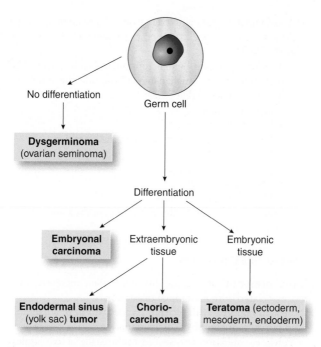

Figure 55.2 Classification of germ cell tumors of the ovary. (Reproduced from Strayer DS, Rubin E, eds. *Rubin's Pathology: Clinicopathologic Foundations of Medicine.* 7th ed. Philadelphia, PA: Wolters Kluwer; 2015.)

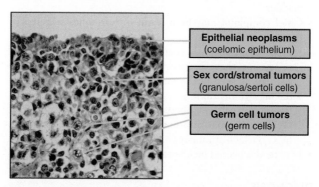

Figure 55.3 Fetal ovary at 18 weeks' gestation. Coelomic epithelium is responsible for epithelial malignancies. This layer is lost in testicular development, thus low frequency of epithelial tumors in testes. Gonadal stromal tumors arise in a specialized stromal layer. (Reprinted with permission from Pizzo PA, Poplack DG, Adamson PC, Blaney SM, Helman L. *Principles and Practice of Pediatric Oncology.* Philadelphia, PA: Wolters Kluwer; 2016.)

- Approximately 75% of ovarian tumors in women up to age 20 years are germ cell tumors; in premenarchal girls, 90% are GCTs.[2]
  - 95% of GCTs are benign teratomas (Table 55.1). The remaining 5% are malignant and include the following major subtypes (Table 55.2):
    - Dysgerminomas
    - Immature teratomas
    - Mature teratomas with somatic malignances
    - Yolk sac tumors
    - Embryonal carcinomas
    - Choriocarcinomas
    - Mixed germ cell tumors
  - Metastatic disease to the ovaries in children and adolescents is very rare.

CLINICAL PRESENTATION

Classic presentation: Abdominal pain then increases over time, associated with abdominal distension.

- **>50% of children with ovarian tumors will have a palpable abdominal mass on physical examination.[3]**
  - Pelvic examination is reserved for sexually active adolescents only.
- Other symptoms include anorexia, nausea or vomiting, and urinary frequency or urgency due to mass effect on the bladder.
- **Chief complaint may be a result of hormones secreted by the tumor:**
  - Precocious puberty is a common chief complaint in stromal cell tumors that secrete estrogen. Virilization is uncommon but can be seen in the rare Sertoli-Leydig or steroid-producing stromal tumors.[3]
  - Pseudoprecocious puberty may be a presenting sign of GCTs that produce β-human chorionic gonadotropin (β-hCG), which stimulates excess estrogen production.[3]
- May be discovered incidentally on imaging.

DIAGNOSIS

Laboratory Findings

- Laboratory tests are used largely to exclude malignancy once a mass is identified on physical examination or imaging.
- Significant laboratory findings differ by the tumor type (Tables 55.1 and 55.2).

TABLE 55.1	
Benign Pediatric Germ Cell Tumor: Mature Teratoma	
	Mature Teratoma (Also Called Dermoid Cyst)
Epidemiology	40%-50% of all ovarian tumors in childhood through adolescence. 95% of ovarian germ cell tumors. **Median age:** 10-15 y old **Rarely bilateral (<10%)**
Etiology and associations	Typically derived from all 3 germ cell layers, although all 3 germ layers do not have to be present within the tumor on pathology inspection.
Clinical presentation	• Pressure on adjacent organs with increasing abdominal pain and distension over time. • May be palpated in the abdomen of infants and children and pelvis of adolescents. • Acute abdominal pain, nausea, and vomiting are possible if the mass ruptures or causes ovarian torsion.
Imaging	• May see calcifications on X-ray. • Positive predictive value of ultrasound approaches 100% with a good technician.

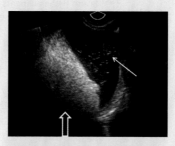

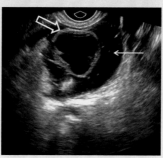

(continued)

TABLE 55.1 (CONTINUED)

Benign Pediatric Germ Cell Tumor: Mature Teratoma

	Mature Teratoma (Also Called Dermoid Cyst)
Pathology	**Gross:**

- Heterogeneous: solid and cystic features.
- May be able to visualize bony structures (eg, teeth), hair, and cartilage.
- Pigmented tissue may be present.

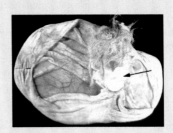

Microscopic:

- Mature tissue elements from all 3 embryonic layers (endoderm, mesoderm, and ectoderm)—most frequent being ectodermal tissue (eg, skin and hair).
- No cytologic atypia.

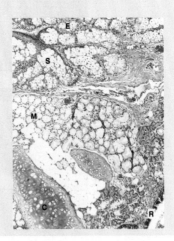

TABLE 55.1 (CONTINUED)
Benign Pediatric Germ Cell Tumor: Mature Teratoma

	Mature Teratoma (Also Called Dermoid Cyst)
Treatment	Surgical resection alone: conservative with cystectomy if possible, oophorectomy may be necessary for large masses.

Data from Sebire N, Malone M, Ashworth M, Jacques T. *Diagnostic Pediatric Surgical Pathology.* Churchill Livingstone; 2009; Orkin SH, Nathan DG, Ginsburg D, Look AT, Fisher DE, Lux S. *Nathan and Oski's Hematology and Oncology of Infancy and Childhood.* 8th ed. Saunders; 2015; Lanzkowsky P, Lipton J, Fish J, eds. *Lanzkowsky's Manual of Pediatric Hematology and Oncology.* 6th ed. Academic Press; 2016; and Coran AG, Adzick NS, Krummel TM, eds, et al. *Pediatric Surgery.* 7th ed. Saunders; 2012. Images reprinted with permission from Daffner RH, Hartman MS. *Clinical Radiology: The Essentials.* 4th ed. Philadelphia, PA: Wolters Kluwer Health/Lippincott Williams & Wilkins; 2014; and Rubin E, Reisner HM. *Essentials of Rubin's Pathology.* 6th ed. Philadelphia, PA: Wolters Kluwer Health/Lippincott Williams & Wilkins; 2014.

- α-Fetal protein (AFP) and β-hCG should be ordered, particularly if there is suspicion of a GCT.
  - AFP is produced by the fetal yolk sac during embryonic development and is therefore secreted by yolk sac tumors. Note that its use is limited in the first month of life, as levels are naturally high in newborns.[3]
  - β-hCG is produced by syncytiotrophoblasts during early embryonic development. If measured greater than 100 ng/mL, one should be concerned about a dysgerminoma, embryonic carcinoma, or choriocarcinoma.[3]
- Lactate dehydrogenase (LDH) may correlate with disease activity because it indicates increased cell turnover.[4]
- CA-125 is the tumor marker most commonly elevated with epithelial ovarian tumors, more common in adults. It can, however, be elevated in pediatric GCTs.[3]
- If signs of precocious puberty are present, the following hormone levels should be assessed: estradiol, inhibin, follicle-stimulating hormone (FSH), luteinizing hormone (LSH), and thyroid-stimulating hormone (TSH). This is rarely required in the pediatric population.[3]

Imaging Findings

- The initial modality of choice is ultrasound (Figure 55.4A).
  - A hypoechoic ovarian mass with defined borders is indicative of a benign lesion.

TABLE 55.2

Malignant Pediatric Germ Cell Tumors

	Dysgerminoma	Yolk Sac Tumor (or Endodermal Sinus Tumor)	Immature Teratoma	Embryonal Carcinoma	Choriocarcinoma
Epidemiology	Most common malignant ovarian GCT in the pediatric population (26%-31%). Median age: 16 y old.	Second most common malignant GCT in children. Median age: 18 y old.	Less than 5% of ovarian teratomas are malignant (ie, immature). Median age: 10-15 y old.	4% of all malignant ovarian tumors. Median age: 14 y old.	Very rare in children. Mean age: 13.9 y old.
Etiology and associations	• Called a "seminoma" when it occurs in the testes. • Can be associated with precocious puberty.	• Often found within immature teratomas.	• May be found within a mature-appearing teratoma. • May be associated with gliomatosis peritonei (ie, glial tissue implants on the peritoneum) that requires biopsy.	• Often found in association with other GCTs, as opposed to being a solitary lesion.	• Typically found in a mixed tumor, eg, within a teratoma.

Clinical presentation	• Rapid development of a large abdominal mass; painless until very large. • Size often leads to GI (constipation) or urinary (urgency) symptoms. • Most patients present in stage I (75%). If advanced, found in regional lymphs nodes.	• Less than 1 mo of increased abdominal girth and pelvic pressure. • Often involves peritoneal surfaces, leading to abdominal pain. • Often late-stage disease at diagnosis with lymphatic spread to liver, lungs, lymph nodes, and other peritoneal structures.	• Chronically increasing abdominal pain and distension.	• Abdominal pain and distension, as tumor size increases. • With hormonal activity, may also lead to pseudoprecocious puberty.	• Abdominal pain. • Anemia and/or bleeding symptoms due to hormonal activity. • Hormonal activity may also lead to pseudoprecocious puberty. • Often presents in late stages with distant metastases.

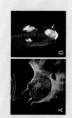

(continued)

TABLE 55.2 (CONTINUED)

Malignant Pediatric Germ Cell Tumors

	Dysgerminoma	Yolk Sac Tumor (or Endodermal Sinus Tumor)	Immature Teratoma	Embryonal Carcinoma	Choriocarcinoma
Laboratory findings	Elevated LDH, other markers negative.	Elevated AFP.	—	May have elevated β-hCG.	Elevated β-hCG.
Pathology	Gross: • Round, nodular—separated into lobules by fibrous bands. • Yellowish.	Gross: • Cystic, with regions of hemorrhage and necrosis. • Yellow • Soft and friable.	Gross: • Heterogeneous: solid and cystic features.	Gross: • Extensive areas of hemorrhage and necrosis.	Gross: • Large, nodular. • Purple, with dark brown areas due to hemorrhage. • Vascular invasion common. Microscopic: • Cytotrophoblastic and syncytiotrophoblastic tissue mixed in random fashion.

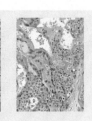

Microscopic:

- Large, epitheliallike cells that may form glandlike structures.
- May have syncytiotrophoblastic cells that secrete β-hCG.
- Many areas of hemorrhage.

Microscopic:

- Immature components of embryonic germ layers present in the form of neuroepithelial rosettes and tubules.
- Graded based on quantity of immature neuroepithelial tissue present:
  <10% = grade I,
  >50% = grade III.

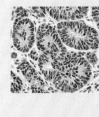

Microscopic:

- Loose myxoid stroma.
- 20% have Schiller-Duval bodies around a central vessel.
- Histologic subtypes: primarily yolk sac/allantois vs lung/liver derivatives.
- 70%-100% will stain positive for AFP.

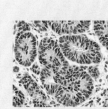

Microscopic:

- Enlarged, uniform cells with big central nuclei and prominent nucleolus.
- Clear cytoplasm.
- May have lymphocytic infiltrate.
- Distinguished from other germinomas by positive Oct4 stain.

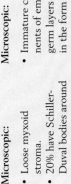

(*continued*)

TABLE 55.2 (CONTINUED)

Malignant Pediatric Germ Cell Tumors

	Dysgerminoma	Yolk Sac Tumor (or Endodermal Sinus Tumor)	Immature Teratoma	Embryonal Carcinoma	Choriocarcinoma
Treatment	• If stage I, unilateral, <10 cm, no evidence of mets or ascites, and 46XX = conservative surgery with unilateral salpingo-oophorectomy and wedge biopsy of the contralateral ovary (95% 5-year survival). • If > stage I, requires combination chemotherapy and surgery. Radiation therapy can be used if unresponsive to chemotherapy.	• If stage I, unilateral salpingo-oophorectomy, with subsequent observation. • If > stage I, tumor debulking with omentectomy, retroperitoneal lymph node sampling, biopsy of uninvolved ovary—or bilateral oophorectomy. Peritoneal washings in all cases.	• Surgical resection: curative for stage I in children. • Chemotherapy typically does not work for these tumors. However, if components of other malignant tumors are present, or a patient relapses, a multimodal approach may be necessary.	• Same as yolk sac tumor.	• If localized (rare), unilateral salpingo-oophorectomy. • Typically, extensive surgery is required with possible hysterectomy, bilateral salpingo-oophorectomy, and metastatic resection. • Platinum-based adjuvant chemotherapy for metastatic disease (82% survival with vs 28% without chemotherapy).

- Requires aggressive platinum-based adjuvant chemotherapy.
- If initially unresectable, 4 cycles neoadjuvant chemotherapy plus "second-look" surgery.

β-hCG, β-human chorionic gonadotropin; AFP, α-fetal protein; GCT, germ cell tumor; GI, gastrointestinal; LDH, lactate dehydrogenase.

Data from Sebire N, Malone M, Ashworth M, Jacques T. *Diagnostic Pediatric Surgical Pathology.* Churchill Livingstone; 2009; Orkin SH, Nathan DG, Ginsburg D, Look AT, Fisher DE, Lux S. *Nathan and Oski's Hematology and Oncology of Infancy and Childhood.* 8th ed. Saunders; 2015; Lanzkowsky P, Lipton J, Fish J, eds. *Lanzkowsky's Manual of Pediatric Hematology and Oncology.* 6th ed. Academic Press; 2016; and Coran AG, Adzick NS, Krummel TM, eds. et al. *Pediatric Surgery.* 7th ed. Saunders; 2012. Images reprinted courtesy of Jonathan R. Dillman, MD, MSc, Cincinnati Children's Hospital Medical Center, Cincinnati, OH; and with permission from Amin MB. *Urological Pathology.* Philadelphia, PA: Lippincott Williams & Wilkins; 2014; Lee EY. *Pediatric Radiology: Practical Imaging Evaluation of Infants and Children.* Wolters Kluwer, PA; 2018; and Strayer DS, Rubin E, eds. *Rubin's Pathology: Clinicopathologic Foundations of Medicine.* 7th ed. Philadelphia, PA: Wolters Kluwer; 2015.

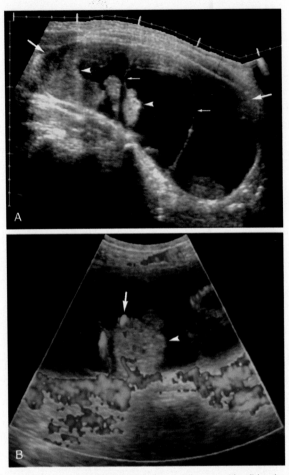

Figure 55.4 Ovarian malignant mixed germ cell tumor with solid and cystic components. A, Extended field-of-view image of ovarian cystic mass (large arrows) containing solid areas (arrowheads) and septations (small arrows). B, Power Doppler image demonstrating flow (arrow) in a solid nodule (arrowhead) within the tumor. (Reprinted with permission from Doubilet PM, Benson CB. *Atlas of Ultrasound in Obstetrics and Gynecology: A Multimedia Reference.* 2nd ed. Philadelphia, PA: Lippincott Williams & Wilkins; 2012.)

- Irregular borders are indicative of a malignant lesion, in addition to increased color flow on Doppler imaging, as malignant masses tend to be more vascular (Figure 55.4B).
- Ultrasound can also assess for pelvic fluid or ascites.[3]

- Follow-up imaging with CT of the abdomen and pelvis, or MRI, can be useful to further define the lesion and allow for staging of malignant disease.
- If a malignant tumor is identified, staging should be performed with at least one of the following[4]:
  - AP and lateral chest X-rays.
  - Chest CT.
  - Bone scan (if known or suspected late-stage disease).
- Staging of ovarian germ cell tumors in children as described by the Children's Oncology Group is as follows[3]:
  - Stage I—limited to the ovary.
  - Stage II—microscopic residual disease, no peritoneal disease identified.
  - Stage III—lymph node involvement, contiguous visceral involvement, or peritoneal disease identified.
  - Stage IV—distant metastasis.

SURGICAL MANAGEMENT

- **Surgical resection is an essential component of the treatment plan.**
- Surgery is the treatment of choice for benign teratomas, immature teratomas, and low-stage malignant disease.[3,4]
  - Benign disease requires ovarian cystectomy or unilateral oophorectomy alone.
  - Malignant disease requires the following:
    - At least unilateral oophorectomy, with salpingo-oophorectomy if the fallopian tube is involved on gross inspection.
    - Inspection of contralateral ovary, with biopsy of suspicious lesions.
    - Biopsy of any suspicious peritoneal, omental, lymph node, or liver lesions. In conjunction with imaging, biopsy will assist in staging disease.
- Chemotherapy is appropriate for known-responsive lesions; neoadjuvant or adjuvant depending on the type of tumor (Table 55.2).
- **The primary goal of surgery is to treat while also preserving fertility.**

Operative Intervention

- The laparoscopic approach is preferred if a simple cystectomy (ie, removal of the tumor without oophorectomy) is required.

- The open approach is preferred for oophorectomy, salpingo-oophorectomy, and advanced-stage disease.
- Hysterectomy is not described here, as it is rarely required in the pediatric population and such radical resection is avoided as often as possible in the pediatric population to ensure future fertility.

Laparoscopic Approach

- The patient is placed supine in the Trendelenburg position.
- Three small incisions are made for laparoscopic instrument ports.
- Port placement varies by surgeon, but most often the camera goes through the umbilicus and the other 2 ports are placed near the anterior superior iliac spine, above the mons pubis, or somewhere in between these 2 sites.
- Once the camera is inserted, the peritoneal and pelvic cavities are inspected.
- If there are no signs of malignancy, the surgeon can proceed with peritoneal fluid sampling and subsequent cystectomy (ie, excision of the mass).
- Initially, the utero-ovarian ligament is grasped for stabilization and held by an assistant.
- Vasopressin is injected into the capsule of the ovary, just before making an incision into the capsule with either electrocautery or a knife.
- With the capsule open, dissection around the mass is completed with blunt instruments.
- When the base of the tumor is visible, it is clamped, coagulated, and excised.
- The tumor should be removed **intact** within a retrieval bag, avoiding spillage, and sent for pathology review.
- The ovary should be reconstructed and the remaining cortical edges are reapproximated with absorbable suture to ensure proper future ovulation (ovum formation and release).[6,7]
- A biopsy of the contralateral ovary is taken if indicated.[5,6]
  - If a malignancy, such as a germ cell tumor, is suspected, the surgeon should proceed with oophorectomy and possible salpingo-oophorectomy through an open approach.[6]

Open Approach

- The patient is placed supine, and a low-transverse abdominal incision is made.
- Pelvic and abdominal washings are obtained to evaluate for malignancy.

- The peritoneal and pelvic cavities are inspected.
- If a cystectomy alone is indicated, it is performed in similar fashion to the laparoscopic approach.
- If oophorectomy is required, resection begins with identification of the suspensory ligament and ureter, so that the peritoneum can be divided parallel to the ovarian artery and vein.
- The round ligament can be divided if necessary for access.
- Blunt dissection is used to open the broad ligament.
- Branches of the ovarian artery should be ligated inferior and lateral to the fallopian tube, allowing for separation of the ovary and fallopian tube.
  - The ovarian artery can then be clearly visualized and ligated. The utero-ovarian ligament is also excised, and the specimen can be removed.
- If salpingo-oophorectomy is required, the same procedure is followed until the point of excision.
  - In this instance, both the utero-ovarian ligament and base of the fallopian tube are ligated, excised, and removed (Figure 55.5).[1]

Complications

- Intraoperative complications include hemorrhage and damage to the ureter, as it passes under the uterine artery.
- As in most surgeries, postoperative complications include continued bleeding or infection and adhesions to the pelvic or abdominal wall.
- Specific to malignant lesions, there is a risk of "spillage"—meaning malignant cells are shed from the specimen and left to seed the abdominal cavity. For this reason, surgeons are careful in resecting the specimen in a bag during laparoscopic procedures, and adjuvant chemotherapy is often used for malignant disease.
- There is a risk of infertility with a unilateral oophorectomy; however, results vary with pregnancy rates ranging from 42% to 88%.[1]

POSTOPERATIVE CARE

- Special postoperative care is as follows[3]
  - If an AFP-producing tumor was excised, an AFP level should be drawn 1-week after surgery to determine response to treatment. As the half-life of AFP is 5 to 7 days, it should return to normal levels. AFP can also be checked if symptoms return, as they may indicate recurrence.

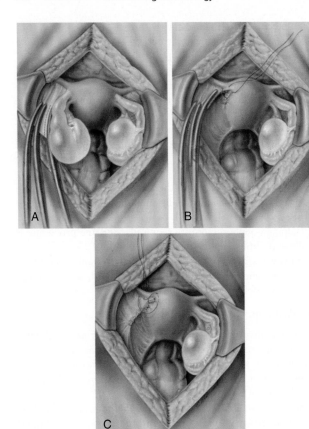

Figure 55.5 Salpingo-oophorectomy. A, The infundibulopelvic ligament is doubly clamped. Another clamp is placed to control back bleeding. Dotted line indicates incision. B, A suture has been placed to ligate the ascending uterine vessels just below the cornual incision. The cornual incision is closed with a figure-of-eight suture of 2-0 delayed absorbable material. C, The infundibulopelvic ligament and the rest of the broad ligament vessels have been ligated. The cornual wound is covered with the round and the broad ligament using a mattress suture of 2-0 delayed absorbable material. (Reprinted with permission from Jones HW, Rock JA. *Te Lindes Operative Gynecology.* 11th ed. Philadelphia, PA: Wolters Kluwer Health; 2015.)

- If a β-hCG-producing tumor was excised, levels should be drawn 1 to 2 days after surgery to determine response to treatment. The half-life of β-hCG is only 20 to 30 hours. β-hCG can also be checked if symptoms return, as they may indicate recurrence.

> ### PEARLS AND PITFALLS
>
> - The most common ovarian tumors in the pediatric population are the GCTs.
> - The single most common germ cell tumor is the benign mature teratoma.
> - No single laboratory value can diagnose ovarian tumors in children, but AFP and β-hCG can give clues to the type of tumor present.
> - Surgical resection plays a role in treatment of all ovarian neoplasms in children, with the goal of preserving fertility.

REFERENCES

1. Valea FA, Mann WJ. Oophorectomy and ovarian cystectomy. *UpToDate*. 2017 [cited October 8, 2018]. Available from https://www.uptodate-com.access.library.miami.edu/contents/oophorectomy-and-ovarian-cystectomy?source=related_link#H15.
2. Frazier AL, Amatruda JF. Pediatric germ cell tumors. In: Orkin SH, Fisher DE, Look AT, et al, eds. *Oncology of Infancy and Childhood*. Philadelphia: Saunders Elsevier; 2009:911-961.
3. Von Allmen D, Fallat ME. Ovarian tumors. In: Coran AG, ed. *Pediatric Surgery*. 7th ed. Philadelphia: Saunders Elsevier; 2012:529-548.
4. Rapkin LB, Olson TA. Germ cell tumors. In: Lanzkowsky P, Lipton JM, Fish JD, eds. *Lanzkowsky's Manual of Pediatric Hematology and Oncology*. 6th ed. San Diego: Elsevier; 2016:555-568.
5. Falcone T, Walters MD. Laparoscopic adnexal surgery. In: Baggish MS, Karram MM, eds. *Atlas of Pelvic and Gynecologic Surgery*. 4th ed. Philadelphia: Saunders Elsevier; 2016:1255-1262.
6. Brandt ML. Laparoscopic ovarian surgery. In: Holcomb GW, Georgeson KE, Rothenberg SS, eds. *Atlas of Pediatric Laparoscopic and Thoracoscopy*. Philadelphia: Saunders Elsevier; 2008:149-155.
7. Sebire NJ, Ashworth M, Malone M, Jacques TS, Rogers BB. Breast and female genital tract pathology. In: Sebire NJ, Ashworth M, Malone M, Jacques TS, Rogers BB, eds. *Diagnostic Pediatric Surgical Pathology*. 1st ed. San Diego: Elsevier; 2010:151-161.

Chapter 56

Pediatric Orthopedic Tumors

Blaze D. Emerson, and Bijan J. Ameri

- The most common malignant bone tumor is osteosarcoma (OS) and the Ewing sarcoma family of tumors (ESFT), which account for 90% to 94% of malignant bone tumors.[1,2]
- OSs are the most common primary bone tumor in children with 56% of cases.
- It is estimated that 3% of all childhood cancers are OSs, whereas ESFTs are responsible for 34% to 36% of childhood bone cancers.[2]
- Eight types of benign bone tumors have been described: osteoma, osteoid osteoma, osteoblastoma, giant cell tumor, aneurysmal bone cyst, fibrous dysplasia, and enchondroma.
- These tumors may be further divided based on the matrix or substance they produce as bone-forming, cartilage-forming, fibrous, and vascular.[3]
- Benign tumors may be static and require no further workup; others may be locally aggressive and require constant supervision and/or treatment.
- In most cases, the age of the child, location of lesion, and radiographic appearance are helpful in determining the underlying pathology.[4]

EPIDEMIOLOGY AND ETIOLOGY

- According to the Surveillance Epidemiology, and End Results (SEER) Cancer Statistics Review of the National Cancer Institute program, 3260 new cases of bone and joint cancer will occur in the United States in 2017.
- This accounts for approximately 0.2% of all cancers.
- Individuals younger than 20 years will account for 26.4% of these cases.
- Furthermore, 1550 cancer deaths or 0.3% of all cancer deaths in 2017 will be caused by cancers of the bone or joint.
- Overall, the 5-year relative survival is 67.7%.[5]

- Primary bone tumors are relatively uncommon, although malignancy of the bone or joints is the third leading cause of cancer deaths in individuals younger than 20 years.[25]
- It is estimated that 3% to 6% of childhood cancer is attributable to malignant bone tumors.[1]
- The incidence of benign bone tumors is higher than malignant lesions; however, benign tumors are difficult to estimate, as most are found incidentally and patients tend to be asymptomatic.[6]

CLINICAL PRESENTATION

History

- Several items in the patient's history may help guide you toward the diagnosis of a bone tumor.
- Variables such as pain, age of patient, location of lesion, and associated symptoms may be useful.

Pain

- Benign lesions are most often asymptomatic, but patients may present with localized pain, swelling, deformity, or a pathologic fracture.
- Aggressive benign bone tumors may cause mild/dull pain that is slowly progressive and worse at night.[7]
- Malignant lesions more commonly present with localized pain of several month's duration that is rapidly progressive.

Age

- Benign bone tumors tend to present during the second decade of life, except for ossifying fibromas, which appear during the first 5 years.
- OSs peak between 13 and 16 years and seem to be associated with the adolescent growth spurt.[8]

Physical Examination

- During examination, it is important to assess bone tenderness, swelling, deformity, joint range of motion, neurologic function, and vascular function.
- Osteochondromas, OSs, ESFT, and periosteal chondromas may sometimes be palpated. Aggressive tumors may compromise neurovascular function.
- Overlying erythema or warmth may indicate an underlying infection, which can confuse clinicians.

DIAGNOSIS

Plain Radiographs

- The best initial modality for suspected primary bone lesions is a plain radiograph.[4]
- It is important to be familiar with the radiographic findings of benign lesions, as 80% to 90% of cases of benign bone tumors may be identified with plain radiographs alone.[7]

Radiographic Characteristics of Benign Lesions (Figure 56.1)[4]

- Well-defined/sclerotic border
- Sharp transitions
- Small size
- Lack of extension into surrounding tissues

Characteristics of Aggressive Lesions (Figure 56.2)[4]

- Poor definition
- Cortical destruction "moth-eaten"

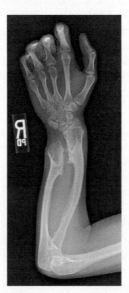

Figure 56.1 In a skeletally mature patient, a radial osteotomy is performed after exostoses excision and ulnar-tether release. (Reprinted with permission from Flynn JM, Wiesel SW. *Operative Techniques in Pediatric Orthopaedics.* Philadelphia, PA: Lippincott Williams & Wilkins, a Wolters Kluwer Business; 2011.)

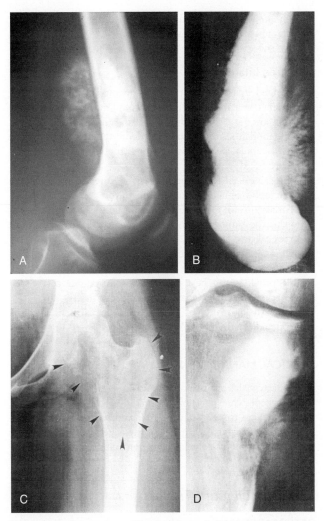

Figure 56.2 Osteosarcoma of the distal femur. A, Plain radiograph of a classic osteosarcoma. Marked sclerosis is present within the intramedullary canal, which represents new bone formation (malignant osteoid formation), in addition to a large posterior extraosseous component that shows osteoid formation. This is the typical appearance of a distal femoral osteosarcoma before treatment. New bone formation within the extraosseous tumor is highly suggestive of an osteosarcoma. The distal femur is the most common site of primary osteosarcoma. B-D, Plain radiographs demonstrate the classic variants of osteosarcoma. C, Arrowheads delineate the approximate margins of the tumor. (Reprinted with permission from DeVita VT, Lawrence TS, Rosenberg SA, eds. *DeVita, Hellman, and Rosenberg's Cancer: Principles and Practice of Oncology.* 9th ed. Lippincott Williams & Wilkins, a Wolters Kluwer business; 2011.)

- Spiculated or interrupted periosteal reaction
- Extension into the soft tissue
- Large size

Advanced Imaging

- Advanced imaging (computed tomography [CT], magnetic resonance imaging [MRI], scintigraphy) may be needed if the lesions are not clearly benign on plain radiographs.
- These modalities may also be needed if the tumors are on the spine, scapula, pelvis, and ribs or if metastasis is suspected (Figure 56.3).[7]
- CT is beneficial for detecting lesions in locations that plain radiographs cannot adequately illustrate.
- CT is also useful for more accurately demonstrating the location of the tumor within the bone and changes within the cortex (Figure 56.4).[4]
- MRI is the most sensitive modality for evaluation of medullary changes and defining the extent of the lesion.
- MRI provides the best contrast resolution for soft tissue masses and tumor extension into adjacent tissues.
- MRI is the modality of choice when a malignant lesion is suspected (Figure 56.5).[4]

SURGICAL MANAGEMENT

- Children with bone tumors should be referred to an orthopedic surgeon who specializes in these lesions.
- Most benign tumors may be followed with serial examinations and imaging; however, locally aggressive or malignant lesions may need surgical resection with possible adjuvant therapy.

Specific Malignant Tumors

OSTEOSARCOMA

- Primary OS is the most common bony malignancy of children accounting for 56% of cases of malignant bone lesions.[2]
- OS has a worldwide annual incidence rate of 1 to 3 per cases per million and when adjusted for age 4.4 per million cases per year.[9]
- OSs are malignant tumors characterized by the overproduction of osteoid (immature bone).

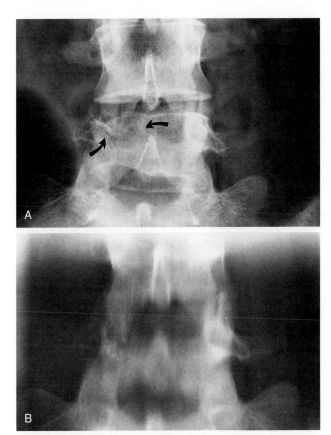

Figure 56.3 Ewing sarcoma: L5. A, AP lumbar spine. B, Tomogram, L5. Observe the lytic destruction of the pedicle of L5 and a portion of the vertebral body (arrows) in this 15-year-old patient. Comment: Ewing sarcoma of the spine is uncommon, occurring in 7% of lesions. When present, the sacrum and lumbar spine are the most common sites. (Reprinted with permission from Yochum TR, Rowe LJ, eds. *Yochum And Rowe's Essentials of Skeletal Radiology.* 3rd ed. Philadelphia, PA: Lippincott Williams & Wilkins; 2004.)

- The tumor is frequently found in the metaphysis of long bones; in decreasing frequency, the femur (75% of cases), proximal tibia, and proximal humerus are the most common locations.[2]
- Most patients have no underlying pathogenesis; however, genetic disposition and exposure to ionizing radiation or chemotherapy are risk factors that have been implicated in the formation of OS.

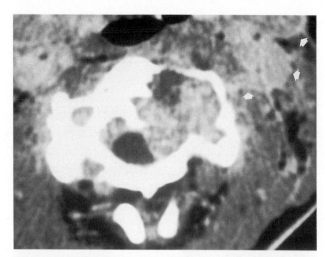

Figure 56.4 Ewing sarcoma in an 18-year-old woman. Axial soft tissue–windowed CT scan showing the tumoral mass arising from the left aspect of the C3 vertebral body and expanding both in the canal and in the prevertebral soft tissues (arrows). Ewing sarcoma was subsequently diagnosed on open biopsy. The patient was submitted to radiation therapy and polychemotherapy. (Reprinted with permission from Benzel EC, Connolly PJ, DiAngelo DJ, et al, eds. *Cervical Spine.* 5th ed. Philadelphia, PA: Lippincott Williams & Wilkins, a Wolters Kluwer business; 2012.)

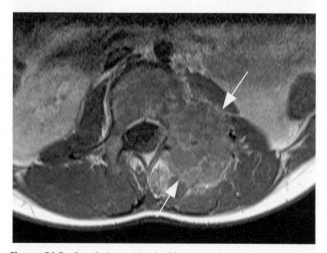

Figure 56.5 Osteolysis associated with metastatic Ewing sarcoma. Axial postcontrast T1-weighted MR image of spine shows a large mass (white arrows) centered in left aspect of L3, consistent with metastatic disease. (Reprinted with permission from Iyer R, Chapman T. *Pediatric Imaging: The Essentials.* Philadelphia, PA: Wolters Kluwer; 2016.)

- Secondary OS due to prior chemotherapy or radiation therapy has been postulated to cause up to 3% of new cases.[10]
- The 2 most common genetic predisposition syndromes related to OS are Li-Fraumeni syndrome and retinoblastoma.
- OS predominately affects young adults and adolescents, appearing to correlate with the pubertal growth spurt.
- Cases of older patients with OS are generally related to prior radiation/chemotherapy exposure or Paget disease.
- A genetic predisposition should be assumed when a child younger than 5 years presents with OS.[1]

Clinical Presentation

- Patients may present after an injury and typically complain of chronic localized pain that waxes and wanes over time.
- Systemic symptoms are generally absent.
- Often, a soft tissue mass is appreciated.
- Laboratory evaluation may demonstrate elevations in alkaline phosphatase, ESR, and LDH.
- At the time of presentation, 10% to 20% of patients have metastatic disease, primarily the lungs; however, micrometastasis is presumed in all patients (Figure 56.6).[11]

Imaging

- Plain radiographs are the initial imaging modality and demonstrate the characteristic "sunburst pattern," which is indicative of new bone formation and extension into nearby tissues (Figure 56.7).
- The cortex may expand lifting the periosteum and forming what is known as a "Codman triangle" (Figure 56.7).
- With rapidly growing tumors, the periosteum cannot produce new bone as fast as the growing lesion, resulting in a pattern of 1 or more concentric shells of new bone over the lesion.
- This pattern is sometimes called lamellated or "onion-skin" periosteal reaction (Figure 56.7).
- OSs may infiltrate neurovascular bundles, nearby soft tissues, and form skip lesions.
- MRI is required to delineate the extent of the tumor and to help the surgeon plan for resection (Figure 56.8).
- A noncontrast CT of the lungs is the test of choice for demonstrating metastatic disease (Figure 56.9).
- Prognosis is directly related to the number and location of pulmonary nodules.[1]

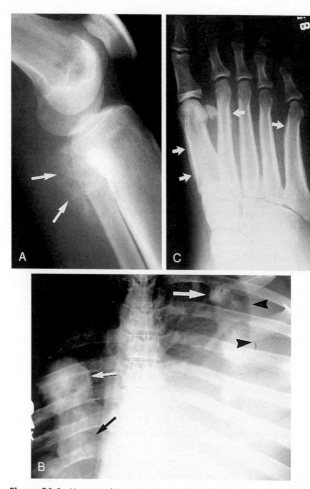

Figure 56.6 Hypertrophic osteoarthropathy developing from osteosarcoma of the tibia. A, Lateral knee. Note the destruction of the posterior surface of the tibia, with a soft tissue mass (arrows). This lesion represents osteosarcoma of the tibia. B, Chest. Observe multiple cannonball metastases in the right and left lungs (arrows). Massive pleural effusion is noted on the left side (arrowheads). C, Foot. (arrows) in the diaphyseal area of all 5 metatarsal bones. Comment: This patient demonstrates an interesting aspect of the pathologic manifestations of osteosarcoma of bone. Metastatic lesions in the lung created hypertrophic osteoarthropathy in the foot. This is somewhat unusual in osteosarcoma because most patients die before osteoarthropathy can develop. (Reprinted with permission from Yochum TR, Rowe LJ, eds. *Yochum And Rowe's Essentials of Skeletal Radiology.* 3rd ed. Philadelphia, PA: Lippincott Williams & Wilkins; 2004.)

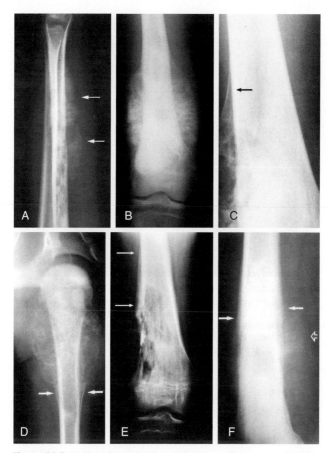

Figure 56.7 Periosteal reaction in osteosarcoma. Three types of periosteal reaction most commonly accompany osteosarcoma. A, The sunburst or perpendicular type of periosteal reaction (arrows) is seen here on the lateral radiograph of the forearm in an 18-year-old woman with tumor in the radius and (B) on the anteroposterior radiograph of the distal femur in a 20-year-old man. C, Codman triangle (arrow) may also be encountered, as seen here in a 15-year-old girl with tumor in the distal femur and (D) in an 11-year-old boy with tumor in the proximal humerus (arrows). E, The onion-skin or lamellated type of periosteal response (arrows) is apparent in a 16-year-old girl with tumor in the distal femur. F, Combination of lamellated (arrows) and sunburst (open arrow) periosteal reaction is present in a 16-year-old girl with osteosarcoma of the femur. (Reprinted with permission from Greenspan A. *Orthopedic Imaging.* 6th ed. Philadelphia, PA: Wolters Kluwer Health; 2014.)

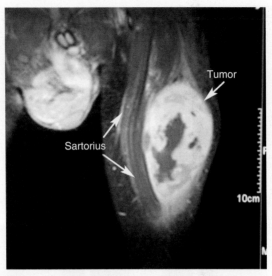

Figure 56.8 MRI of a large thigh high-grade (stage IIB) soft tissue sarcoma. The thigh is the most common site for extremity soft tissue sarcomas. MRI evaluation is the most useful study in determining the extent of soft tissue sarcomas. (Reprinted with permission from Wiesel SW, Parvizi J, Rothman RH, et al, eds. *Operative Techniques in Orthopaedic Surgery.* Vol 2. Philadelphia, PA: Lippincott Williams & Wilkins; 2011.)

Treatment

- Thirty years ago, survival has increased from 15% owing to the use of chemotherapy and improved surgical techniques.
- In the United States, treatment consists of 10 weeks of MAP therapy (methotrexate, doxorubicin, and cisplatin) followed by surgical resection.
- The prognosis for patients is good with 65% to 70% of patients surviving the disease.[1]

EWING SARCOMA FAMILY OF TUMORS

- Ewing sarcoma (EWS) of bone, extraskeletal EWS, peripheral primitive neuroectodermal tumors of bone and soft tissue (PNET), and Askin tumors are malignant tumors that are recognized as the ESFT.[1]
- ESFTs have an incidence of 2.5 to 3 cases per million per year and accounts for 2.9% of all childhood cancers.[2,9]
- ESFTs primarily affect adolescents and young adults with few cases being reported in infants.[3]

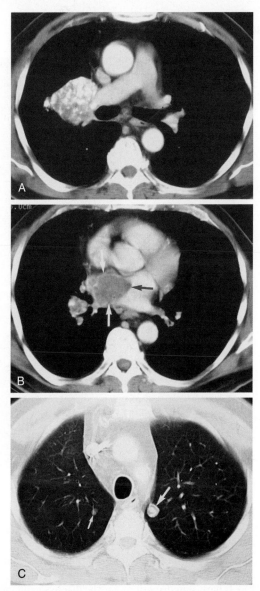

Figure 56.9 Metastatic osteosarcoma. A, CT scan shows coarse areas of calcification within the mass. B, CT at a level inferior to (A) shows that the tumor extends into the left atrium (arrows). C, CT with lung windowing shows a small pulmonary metastasis in the right upper lobe (small arrow) and a larger, densely calcified metastasis in the left upper lobe (large arrow). D, Magnetic resonance (MR) imaging, coronal view, shows that the tumor (large arrows) is growing through the right superior pulmonary vein into the left atrium (small arrows). E, MR axial view shows low-signal tumor (large arrows) invading the normal high-signal-intensity left atrium (LA). Note the high signal within left inferior pulmonary vein (small arrows). (Reprinted with permission from Collins J, Stern EJ, eds. *Chest Radiology: The Essentials*. 3rd ed. Philadelphia, PA: Wolters Kluwer Health; 2015.)

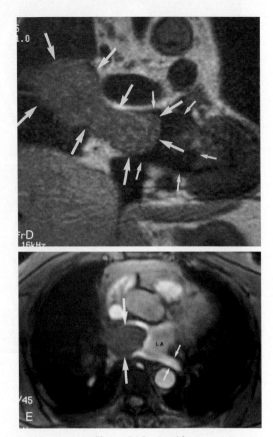

Figure 56.9—cont'd

- ESFTs are destructive lesions believed to originate from mesenchymal tissue and are related to specific genetic aberrations.
- The t(11; 22) (q24; q12) translocation is present in approximately 85% of cases.[1]
- ESFTs have a predisposition for the diaphysis and metaphysis of long bones, particularly the femur and tibia, followed by the pelvis, chest wall, and spine Table 56.1.[1]
- A unique feature of ESFTs is that 20% originate in soft tissue.[3]

Clinical Presentation

- Clinical presentation varies, but most patients note localized pain and symptoms associated with the site of the tumor, which is worse at night.

TABLE 56.1

Common Locations of Long Bone Tumors

	Epiphysis	Metaphysis	Diaphysis
Benign Tumors	Chondro-blastoma	Osteoblastoma	Enchondroma
	Giant Cell Tumor	Osteochondroma	Fibrous Dysplasia
		Non-ossifying Fibroma	
		Osteoid Osteoma	
		Chondromyxoid Fibroma	
		Giant Cell Tumor	
Malignant Tumors		Osteosarcoma	Ewing Sarcoma
		Juxtacortical Osteosarcoma	Chondro-sarcoma

- Patients may also have constitutional symptoms, such as fever, fatigue, and weight loss.[12]
- Laboratory abnormalities include elevated LDH and anemia. ESFTs are common in the axial skeleton; neurologic symptoms, such as sciatica, neuropathy, and bladder outlet obstruction, may be present.
- 80% of patients present with clinically localized disease; however, subclinical metastatic disease is assumed in all cases, especially to the lung.[13]
- Pathologic fractures occur in 10% to 15% of cases.[12]

Imaging

- Plain radiographs of the area demonstrate a poorly marginated destructive lesion accompanied by a soft tissue mass (Figure 56.10).
- The appearance on X-ray is described as "moth-eaten" due to the confluence of many fine destructive lesions (Figure 56.10).
- A "Codman triangle" is sometimes apparent (Figure 56.11).
- The characteristic "onion peel" may be evident and is formed by the deposition of new periosteum (Figure 56.11).
- CT is as accurate as MRI for detecting ESFTs; however, MRI is preferred, as it is better able to delineate tumor size, extra/intraosseous extension, and the tumor's relationship to surrounding anatomy (Figure 56.12).[14]

Treatment

- Currently, the 5-year overall survival for patients with localized disease at presentation is 85% and the 5-year event-free survival is 73%.[15]

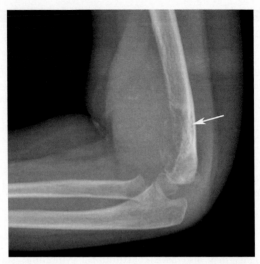

Figure 56.10 Ewing sarcoma in a 5-year-old male child. Lateral elbow radiograph demonstrates an aggressive lytic lesion in the distal humerus (arrow) with cortical breach and a soft tissue component anteriorly. (Reprinted with permission from Iyer R, Chapman T. *Pediatric Imaging: The Essentials.* Philadelphia, PA: Wolters Kluwer; 2016.)

- Complete surgical resection followed by chemotherapy is the treatment of choice.
- Radiation therapy is implemented if tumor free margins cannot be achieved.
- Chemotherapy consists of a 5-drug backbone of vincristine, doxorubicin, cyclophosphamide (VDC) alternating with ifosfamide and etoposide (IE).[1]

Specific Benign Tumors

OSTEOCHONDROMA

Pathophysiology

- Osteochondromas are bony outgrowths with a cartilaginous cap (Figure 56.13).
- These cartilaginous tumors comprise approximately 30% of benign bone tumors.[16]
- The tumor has a predilection for the metaphysis and diaphysis of long bones; the femur and then tibia are the most common locations.
- Osteochondromas are known to occur spontaneously, but radiation therapy is known to be a risk factor.

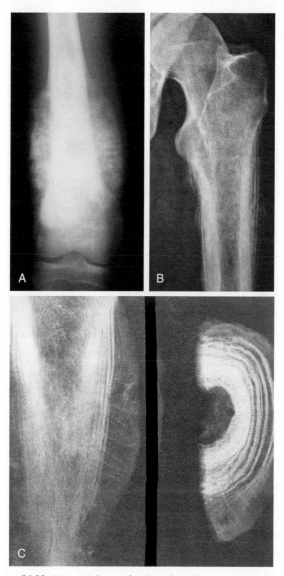

Figure 56.11 Interrupted type of periosteal reaction. A, Highly aggressive and malignant lesions may present radiographically with a sunburst pattern of periosteal reaction, as seen in this case of osteosarcoma. B, Another pattern of interrupted periosteal reaction is the lamellated or onion-skin type, as seen here in Ewing sarcoma involving the proximal left femur. C, Radiograph of the slab sections (coronal at left and transverse at right) of the resected specimen from Ewing sarcoma demonstrates lamellated type in more detail. Codman triangle (arrows) also reflects an aggressive, usually malignant type of periosteal reaction, as seen here (D) in a patient with Ewing sarcoma and (E) in a patient with osteosarcoma. (A, B, D-F, Reprinted with permission from Greenspan A. *Orthopedic Imaging*. 6th ed. Philadelphia, PA: Wolters Kluwer Health; 2014. C, Reprinted with permission from Greenspan A, Remagen W. *Differential Diagnosis of Tumors and Tumor-like Lesions*. Philadelphia, PA: Lippincott-Raven Publishers; 1998.)

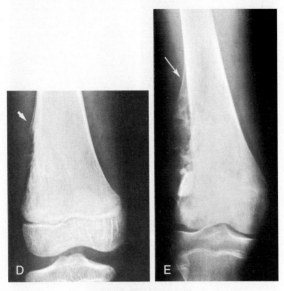

Figure 56.11—cont'd

Clinical Presentation

- OSs commonly present as a painless mass near a joint or as a painful mass associated with local trauma.
- They may cause pain, decreased range of motion, deformity, and pathologic fracture.

Imaging

- Radiographic features include a bony spur that arises from the surface of the cortex and usually points away from the joint (Figure 56.13).
- The cortex of the spur is continuous with the cortex of the underlying bone.
- If the cartilaginous cap is >2 cm in an adult, chondrosarcoma should be considered.[17]

Treatment

- Most osteochondromas may be observed and radiographed yearly.
- If the tumors cause irritation or deformity, they may be excised.
- If lesions increase in size after skeletal maturity, if they cause growth disturbance, or if cartilage cap is >2 cm, they should be removed.[7]

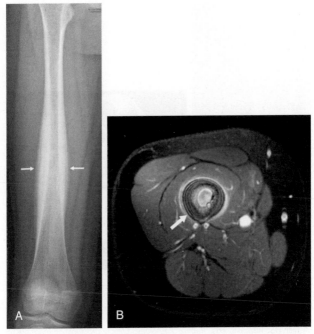

Figure 56.12 Multilamellar periosteal reaction (arrows) in a plain radiograph (A) and MRI axial T2-weighted image (B) of the femur of a young girl who presented with intermittent leg pain. Diagnostic considerations included Ewing sarcoma, osteomyelitis, osteosarcoma, and Langerhans cell histiocytosis. Open biopsy of the lesion revealed Ewing sarcoma. (Reprinted with permission from DeVita VT, Lawrence TS, Rosenberg SA, eds. *DeVita, Hellman, and Rosenberg's Cancer: Principles and Practice of Oncology.* 10th ed. Philadelphia, PA: Wolters Kluwer; 2015.)

GIANT CELL TUMORS

Pathophysiology

- Giant cell tumors (GCTs) are generally benign lytic lesions; however, their behavior may be erratic; GCTs can be locally aggressive and recur after curettage, and some tumors, 3%, metastasize to the lungs.[18]
- GCTs are the second most common cause of benign bone tumors accounting for 20% of these lesions.[16]
- Their peak incidence is between the ages of 20 and 40.[19] GCTs and chondroblastomas are unique in the fact that the most commonly effected areas are the epiphysis.
- Most lesions occur at the long bones with approximately 50% of cases being identified at the distal femur/proximal tibia.[16]

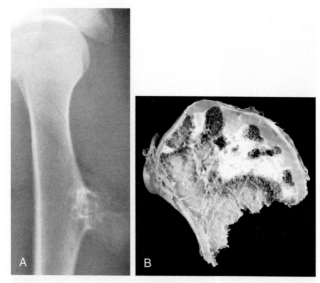

Figure 56.13 Osteochondroma. A, A radiograph of an osteochondroma of the humerus shows a lesion that is directly contiguous with the marrow space. B, The cross-section of an osteochondroma shows the cap of calcified cartilage overlying poorly organized cancellous bone. (Reprinted with permission from Strayer DS, Rubin E, eds. *Rubin's Pathology: Clinicopathologic Foundations of Medicine.* 7th ed. Philadelphia, PA: Wolters Kluwer; 2015.)

Clinical Presentation

- Patients with GCTs present with pain, swelling, and limited range of motion. 11% to 37% of patients may have a pathologic fracture.[16]

Imaging

- On plain X-rays, GCTs appear as lytic cystic lesions, due to intratumoral hemorrhage, near the epiphysis/metaphysis.
- Cortical thinning, bone destruction, and pathologic fractures are common (Figure 56.14).
- CT is useful for determining tumor margins, cortical changes, and periosteal reaction.

Treatment

- Previously the treatment of GCTs consisted of curettage followed by bone cement.

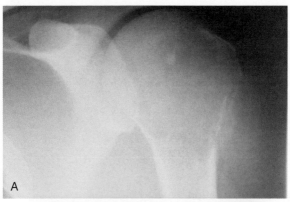

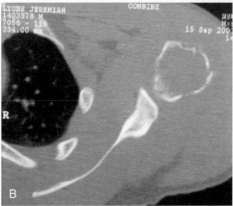

Figure 56.14 Giant cell tumor of the proximal humerus. A, Plain radiograph demonstrating a lytic lesion of the proximal humerus with poorly defined borders and with cortical destruction. There is no matrix formation. B, Computed tomography scan showing marked cortical thinning and destruction. Needle biopsy shows a giant cell tumor. Giant cell tumors of the proximal humerus are very rare and represent less than 1% to 2% of all giant cell tumors. (Reprinted with permission from Iannotti JP, Williams GR, Miniaci A, Zuckerman JD, eds. *Disorders of the Shoulder: Reconstruction.* 3rd ed. Philadelphia, PA: Lippincott Williams & Wilkins; 2014.)

- However, owing to reoccurrence and possible metastasis, adjuvants have been used. Zinc chloride, bisphosphonates, phenol, liquid nitrogen, and alcohol have been used in addition to curettage to prevent local reoccurrence.
- Denosumab, a monoclonal antibody, has been used, as it inhibits GCT's osteoclastic abilities.[19]

OSTEOBLASTOMA

Pathophysiology

- Osteoblastoma is a benign bone-forming tumor that most commonly affects people in the second decade of life.
- It is the third most common benign bone tumor comprising 14% of cases.[20]
- Osteoblastomas prefer the axial skeleton with one-third of cases involving the spine.[21]
- Osteoblastomas tend to stay confined to the bone, do not penetrate the cortex, and have a relatively low instance of reoccurrence.

Clinical Presentation

- Patients typically present with chronic pain, which is not responsive to nonsteroidal anti-inflammatory drugs (NSAIDs). Children with spinal lesions may present with limp or neurologic impairments if a tumor impinges upon a nerve root.

Imaging

- CT is the study of choice, as most tumors are located on the axial skeleton.
- Imaging characteristics are variable, but osteoblastomas are generally large (2-15 cm) and have a nidus of sclerotic bone (Figure 56.15).[22]
- The tumors rarely extend into the soft tissues and do not penetrate the cortex.

Treatment

- Untreated osteoblastoma will continue to enlarge and damage bone and soft tissue.
- Treatment consists of curettage and bone grafting; en bloc excision may be considered with locally aggressive tumors.
- Radiation may be required for spinal lesions that cannot be resected.[23]
- Recurrence rates are approximately 20% if the lesion has spread beyond the bone.[24]

OSTEOID OSTEOMA

- Osteoid osteomas are common benign bone-forming tumors typically presenting during the second decade.
- The tumors account for 12% of benign bone tumors.[16]

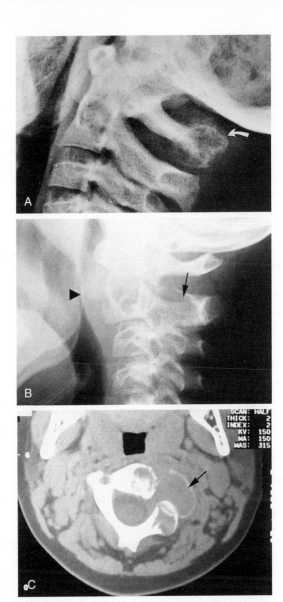

Figure 56.15 Osteoblastoma: upper cervical spine. A, Posterior tubercle, atlas. Observe the expansile lytic lesion of the posterior tubercle of the atlas (arrow). The geographic destruction leaves a clearly defined peripheral cortical margin, suggesting the benign nature of the tumor. B, Axis. Note the destruction of the lamina and lucency of C2 body (arrow). Also note the prevertebral soft tissue swelling (arrowhead). C, CT, Axis. Note the expansile nature of the lesion (arrow). (Reprinted with permission from Yochum TR, Rowe LJ, eds. *Yochum And Rowe's Essentials of Skeletal Radiology*. 3rd ed. Philadelphia, PA: Lippincott Williams & Wilkins; 2004. A, Courtesy of Paul E. Siebert, MD, Denver, Colorado.)

- Boys are more often affected than girls with a ratio of 2:1.
- Osteoid osteomas typically affect the subperiosteal region of long bones of the lower extremities; the proximal femur and tibia account for >50% of cases.
- Spinal lesions account for 10% to 25% of osteoid osteomas, which can contribute to scoliotic curves within the region.[25,26]
- Osteoid osteomas are generally small radiolucent lesions with a nidus <1.5 cm in diameter.
- Unique to osteoid osteomas is the production of high levels of prostaglandins.

Clinical Presentation

- Patients with osteoid osteomas typically present with progressive pain that is worse at night and unrelated to activity.
- It is important to note that pain may rapidly resolve after administration of NSAIDs, which block prostaglandin production by the tumor.
- Children may present with limp, muscular atrophy, tenderness, and muscle contractures.

Imaging

- On plain radiographs, osteoid osteomas appear as small (1.5 cm) radiolucent nidus surrounded by a zone of sclerotic bone (Figure 56.16).
- CT is the imaging study of choice to detect osteoid osteomas on the spine or when the lesions are obscured by sclerotic bone.[26]

Treatment

- Patients whose symptoms are tolerable may be treated with NSAIDs and followed with examinations and imaging every 4 to 6 months.
- Treatment for lesions causing intractable pain, limp, or scoliosis requires surgical resection.
- However, osteoid osteomas will completely resolve over the course of several years.[24]

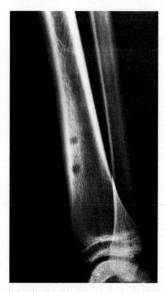

Figure 56.16 Multifocal osteoid osteoma. A 17-year-old boy presented with pain in the left lower leg for 3 months. It was promptly relieved by aspirin. Lateral radiograph of the lower leg shows 2 well-defined radiolucencies within a sclerotic area in the anterior aspect of the distal tibia. A resected specimen showed 3 nidi of osteoid osteoma, the 2 most distal of which were fairly close to one another, creating a single radiolucency on the radiograph. (From Greenspan A, Elguezabel A, Bryk D. Multifocal osteoid osteoma: a case report and review of the literature. *Am J Roentgenol.* 1974; 121:103-106. Reprinted with permission from the American Journal of Roentgenology.)

PEARLS AND PITFALLS

- OS and ESFT are the most common malignant bone tumors.
- There are also many benign tumors that affect children, which may, although benign, be locally aggressive.
- Children with bone tumors should be referred to an orthopedic surgeon.

REFERENCES

1. Jackson T, Bittman M, Granowetter L. Pediatric malignant bone tumors: a review and update on current challenges, and emerging drug targets. *Curr Probl Pediatr Adolesc Health Care.* 2016;46:213-228.
2. Mirabello L, Troisi RJ, Savage SA. Osteosarcoma incidence and survival rates from 1973 to 2004: data from the Surveillance, Epidemiology, and End Results Program. *Cancer.* 2009;115:1531.

3. Woertler K. Benign bone tumors and tumor-like lesions: value of cross-sectional imaging. *Eur Radiol.* 2003;13(8):1820-1835.

4. Wyers MR. Evaluation of pediatric bone lesions. *Pediatr Radiol.* 2010;40:468.

5. Howlader N, Noone AM, Krapcho M, et al, eds. *SEER Cancer Statistics Review, 1975-2014.* Bethesda, MD: National Cancer Institute. https://seer.cancer.gov/csr/1975_2014/, based on November 2016 SEER data submission, posted to the SEER web site, April 2017, last updated on 2018.

6. Franchi F. Epidemiology and classification of bone tumors. *Clin Cases Miner Bone Metab.* 2012;9(2):92-95.

7. Springfield DS, Gebhardt MC. Bone and soft tissue tumors. In: Morrissy RT, Weinstein SL, eds. *Lovell and Winter's Pediatric Orthopaedics.* 6th ed. Philadelphia: Lippincott Williams & Wilkins; 2006:493.

8. Gurney JG, Swensen AR, Bulterys M. Malignant bone tumors. In: Reis LAG, Smith MA, Gurney JG, et al, eds. Cancer Incidence and Survival Among Children and Adolescents: United States SEER Program, 1975-1995. NIH Pub. No. 99-4649. Bethesda. National Cancer Institute SEER Program:99-110; 1999.

9. Bleyer A, O'Leary M, Barr R, Ries L. *Cancer Epidemiology in Older Adolescents and Young Adults 15 to 29 Years of Age, Including SEER Incidence and Survival: 1975–2000.* NIH Pub. No. 06-5767:1-14-173-190. Bethesda, MD: National Institutes of Health, National Cancer Institute; 2006.

10. Thomas DM, Ballinger ML. Etiologic, environmental, and inherited risk factors in sarcomas. *J Surg Oncol.* 2015;111(5):490-495.

11. Mialou V, Philip T, Kalifa C, et al. Metastatic osteosarcoma at diagnosis: prognostic factors and long term outcome the French pediatric experience. *Cancer.* 2005;104:1100.

12. Rud NP, Reiman HM, Pritchard DJ, et al. Extraosseous Ewing's sarcoma. A *study of 42 cases. Cancer. 1989;64:1548.*

13. Nesbit ME Jr, Gehan EA, Burgert EO Jr, et al. Multimodal therapy for the management of primary, nonmetastatic Ewing's sarcoma of bone: a long term follow up of the First Intergroup study. *J Clin Oncol.* 1990;8:1664.

14. Panicek DM, Gatsonis C, Rosenthal DI, et al. CT and MR imaging in the local staging of primary malignant musculoskeletal neoplasms: report of the Radiology Diagnostic Oncology Group. *Radiology.* 1997;202:237.

15. Hamilton SN, Carlson R, Hasan H, Rassekh SR, Goddard K. Long-term outcomes and complications in pediatric Ewing sarcoma. *Am J Clini Oncol.* 2017;40(4):423-428.

16. Hakim DN, Pelly T, Kulendran M, Caris JA. Benign tumours of the bone: a review. *J Bone Oncol.* 2015;4(2):37-41.

17. Bernard SA, Murphey MD, Flemming DJ, Kransdorf MJ. Improved differentiation of benign osteochondromas from secondary chondrosarcomas with standardized measurement of cartilage cap at CT and MR imaging. *Radiology.* 2010; 255:857.

18. Balke M, Schremper L, Gebert C, et al. Giant cell tumor of bone: treatment and outcome of 214 cases. *J Cancer Res Clin Oncol.* 2008;134(9):969. Epub March 6, 2008.

19. Chakarun CJ, Forrester DM, Gottsegen CJ, et al. Giant cell tumor of bone: review, mimics, and new developments in treatment. *Radiographics.* 2013;33(1):197-211.

20. Lucas DR. Osteoblastoma. *Arch Pathol Lab Med.* 2010;134(10):1460-1466.
21. Greenspan A. Benign bone-forming lesions – osteoma, osteoid osteoma, and osteoblastoma – clinical, imaging, pathological, and differential considerations. *Skelet Radiol.* 1993;22(7):485-500.
22. Dias LDS, Frost HM. Osteoidosteoma–osteoblastoma. *Cancer.* 1974;33(6):1075-1081.
23. Boriani S, Capanna R, Donati D, et al. Osteoblastoma of the spine. *Clin Orthop Relat Res.* 1992:37.
24. Aboulafia AJ, Kennon RE, Jelinek JS. Benign bone tumors of childhood. *J Am Acad Orthop Surg.* 1999;7:377.
25. Horvai A, Klein M. Osteoid osteoma. In: *WHO Classification of Tumours of Soft Tissue and Bone.* 4th ed. Fletcher CD, Bridge JA, Hogendoorn PC, Mertens F, eds. *International Agency for Research on Cancer Lyons.* 2013:277.
26. Papathanassiou ZG, Megas P, Petsas T, et al. Osteoid osteoma: diagnosis and treatment. *Orthopedics.* 2008;31:1118.

Chapter 57

CNS Tumors in Children

Lukas Gaffney

- Brain and central nervous system (CNS) tumors are the most common pediatric solid organ tumor and second most common malignancy overall behind leukemia.[1]
- CNS tumors are the leading cause of cancer death in children aged 0 to 14 years.[2]
- Associated morbidity and mortality have improved with more advanced treatment but are still significant.

RELEVANT ANATOMY

- The base of the skull contains 3 fossae: anterior, middle, and posterior.
- The posterior fossa is the most inferior fossa and houses the cerebellum, medulla, and pons (Figure 57.1).
- The cerebellum is separated from the cerebrum by the tentorium cerebelli, an extension of the dura mater.
- Structures in or adjacent to the posterior fossa include the foramen magnum, jugular foramen, internal acoustic meatus, and the ventricular system distal to the third ventricle (Figure 57.2).

EPIDEMIOLOGY AND ETIOLOGY

Incidence: According to the Central Brain Tumor Registry of the United States, the estimated incidence of primary nonmalignant and malignant CNS tumors is 5.4 cases/100 000 person-years for children and adolescents ≤19 years of age.[3]

- Males are diagnosed more frequently than females.
- Incidence decreases with age, with newborns (<1 year old) diagnosed at an annual age-adjusted rate of 6.22/100 000; 1- to 4-year-olds at 5.53/100 000; and both 5- to 9-year-olds and 10- to 14-year-olds at 5/100 000.[4]
- CNS tumors are more common in Asian/Pacific Islanders (6.05/100 000) and whites (5.46/100 000) than Hispanics (4.36/100 000) or blacks (4.12/100 000).[4]

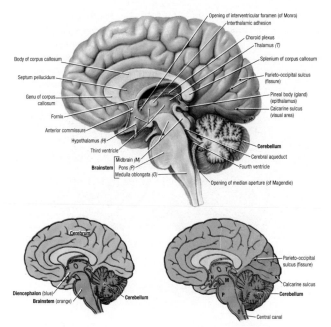

Figure 57.1 Medial views of the brain. (Reprinted with permission from Agur AMR, Dalley AF. *Grant's Atlas of Anatomy.* 14th ed. Philadelphia, PA: Wolters Kluwer Health; 2017.)

Etiology: The etiology of most pediatric CNS tumors is unknown.
- Exposure to ionizing radiation, particularly cranial irradiation for ALL treatment, increases risk.
- A minority of cases are associated with genetic conditions, such as neurofibromatosis, tuberous sclerosis, and Turcot syndrome.

CLINICAL PRESENTATION

Classic presentation: Symptoms depend on tumor location and patient age. They are often nonspecific and may be confused for more common childhood conditions, leading to a median delay in diagnosis of ~3 months.[5]
- Headaches are the most common symptom, classically presenting in the early morning and relieved by vomiting.
- Tumors occupying the fourth ventricle or cerebral aqueduct are likely to cause symptoms of elevated intracranial pressure (ICP), such as headache, papilledema, nausea, or vomiting.

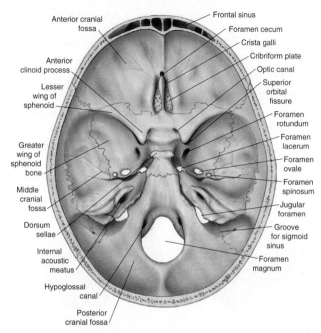

Figure 57.2 Base of the skull (inner surface). (Reprinted with permission from Anatomical Chart Company. *Human Skull Anatomical Chart.* Lippincott Williams & Wilkins, PA; 2000.)

- CNS tumors in children most commonly arise in the posterior fossa. Tumors in this region are likely to cause symptoms of increased ICP, gait abnormalities, and coordination deficits.
- Owing to unfused fontanelles, infants often present with macrocephaly instead of increased ICP. They may also demonstrate developmental delays.
- Brainstem tumors may cause cranial nerve palsies (diplopia, facial palsy, drooling, difficulty swallowing) and issues with gait or coordination.
- Seizures are likely indicative of a supratentorial tumor.

DIAGNOSIS

Laboratory Findings

- Children with CNS tumors often will have normal laboratory findings.

- Certain tumors—craniopharyngiomas, in particular—may impact the function of the pituitary, leading to endocrine abnormalities.

Imaging Findings

- Magnetic resonance imaging (MRI) is the preferred imaging modality, as it can indicate specific tumor type and help stage tumors.
- Computed tomography (CT) is often performed first as part of the workup for symptoms. However, normal CT does not exclude the possibility of a brain lesion.
- Masses on neuroimaging need to be biopsied for histologic diagnosis.
- **Astrocytomas** are one of the most common pediatric CNS tumors. They generally arise in the cerebellum and contain both cystic and solid components. On histology, they may show eosinophilic Rosenthal fibers (Figure 57.3A).
- **Medulloblastomas** are the most common malignant solid tumor in children.[6] They most commonly arise in the vermis filling the fourth ventricle. On histology, they classically appear as small blue cells forming Homer-Wright rosettes (Figure 57.3B).
- **Ependymomas** represent 10% of all pediatric brain tumors.[6] They commonly arise in the fourth ventricle but can arise in the spinal cord as well. Histologically they form perivascular rosettes (Figure 57.3C).

SURGICAL MANAGEMENT

- Surgery is a mainstay of treatment for pediatric CNS tumors and is often paired with radiotherapy and chemotherapy.
- The greater the extent of resection, the better the outcome.
- An open approach with a **craniotomy** is used to obtain tissue for diagnosis as well as bulk removal of the mass.
- Complete resection is the goal, but it is often not possible in cases where obtaining clear margins risks damage to nearby structures.
- Surgery often causes new or worsening neurological deficits. These can be minimized by using preoperative stereotactic imaging, intraoperative functional MRI, and/or intraoperative neurophysiologic monitoring.
- Operative approach depends on the precise location and size of the individual tumor.

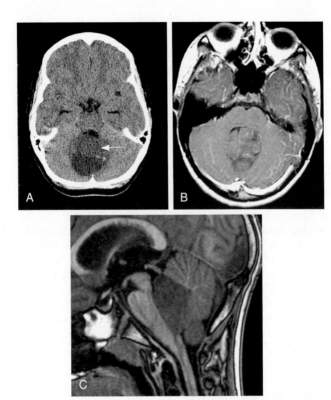

Figure 57.3 Imaging and histologic views of characteristic findings from pediatric CNS tumors. A, MRI of cerebellar pilocytic astrocytoma (arrow). B, MRI of desmoplastic medulloblastoma. C, MRI of ventricular ependymoma. D, Histologic view of Rosenthal fibers. E, Histologic view of Homer-Wright rosette. F, Histologic view of perivascular rosette. (A, Reprinted with permission from Iyer R, Chapman T. *Pediatric Imaging: The Essentials.* Philadelphia, PA: Wolters Kluwer Health; 2016. B, Barkovich AJ, Raybaud C. *Pediatric Neuroimaging.* Philadelphia, PA: Wolters Kluwer Health; 2019. C, Zamora C, Castillo M. *Neuroradiology Companion.* Philadelphia, PA: Wolters Kluwer Health; 2017. D, Husain AN, Stocker JT, Dehner LP. *Stocker and Dehner's Pediatric Pathology.* Philadelphia, PA: Wolters Kluwer Health; 2016. E, Schniederjan MH, Brat DJ. *Biopsy Interpretation of the Central Nervous System.* Philadelphia, PA: Wolters Kluwer Health; 2012. F, Kini SR. *Color Atlas of Differential Diagnosis in Exfoliative and Aspiration Cytopathology.* Philadelphia, PA: Wolters Kluwer Health; 2012.)

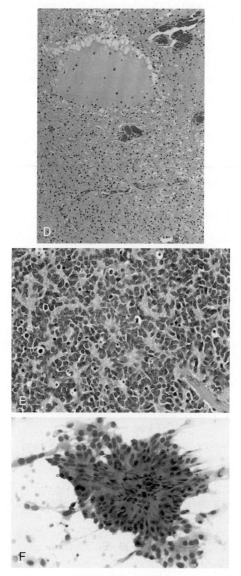

Figure 57.3—cont'd

PREOPERATIVE/PERIOPERATIVE CONSIDERATIONS

- Various common conditions need to be managed both before and during the performance of the craniotomy and resection.
- The 2 most common are elevated ICP and seizures.
- Patients with **elevated ICP** can be given corticosteroids to reduce edema pre-, peri- and postoperatively. If the increase in ICP is secondary to obstructive hydrocephalus, preoperative shunting with an external ventricular drain can reduce the risk of herniation and will allow postsurgical drainage of debris.
- Patients with preoperative **seizures** should continue anticonvulsant therapy leading up to surgery. Prophylactic anticonvulsant therapy is not recommended for patients who have not had preoperative seizures.

POSTOPERATIVE CARE

- Depending on the tumor type and location, as many as one-third of patients may experience postoperative neurologic deficits, although some of these may be transient.[6]
- For patients with preoperative elevated ICP, ventricular drains should be kept in place for at least a few days postoperatively.
- MRI should be obtained within 24 to 72 hours postoperatively to assess for extent of resection and the need for repeat surgery.
- Adjuvant radiotherapy is generally utilized for patients older than 3 years but should be avoided in those younger owing to increased radiation-induced morbidity. There are various approaches depending on histology, age, location, stage, and spread.
- Radiotherapy can cause many complications, including edema, focal neurologic deficits, necrosis, secondary malignancy, and vasculopathy.
- Chemotherapy is used as an adjunctive therapy in older children with embryonal tumors or as a replacement for radiotherapy in infants.
- Penetration of the blood-brain barrier limits the majority of systemically administered agents. Most are given intrathecally, intratumorally, or systemically if paired with an agent that can disrupt the blood-brain barrier.

PEARLS AND PITFALLS

- Diagnosis of CNS tumors is often delayed. Index of suspicion should be raised if children have refractory headaches, elevated ICP, seizures, and cranial nerve palsies.
- Management is very specific to the specific tumor based on size, location, and histology.
- The greater the extent of resection, the better the outcome.
- CNS tumors are not a death sentence—5-year survival is 73% and is largely dependent on tumor histology.

REFERENCES

1. Johnson KJ, Cullen J, Barnholtz-Sloan JS, et al. Childhood brain tumor epidemiology: a brain tumor epidemiology consortium review. *Cancer Epidemiol Biomarkers Prev.* 2014;23:2716-2736.
2. Linaberry AM, Ross JA. Trends in childhood cancer incidence in the U.S. (1992-2004). *Cancer.* 2008;112:416-432.
3. Ostrom QT, Gittleman H, Liao P, et al. CBTRUS statistical report: primary brain and central nervous system tumors diagnosed in the United States in 2007-201. *Neuro Oncol.* 2014;16(suppl 4):iv1-63.
4. Ostrom QT, de Blank P, Krucho C, et al. Alex's Lemonade Stand Foundation infant and childhood primary brain and central nervous system tumors diagnosed in the United States in 2007-2011. *Neuro Oncol.* 2015;16(suppl 10):x1-x36.
5. Wilne S, Koller K, Collier J, et al. The diagnosis of brain tumours in children: a guideline to assist healthcare professionals in the assessment of children who may have a brain tumour. *Arch Dis Child.* 2010;95:534-539.
6. Holcomb GW, Murphy JP, eds. *Ashcraft's Pediatric Surgery.* 5th ed. Philadelphia: Saunders, Elsevier Inc; 2010.

Chapter 58

Rhabdomyosarcoma

Courtland Polley

- Rhabdomyosarcomas (RMSs) are primary malignant soft tissue tumors that arise from embryonic mesenchyme with the potential to differentiate into skeletal muscle.[1]
- They are rare overall but account for over half of all soft tissue sarcomas in children.
- This is the third most common solid tumor in infants and children, behind neuroblastoma and Wilms tumor.[1]
  - 250 to 300 new cases per year
  - 75% of cases are diagnosed in children younger than 6 years

EPIDEMIOLOGY AND ETIOLOGY

- RMSs can occur in any anatomical location in the body except for bone, even in places where there is no skeletal muscle (eg, the bladder, biliary tree) (Figure 58.1).
- Most cases of RMS appear to be sporadic, but they have been associated with familial syndromes such as neurofibromatosis, Li-Fraumeni, Beckwith-Wiedemann, and Costello syndromes).[2]

CLINICAL PRESENTATION

- The presenting signs and symptoms are variable and influenced by the site of origin, age of the patient, and presence or absence of distant metastases.
- In general, the primary lesion has the appearance of a nontender mass, occasionally with overlying skin erythema[3] (Figures 58.2 and 58.3).

DIAGNOSIS

- Diagnosis is usually made by direct open biopsy.
- There are no helpful markers or specific imaging studies.

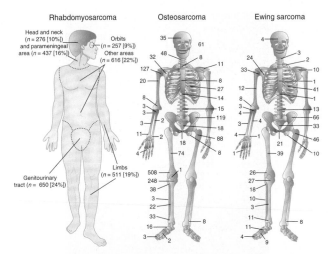

Figure 58.1 Primary sites of rhabdomyosarcoma, osteosarcoma, and Ewing sarcoma, showing numbers of patients with primary tumors at specific sites. (Reprinted with permission from Abraham J, Gulley JL, Allegra CJ. *Bethesda Handbook of Clinical Oncology.* Philadelphia, PA: Wolters Kluwer Health; 2014.)

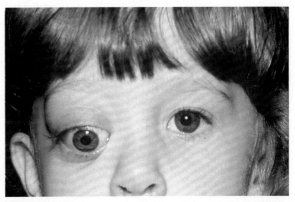

Figure 58.2 Rhabdomyosarcoma. An 8-year-old girl with a 3-week history of progressive swelling of the right eye. (Reprinted with permission from Penne R. *Oculoplastics.* Philadelphia, PA: Wolters Kluwer Health; 2019.)

- Several grams of tissue are usually needed for the pathologist to identify histologic subgroups and subsequently provide adequate staging and to direct therapy.[3]
  - Trunk and extremity RMS should have excisional or incisional biopsy.

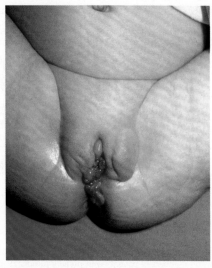

Figure 58.3 Botryoid rhabdomyosarcoma on the vulva of a newborn girl. (Reprinted with permission from Requena L, Kutzner H. *Cutaneous Soft Tissue Tumors.* Philadelphia, PA: Wolters Kluwer Health; 2015.)

- The incision should be placed so that it will not interfere with the incision needed for subsequent wide local excision.
  - The ultimate goal is wide local excision with clear margins.
  - Biopsies of genitourinary primaries are frequently performed endoscopically.
- Regional lymph nodes are evaluated depending on location of the primary.
  - Sentinel lymph node mapping is advised for trunk and extremity lesions, as they have a high incidence of lymph node involvement.[3]

Staging and Clinical Grouping

- Pretreatment staging for RMS is performed to stratify the extent of the disease for different treatment regimens as well as to compare outcome (Table 58.1).
  - It is a variation on the TNM staging system, and it is based on primary tumor site, primary tumor size, clinical regional node status, and distant spread.[3]
- The initial radiologic evaluation should include plain radiographs of the affected area, as well as CT scan or MRI of the primary site and surrounding structures.

- MRI is increasingly considered the imaging method of choice for certain primary locations, such as the head and neck, extremity, parameningeal, and pelvic tumors.
- Ultrasonography may provide additional information in patients with pelvic tumors (particularly the bladder) because the characteristic water density of urine helps in tumor localization.[4]
- The clinical grouping system was developed by the Intergroup Rhabdomyosarcoma Group (IRS) and is based on the pre-treatment and operative outcome (Table 58.2).
- The underlying premise is that total tumor extirpation is the best hope for cure and it allows for risk stratification.[3]
- The IRS-V study combines group, stage, and histology sub-type to allocate patients to 3 different therapeutic protocols according to risk of recurrence.[1]
  - Low risk includes patients with stage 1 or 2 disease and no nodal spread, or patients with orbital involvement with incomplete resection.
    - Estimated 3-year failure-free survival (FFS) rate of 88%
  - High risk constitutes patients with metastatic disease.
    - FFS <30%
  - Intermediate risk includes all other patients.
    - FFS 55% to 76%

MEDICAL AND SURGICAL MANAGEMENT

- The approach to treatment of RMS is multimodal in nature, and specific surgical treatment has been progressively less aggressive and less mutilating, while maintaining excellent survival statistics.
- General principles of surgical treatment include complete wide excision of the primary tumor and surrounding uninvolved margins while preserving cosmesis and function.[3]
- Initial biopsy is generally incisional except for small lesions that can be safely excised (Figure 58.4).
  - At many anatomic sites, there will be gross or microscopic residual, and pretreatment re-excision is warranted if this can be done without disfigurement.
  - Longitudinal incisions are frequently better than horizontal incisions on areas such as an extremity.
  - Ideally excisional biopsies will leave behind only negative biopsies; however, margins should be carefully marked with sutures or clips to allow re-resection should the biopsy reveal a positive margin.[3]
  - Any question of margin status should warrant re-resection.

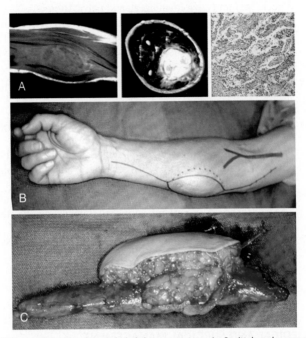

Figure 58.4 Resection of rhabdomyosarcoma. A, Sagittal and coronal magnetic resonance imaging sequences show a well-localized tumor within the flexor pronator muscle group in this 32-year-old mother of 5 children. The histology was consistent with a low-grade rhabdomyosarcoma. The ulnar nerve and artery were adjacent to the tumor. B, The planned incision is placed on the ulnar side of the forearm. The biopsy scar is widely excised in continuity with the tumor. The ulnar nerve and artery were also excised and reconstructed immediately. Sural nerve cable grafts were used for the nerve and a reversed cephalic vein for the artery. After tumor excision, intraoperative radioactive seeds were placed within the wound and removed 2 weeks later. C, A gracilis myocutaneous flap has been harvested from the thigh. The suture markings at 5-cm intervals were used to adjust the final tension of the muscle inset. D, The forearm and flexed digits are seen 1 year later. She has regained full digital flexion through the profundus tendons. The long flexor to the thumb was not removed. E, Despite multiple thoracotomies for isolated resection of pulmonary metastases and multiple resections of soft tissue nodules, the patient has remained alive and well. The skin paddle was debulked and reduced. (Reprinted with permission from Fischer JF, Bland KI, Callery MP, et al, eds. *Mastery of Surgery.* 5th ed. Philadelphia, PA: Lippincott Williams & Wilkins; 2007.)

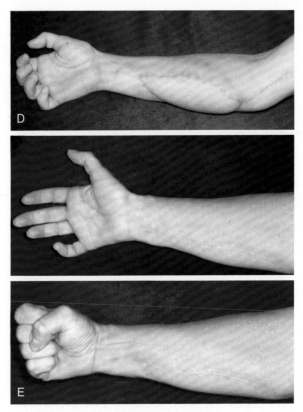

Figure 58.4—cont'd

- Secondary excision after initial biopsy and neoadjuvant therapy has better outcomes than does partial or incomplete excision.
  - Chemotherapy followed by delayed or second-look surgery has allowed for better prognosis with less mutilating surgery.[1]
- Primary chemotherapy followed by radiation therapy is the recommended approach for neoadjuvant and adjuvant therapy.
- There is a direct relationship between age at diagnosis and likelihood of regional lymph node involvement in boys with nonmetastatic paratesticular RMS.

- A modified ipsilateral retroperitoneal lymph node dissection is recommended in older boys (age 10 years) who have no clinical evidence of regional node involvement.[3]
- Testicular masses should be approached through an inguinal rather than scrotal incision, so that proximal control of the cord can be obtained and a wide local excision performed without seeding the scrotum.[5]

Metastatic Disease

- Metastatic disease most commonly involves the lung, bone, regional lymph nodes, liver, and brain.[3]
- Metastatic disease is the single most important predictor of clinical outcome, with a 3-year FFS of only 25%.[3]
- Sentinel lymph node mapping with a vital dye such as isosulfan blue, along with radiolabeled technetium sulfur colloid, can localize the regional node most likely to contain tumor cells.
  - If the node is positive, then the nodal basin can be irradiated.[3]

POSTOPERATIVE CARE

- The development of adjuvant and neoadjuvant chemotherapy has led to a marked increase in survival.
- Agents with known activity in the treatment of RMS include vincristine, actinomycin, doxorubicin, cyclophosphamide, ifosfamide, and etoposide.
- Complications of treatment for rhabdomyosarcoma are varied and include chemotherapy toxicity, acute and long-term complications related to radiation therapy, and standard surgical complications.[6]
- Long-term follow-up for delayed complications and second malignancies is warranted in all patients.[3]

PEARLS AND PITFALLS

- Longitudinal incision for biopsies to facilitate inclusion in reoperations
- Wide excision of the primary lesion to remove microscopic residual tumor
- Orient and mark excision in specimen and in tumor site to allow for re-excision if necessary
- Reoperation for complete resection of tumor has led to improved survival

TABLE 58.1					
Pretreatment Stage Classification[3]					
Stage	**Sites**	**T**	**Size**	**N**	**M**
1	Orbit, head, and neck (not para-meningeal), bladder/nonprostate	T1 or 2	A or B	N0 or Nx	M0
2	Bladder and prostate, extremity, cranial paramenin-geal, trunk, perineal, thoracic	T1 or 2	A	N0 or Nx	M0
3	Same as 2	T1 or 2	A B	N1 N0/N1/Nx	M0
4	All	T1 or 2	A or B	N0/N1/Nx	M1

Reprinted by permission from Springer: Radhakrishnana RS, Andrassy RJ. Rhabdomyosarcoma. In: Mattei P, Nichol PF, Rollins MD, Muratore CS, eds. *Fundamentals of Pediatric Surgery*. 2nd ed. New York, NY: Springer; 2010. Copyright © 2011 Springer Science+Business Media, LLC.

Additional Classification:

Tumor:

T1: confined to the anatomic site of origin

A: ≤5 cm diameter

B: >5 cm diameter

T2: extension and/or fixation to surrounding tissue

A: ≤5 cm diameter

B: >5 cm diameter

Regional node:

N0: regional nodes not clinically involved

N1: regional nodes clinically involved

Nx: clinical status of regional nodes unknown

Metastasis:

M0: no distant metastasis

M1: distant metastasis

TABLE 58.2	
Clinical Grouping of Rhabdomyosarcoma[3]	
Group I	Tumor completely excised with microscopic negative margins
Group II	Tumor completely excised with microscopic positive margins
Group III	Tumor excised with gross residual tumor
Group IV	Distant metastases

Reprinted by permission from Springer: Radhakrishnana RS, Andrassy RJ. Rhabdomyosarcoma. In: Mattei P, Nichol PF, Rollins MD, Muratore CS, eds. *Fundamentals of Pediatric Surgery.* 2nd ed. New York, NY: Springer; 2010. Copyright © 2011 Springer Science+Business Media, LLC.

REFERENCES

1. Dagher R, Helman L. Rhabdomyosarcoma: an overview. *Oncologist.* 1999;4(1):34-44.
2. Li FP, Fraumeni Jr JF. Rhabdomyosarcoma in children: epidemiologic study and identification of a familial cancer syndrome. *J Natl Cancer Inst.* 1969;43:1365-1373.
3. Radhakrishnana RS, Andrassy RJ. Rhabdomyosarcoma. In: Mattei P, ed. *Fundamentals of Pediatric Surgery.* Springer Science & Business Media; 2011.
4. Crist W, Gehan EA, Ragab AH, et al. The third intergroup rhabdomyosarcoma study. *J Clin Oncol.* 1995;13(3):610-630.
5. Wiener ES, Anderson JR, Ojimba JI, et al. Controversies in the management of paratesticular rhabdomyosarcoma: is staging retroperitoneal lymph node dissection necessary for adolescents with resected paratesticular rhabdomyosarcoma? *Semin Pediatr Surg.* 2001;10:146.
6. Miller SD, Andrassy RJ. Complications in pediatric surgical oncology. *J Am Coll Surg.* 2003;197:832-837.

SUGGESTED READING

Fletcher CDM, Chibon F, MErtens F. Undifferentiated/unclassified sarcomas. In: Fletcher CDM, Bridge JA, Hogendoorn PCW, Mertens F, eds. *WHO Classification of Tumours of Soft Tissue and Bone.* Lyons: IARC; 2013:236.

Stevens MC, Rey A, Bouvet N, et al. Treatment of nonmetastatic rhabdomyosarcoma in childhood and adolescence: third study of the International Society of Paediatric Oncology–SIOP Malignant Mesenchymal Tumor 89. *J Clin Oncol.* 2005;23(12):2618-2628.

Andrassy RJ. Chapter 14. Soft tissue sarcomas. In: Carachi R, Azmy A, Grosfeld JL, eds. *The Surgery of Childhood Tumors.* Berlin: Springer; 2008.

Crist WM, Anderson JR, Meza JL, et al. Intergroup rhabdomyosarcoma study IV: results for patients with nonmetastatic disease. *J Clin Oncol.* 2001;19:3091.

Chapter 59

Nevi and Melanoma in Children

Gina Prado

- Pigmented lesions in childhood can pose diagnostic and therapeutic challenges for pediatric surgeons.
- This chapter examines the common pigmented lesions encountered in childhood.

RELEVANT ANATOMY

- The skin is the largest organ in the body and is composed of 3 layers: the epidermis, dermis, and subcutaneous fat. It serves many functions including thermoregulation, sensory perception, and protection microbial invasion.
- The epidermis originates from ectodermal cells and consists of several layers: stratum basalis (inner layer), stratum spinosum, stratum granulosum, stratum lucidum, and stratum corneum (outer layer) (Figure 59.1).
- Cell types found in the epidermis includes keratinocytes, melanocytes, and Langerhans (dendritic) cells.
  - Keratinocytes are the stem cells that will repopulate the other layers over an individual's lifetime.
  - They progress from the stratum basale to the stratum corneum.
  - Melanocytes are derived from neural crests cells and are found in the stratum basale.
  - Their primary function is to produce the pigment melanin for defense against UV injury.
  - Melanin accumulates in melanosomes, which are then phagocytosed by neighboring keratinocytes for melanin storage.[1]
  - Skin color results from the variable production and degradation of melanosomes and not on numbers of melanocytes.
  - Langerhans (dendritic) cells are bone marrow–derived, antigen-presenting cells that detect and present foreign antigen to T cells.

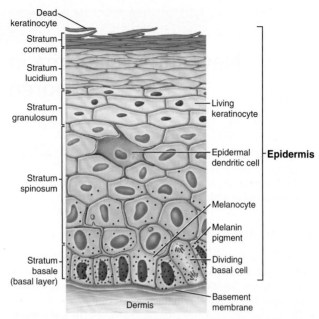

Figure 59.1 Layer of the epidermis. (Reprinted with permission from McConnell TH, Hull KL. *Human Form, Human Function.* Philadelphia, PA: Lippincott Williams & Wilkins, a Wolters Kluwer Business; 2011.)

- The dermis is of mesodermal origin and consists of consist of connective tissue, nerve endings, blood and lymphatic vessels, and adnexal structures (eg, hair shafts, sweat glands, and sebaceous glands).
- It is divided into a superficial papillary layer and a deeper reticular layer.

COMMON DERMATOLOGIC TERMS

- Common terminologies to be familiar with are shown in **Table 59.1**.

Nevi

- Nevus skin lesions are collections of well-differentiated cells within the tissue of origin.
- Classified based on the cell of origin (melanocytic and nonmelanocytic).
- Melanocytic nevi are derived from melanocytes or their precursors.

TABLE 59.1

Common Dermatologic Terminology

	Definition
Macule	Flat lesion with well-circumscribed skin color change <1 cm
Patch	Flat lesion >1 cm
Papule	Elevated solid skin lesion <1 cm
Plaque	Raised lesions >1 cm
Nodule	Lesion arising from the dermis or subcutaneous tissues
Nevus	Proliferation of cells within their own tissue of origin
Hyperkeratosis	Increased thickness of stratum corneum
Melanocytosis	Increased number of melanocytes
Acanthosis	Epidermal hyperplasia due to increased spinosum
Papillomatosis	Hyperplasia of dermal papillae

- Vary in their location within the dermis and epidermis and in their content of melanin.
- Nonmelanocytic nevi are derived from keratinocytes and are also referred to as epidermal nevi.
- Can be primarily keratinocytic or organoid, which originate from adnexal structures.

MELANOCYTIC NEVI

- Melanocytic nevi are divided into acquired nevi (those that appear after birth) and congenital nevi (those that are present at birth) (Figure 59.2).
- They are then further subclassified as junctional, compound, or dermal according to the location of the nevus cells in the skin.
- Junctional nevi are at the junction of the epidermis/dermis.
- Compound nevi involve both the epidermis and dermis.
- Dermal nevi are confined to the dermis.
- In childhood, >90% of nevi are junctional.[2]
- Most nevi then become compound or dermal nevi as they migrate into the papillary dermis.
- In general, the deeper the nests of nevus cells, the more raised and less pigmented the lesion (ie, dark flat lesions vs raised tan lesions).
- The common variants of melanocytic nevi are shown in Table 59.2.

TABLE 59.2			
Common Melanocytic Nevi			
	Onset of Lesion	**Appearance**	**When to Biopsy**
Acquired nevus	After age 6 mo; sun-exposed areas	Small (<5 mm) Flat, symmetric, well-demarcated, dark pigmentation	Not indicated
Atypical nevus	Adolescence; sun-exposed areas, posterior trunk	5-15 mm Irregular outline and uneven dark pigmentation, partially raised with a "fried-egg" appearance	Atypical change
Congenital nevus	At birth or within 6 mo of life; trunk	Variable size Uniform and flat, may grow hair; various shades of blue, black, brown	Large lesions (>40 cm) should undergo biopsy
Halo nevus	6-15 y; trunk, extremities	Central area of brown pigmentation with a rim of depigmentation, flat to slightly raised	Atypical change in center of lesion
Blue nevus	Childhood, dorsum of hands/feet	<5 mm Smooth, blue-gray nodules	Not indicated
Cellular blue nevus	Any time Scalp, sacrum, face	5-15 mm Well-demarcated blue-gray nodule	Atypical change
Spitz nevus	Face, lower extremities	5-15 mm Dome-shaped, smooth Pink to red lesions	Atypical change
Becker nevus	Young male; upper torso and arm	Irregular hyperpigmented plaque Brown pigmentation	Not indicated

Adapted from Holcomb GW, Murphy JD, Ostlie DJ, eds. *Ashcraft's Pediatric Surgery*. 6th ed. New York, NY: Saunders; 2014.

Acquired Melanocytic Nevi

- Appear after 6 months of age and persist through the fourth decade, after which many disappear.[1]
- They are most frequently found on sun-exposed areas.
- They are less than 6 to 8 mm in diameter, are symmetric in shape, have an even pigmentation, and have a regular contour with a sharply demarcated border.
- These nevi undergo natural evolution in appearance and should not be mistaken for malignant progression.

Atypical Melanocytic Nevi

- Previously referred to as dysplastic nevi or Clark nevi.
- May occur sporadically or in a familial pattern.[1]
- The onset is usually during adolescence on sun-exposed areas of skin and continues to increase in number and size with age.
- Unlike the acquired nevi, these lesions tend to be larger (5-15 mm).
- They have irregular edges with raised portions and dark and uneven pigmentation, giving it a "fried-egg" appearance.
- Atypical nevi are not necessarily removed but should be biopsied if melanoma is suspected.
- Children with atypical nevi should undergo a routine complete skin examination with photo documentation every 6 to 12 months.

Congenital Melanocytic Nevi

- Pigmented lesions that develop within the first few months of life.[1]
- These lesions are classified according to size: small (<1.5 cm), medium (1.5-20 cm), and large (>20 cm).
- They most commonly occur in the lower trunk, upper back, shoulders, chest, and proximal limbs.
- The lesions may initially be homogenous and flat but can evolve into thick and hair-covered lesions of various shades of brown, black, or blue.
  - The especially large lesions (>40 cm) are referred to as a giant hairy nevus and tend to cover large truncal areas (Figure 59.3).
  - These nevi are of clinical implication because of their association with leptomeningeal melanocytosis (neurocutaneous melanocytosis) and their predisposition for malignant melanoma.[3]

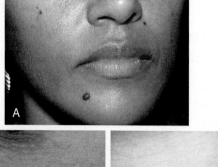

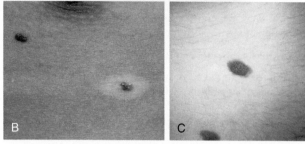

Figure 59.2 Melanocytic nevi. A, Acquired nevus. B, Halo nevus. C, Atypical nevus. Note the raised center and indistinct border giving a "fried-egg" appearance of the atypical nevus. (Reprinted with permission from Goodheart HP. *Goodheart's Photoguide of Common Skin Disorders: Diagnosis and Management.* 2nd ed. Philadelphia, PA: Lippincott Williams & Wilkins; 2003)

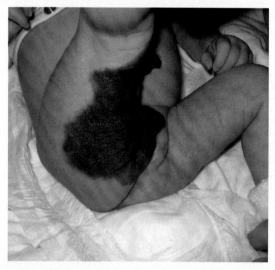

Figure 59.3 Giant congenital melanocytic nevus (CMN) on the thigh of a neonate. Giant CMN have an increased risk of developing melanoma. (Reprinted with permission from Goodheart HP, Gonzalez ME. *Goodheart's Photoguide to Common Pediatric and Adult Skin Disorders.* 4th ed. Philadelphia, PA: Wolters Kluwer Health; 2016.)

- The overall incidence of malignant melanoma has been estimated to be 5% to 10%. Risk factor for malignant transformation includes a nevus of predicted adult size >40 cm, lesions on posterior trunk, and presence of satellite lesions.
- Removal of small congenital nevi is not warranted; rather, lifelong observation is preferred.
- In the case of giant congenital nevi, close medical surveillance is necessary.
- If the nevus lies over the head or spine, an MRI is indicated for detection of leptomeningeal melanocytosis.
- Early excision of the nevus may reduce the potential for melanoma development.
- Biopsy of newly expanding nodules is indicated.

Nonmelanocytic Nevi

- Epidermal nevi are skin lesions characterized by proliferation of the epidermis and/or adnexal structures.
- Keratinocytic nevi involve the epidermal layer only, whereas the organoid nevi involve the adnexal sebaceous, apocrine, eccrine, and follicular structures.
- Various syndromes are associated with these epidermal nevi, including Proteus syndrome, Becker nevus syndrome, and congenital hemidysplasia with ichthyosiform erythroderma and limb defects syndrome.
- Abnormalities affect the skin and soft tissues, eyes, central nervous system (CNS), and musculoskeletal system.[1]
- The common variants of epidermal nevi are shown in Table 59.3.

Nevus Sebaceous

- A relatively small, sharply demarcated, oval or linear, elevated yellow plaque[1] (Figure 59.4).
- Most commonly found on the scalp, temple, or preauricular region of infants.
- The lesion is frequently flat and distinct early on and with maturity become stippled with rubbery nodules.
- Sebaceous nevi can be associated with CNS, skeletal, and ocular defects as part of the epidermal nevus syndrome.
- Progression to basal cell carcinoma (BCC) reported in 6% to 22% of adults.[2]
- Treatment of choice is total excision before adolescence.

TABLE 59.3			
Common Epidermal Nevi			
	Appearance	Histology	Clinical Features
Sebaceous nevus	Well-circumscribed yellow plaque, usually less than 2-3 cm in diameter	Hyperkeratosis, malformed hair follicles, abundance of sebaceous glands	Developmental delay, seizures, central nervous system (CNS) and eye abnormalities
Nevus comedonicus	Linear well-circumscribed plaque that appear like comedones	Dilated hair follicles containing keratotic plug	Cataracts, CNS and spinal abnormalities
Linear epidermal nevus	Nonpruritic warty brown plaque, scaly discoloration, or linear lesions	Hyperkeratosis, acanthosis, papillomatosis	Significant involvement of CNS, ophthalmic, and skeletal systems
Inflammatory linear verrucous epidermal nevus	Warty or scaling pruritic plaque, tends to group together in a linear pattern	Inflammatory infiltrate, hyperkeratosis	Female predisposition (4:1 female:male ratio)

Adapted from Holcomb GW, Murphy JD, Ostlie DJ, eds. *Ashcraft's Pediatric Surgery.* 6th ed. New York, NY: Saunders; 2014.

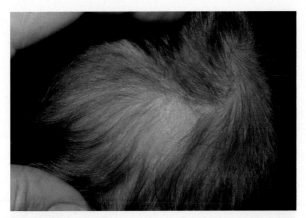

Figure 59.4 Typical yellow-tan color, oval shape, and finely papulated appearance of a nevus sebaceous. (Reprinted with permission from Goodheart HP, Gonzalez ME. *Goodheart's Photoguide to Common Pediatric and Adult Skin Disorders*. 4th ed. Philadelphia, PA: Wolters Kluwer Health; 2016.)

Nevus Comedonicus

- A rare organoid nevus of epithelial origin that consists of linear plaques of plugged follicles that simulate comedones; the horny plugs represent keratinous debris within dilated, malformed pilosebaceous follicles (Figure 59.5).[1]
- These lesions may be present at birth or appear during childhood and may develop at any site.
- They are usually unilateral and asymptomatic.
- Symptomatic individuals may experience recurrent inflammation, resulting in cyst formation, fistulas, and scarring.
- Rarely, they are associated with other congenital malformations, including skeletal defects, cerebral anomalies, and cataracts.
- Effective treatment consists of full-thickness excision; keratolytic agents such as retinoic acid may be moderately effective for larger lesions in reducing scaling.[2]

Melanoma

- Malignant melanoma accounts for 1% to 3% of all pediatric malignancies and approximately 2% of all melanomas occur before 20 years of age.[1]
- Annual incidence is 0.8/million in the first decade of life.[1]
- The incidence and mortality rate increase with age.
- About half of the time, melanoma develops at a site where there was no apparent nevus.

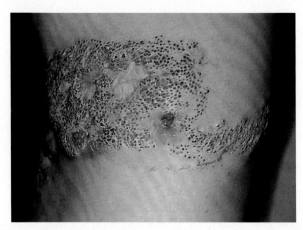

Figure 59.5 Nevus comedonicus on the abdomen. Note the keratin-plugged hair follicles. (Reprinted with permission from Hall BJ, Hall JC, eds. *Sauer's Manual of Skin Diseases.* 11th ed. Philadelphia, PA: Wolters Kluwer; 2017.)

- Sites of involvement include extremities > trunk > head and neck.
- The extent of disease is localized in most pediatric patients, but some patients may present with nodal involvement or metastases such as lung, liver, and brain.

RISK FACTORS

- Presence of the familial atypical mole melanoma syndrome or xeroderma pigmentosum; increased number of acquired melanocytic nevi; presence of atypical nevi; fair complexion; excessive sun exposure; a personal or family (first-degree relative) history of a previous melanoma; giant congenital nevus; and immunosuppression

DIAGNOSIS

- Unfortunately, diagnosis is often delayed in pediatric melanomas.
- The *ABCDE* (asymmetry, border irregularities, color variability, diameter >6 mm, evolution) rule has not been shown to be useful for children.
- Most common presenting features include recent growth, ulceration, bleeding, and change in color.[4]

TABLE 59.4

American Joint Committee on Cancer (AJCC) Guideline for Surgical Management of Cutaneous Melanoma

Tumor Thickness	Margins (cm)	Sentinel Node Biopsy
In situ	0.5	No
<1 mm	1.0	No
1.01-2 mm	1.0-2.0	Yes
>2 mm	2.0	Yes

Adapted from Holcomb GW, Murphy JD, Ostlie DJ, eds. *Ashcraft's Pediatric Surgery*. 6th ed. New York, NY: Saunders; 2014.

- Less frequent signs or symptoms included a subcutaneous mass, pruritic, and regional lymphadenopathy.
- In some cases, the patient may be asymptomatic.
- Frequent clinical skin examinations of patients at risk and prompt workup to acute changes in nevi may aid in early detection.

SURGICAL APPROACH

- Full-thickness biopsy with an adequate margin is recommended.[5]
- As such, young children may benefit from excision under general anesthesia.
- The American Joint Committee on Cancer (AJCC) guideline for surgical management of melanoma should guide biopsy (Table 59.4).
- During excision, any suspicious lesion should be marked in case re-excision is deemed necessary. Additionally, specimens should be acquiesced for permanent section.

POSTOPERATIVE CARE

- Patients should be examined at 3-month intervals during the first 5 years and every 6 months for the next 5 years.[1]
- Prognosis
  - Patients younger than 20 years had an overall 5-year survival of 93.6%.[1]
  - Worse prognosis associated with male gender, increased age, more advanced disease, and location other than trunk or extremity.
  - The most important prognostic parameters remain tumor thickness and the level of invasion into the skin

PEARLS AND PITFALLS

- Melanoma remains a challenge for diagnosis and treatment.
- Keen clinical observation is necessary.
- Atypical changes of pigmented lesions include rapid increase in size, development of satellite lesions, variegation of color, irregularity of the borders, and changes in texture such as scaling, erosion, ulceration.
- Skin safety is key. Emphasis should be given in avoiding midday sun exposure between 10 am and 3 pm; wearing of protective clothing such as a hat, long sleeves, and pants; and use of sunscreen.

REFERENCES

1. Kurkchubasche AG, Tracy TF. Chapter 71: nevus and melanoma. In: Holcomb GW, Murphy JP, eds. *Ashcraft's Pediatric Surgery*. 6th ed. N.p.:Elsevier Health Sciences; 2014:991-1006.
2. Martin KL. Chapter 651: cutaneous nevi. In: Kliegman RM, Stanton BM, St. Geme J, Schor NF, eds. *Nelson Textbook of Pediatrics*. 20th ed. Philadelphia: Elsevier; 2016:3129-3133.e1.
3. Ramaswamy V, Delaney H, Haque S, et al. Spectrum of central nervous system abnormalities in neurocutaneous melanocytosis. *Dev Med Child Neurol*. 2012;54:563-568.
4. Garbe C, Eigentler TK. Diagnosis and treatment of cutaneous melanoma: state of the art 2006. *Melanoma Res*. 2007;17:117-127.
5. Neier M, Pappo A, Navid F. Management of melanomas in children and young adults. *J Pediatr Hematol Oncol*. 2012;34:S51-S54.

Index

Note: Page numbers followed by "f" indicate figures and "t" indicate tables.